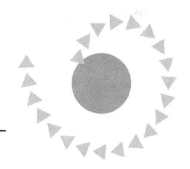

Recent Advances in

Surgery
26

D1424204

Edited by

I. Taylor MD ChM FRCS FMedSci FRCPS(Glas)Hon

David Patey Professor of Surgery
Royal Free and University College London Medical School
University College London, London, UK

C. D. Johnson MChir FRCS

Reader and Consultant Surgeon
University Surgical Unit, Southampton General Hospital, Southampton, UK

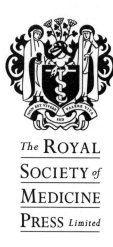

The ROYAL
SOCIETY *of*
MEDICINE
PRESS Limited

1 Wimpole Street, London W1G 0AE, UK
http://www.rsmpress.co.uk/agents.htm

Customers in North America should order via:
c/oJamco Distribution Inc., 1401 Lakeway Drive, Louisville, Texas 75057, USA
Email: jamco@majors.com; Tel: +1 800-538-1287 (toll free); Fax: +1 972-353-1303

British Library Cataloguing in Publication Data
A catalogue record for this book is available from the British Library
ISBN 1-85315-551–9
ISSN 0143 8395

Commissioning editor - Peter Richardson
Editorial assistant - Gabrielle Mills
Production by GM & BA Haddock, Midlothian, UK
Printed in Great Britain by Bell & Bain, Glasgow, UK

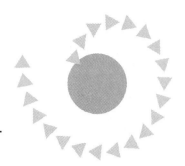

Contents

Contributors

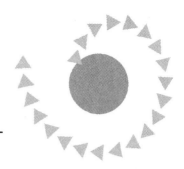

Timothy G. Allen-Mersh BSc MD FRCS
Professor of Gastrointestinal Surgery, Imperial College School of Science, Technology and Medicine, Chelsea and Westminster Hospital, London, UK

Wendy Atkin MPH PhD
Deputy Director, Colorectal Cancer Unit, Cancer Research UK; and Honorary Reader in Epidemiology, Imperial College of Science, Technology and Medicine, St Mark's Hospital, Harrow, Middlesex, UK

Simon V. Baudouin MBBS MD FRCP
Senior Lecturer, University Department of Anaesthesia and Critical Care, Royal Victoria Infirmary, Newcastle upon Tyne, UK

Michael Baum MD ChM FRCS
Professor of Surgery, University College London, London, UK

Simon R. Bramhall MD FRCS
Consultant Hepatobiliary and Liver Transplant Surgeon, University Hospital Birmingham NHS Trust, Liver Unit, The Queen Elizabeth Hospital, Birmingham, UK

Karim Brophy BSc FRCA FRCS
Specialist Registrar, The Royal London Hospital, Whitechapel, London, UK

Eddie Chaloner FRCS
Consultant Vascular Surgeon, University College Hospitals NHS Trust, London, UK

Simon G. Darke MS FRCS
Consultant Surgeon, The Royal Bournemouth Hospital, Bournemouth, UK

Michael Douek MD FRCS
Lecturer in Surgery, Royal Free and University College Medical School, University College London, London, UK

Dominic Errington MBBS MRCP(UK) FRCA
Research Fellow, University Department of Anaesthesia and Critical Care, Royal Victoria Infirmary, Newcastle upon Tyne, UK

Majid Hashemi FRCS(Gen)
Consultant Surgeon/Senior Lecturer in Surgery, Royal Free and University College Medical School, University College London, Whittington Campus, London, UK

Colin D. Johnson MChir FRCS
Reader and Consultant Surgeon, University Surgical Unit, Southampton General Hospital, Southampton, UK

Charles H. Knowles PhD FRCS
Specialist Registrar and Clinical Lecturer in Surgery, Academic Department of Surgery, Te Royal London Hospital, London, UK

Constantinos Kyriakides MD FRCS
Senior Clinical Vascular Fellow, Regional Vascular Unit, St Mary's Hospital, London, UK

Peter J. Lunniss MS FRCS
Senior Lecturer and Honorary Consultant Surgeon, Academic Department of Surgery, The Royal London and Homerton Hospitals, London, UK

Matthew Mattson BSc FRCR
Consultant Radiologist, The Royal London Hospital, Whitechapel, London, UK

Brendan J Moran MCh FRCSI(Gen) FRCS, Consultant Surgeon, Director NSCAG Pseudomyxoma Peritonei Centre, The North Hampshire Hospital, Basingstoke, Hampshire, UK

Timothy K. McCullough BSc MBBS MRCS
Research Fellow, Department of Surgery, Imperial College School of Science, Technology and Medicine, Chelsea and Westminster Hospital, London, UK

John Northover MS FRCS
Professor of Intestinal Surgery, Imperial College of Science, Technology and Medicine, London; Director, Colorectal Cancer Unit, Cancer Research; and Chair, Department of Surgery, St Mark's Hospital, Harrow, Middlesex, UK

Timothy A. Rockall MD FRCS
Senior Lecturer/Honorary Consultant, Department of Surgical Oncology and Technology, Division of Surgery Anaesthetics and Intensive Care, Faculty of Medicine, Imperial College of Science, Technology and Medicine, St Mary's Hospital, London, UK

Richard Sainsbury MBBS MD FRCS
Senior Lecturer in Surgery, University College London, London, UK

Sanjeev Sarin MS FRCS
Consultant Surgeon, Department of Surgery, Watford General Hospital, Watford, Hertfordshire, UK

Richard J. Sutton FRCS
Specialist Registrar, Department of Surgery, Watford General Hospital, Watford, Hertfordshire, UK

Irving Taylor MD ChM FRCS
Professor of Surgery, Head of Department of Surgery, Royal Free and University College Medical School, University College London, London, UK

Jayant S. Vaidya MBBS MS DNB FRCS PhD
Honorary Lecturer and Specialist Registrar, Department of Surgery, The Middlesex and Whittington Hospitals, University College London, London, UK

Carolynne Vaizey MD FRCS(Gen) FCS(SA)
Consultant Colorectal Surgeon, The Middlesex Hospital, London, UK

John H.N. Wolfe MS FRCS
Consultant Vascular Surgeon, Regional Vascular Unit, St Mary's Hospital, London, UK

Dominic Errington Simon V. Baudouin

1

Fluid resuscitation and pre-optimisation before abdominal surgery

The management of the shocked patient with an acute abdominal catastrophe remains a major challenge for surgeons, anaesthetists and intensivists. In the UK, hospital mortality in patients undergoing emergency surgery for acute lower gastrointestinal conditions is at least 10% and, in some series, considerably higher.[1]

Modern resuscitation of the acutely ill began during the conflicts which occurred in the early and middle parts of the 20th century. It was rapidly established that emergency surgery in trauma patients with little or no resuscitation carried a very high mortality. Laboratory experiments sub-sequently demonstrated that intravenous volume replacement, given before, during and after surgery, significantly reduced mortality. These results were rapidly transferred into clinical practice. However, this occurred in the era before clinical trials were conducted and many important issues still remain in terms of fluid resuscitation. These include questions about the type and volume of fluid to be used and the monitoring of clinically relevant end-points of resuscitation. This article will consider recent work in the field of fluid resuscitation with particular relevance to abdominal surgery.

An ageing population with significant cardiac and respiratory co-morbidity also presents a major problem to those delivering peri-operative care. Very major elective surgical procedures are now routinely performed on this group of patients. This has led a number of research groups to study methods of so-called pre-optimisation.[2–4] These are interventions that aim to reduce operative risk and usually commence pre-operatively. This review will consider two approaches to pre-optimisation, which have been extensively investigated, in the last decade: (i) supra-normalisation strategies that deliberately drive tissue

Dr D. Errington MBBS MRCP(UK) FRCA, Research Fellow, University Department of Anaesthesia and Critical Care, Royal Victoria Infirmary, Queen Victoria Road, Newcastle upon Tyne NE1 4LP, UK

Dr S.V. Baudouin MBBS MD FRCP, Senior Lecturer, University Department of Anaesthesia and Critical Care, Royal Victoria Infirmary, Queen Victoria Road, Newcastle upon Tyne NE1 4LP, UK (for correspondence)

oxygen delivery above the normal range; and (ii) β-blockade that reduces heart rate and may decrease cardiac output.

FLUID RESUSCITATION OF THE PATIENT FOR ABDOMINAL SURGERY

The crystalloid *versus* colloid debate has been with us for more than 20 years.[5] A huge research literature has been generated over this time and, on occasions, extreme views on the use of one or the other alternative have been put forward. This debate has been coloured by transatlantic differences in practice – crystalloid in North America, colloids in the UK. In addition, the significant expense of resuscitation fluids and the willingness of manufacturers to fund studies and trials have also had a major impact on the debate. One of the main drives in the crystalloid *versus* colloid debate may have been a desire by manufacturers to increase market share. While this is probably an extreme view, the debate may have deflected the research community away from potentially more interesting and important questions in resuscitation.

In simple terms, the fluids available are: (i) iso-osmolar crystalloid solutions; (ii) hypertonic crystalloid solutions; (iii) colloid solutions; and (iv) blood products and synthetic haemoglobins.

Crystalloid solutions provide water and a variable amount of electrolytes and glucose. Intravenous solutions, which would be hypo-osmolar, have dextrose added to ensure they are iso-osmolar with blood to prevent an osmotic haemolysis at their site of administration. Hartmann's solution contains sodium, potassium, chloride and calcium at concentrations very similar to those found in the plasma of healthy individuals. It is not possible to store bicarbonate in solution with calcium; instead lactate is used which is metabolised to bicarbonate by the liver. A major disadvantage of crystalloid solutions is that relatively large volumes have to be infused to restore an intravascular volume deficit (the classical 3:1 replacement rule). This can lead to interstitial oedema which may worsen gas exchange in the lungs and impair wound healing in the skin.

Recently, attention has focused on the use of hyper-osmolar crystalloid fluids in the resuscitation of critically ill patients.[6] These have the advantage of needing only small volumes (and consequently shorter infusion times) to achieve resuscitation end-points. They act by drawing fluid from the intracellular and interstitial space to the intravascular volume.

Colloid solutions can be synthetic or derived from blood products.[7,8] A variety of solutions are available with different characteristics. These are essentially crystalloid solutions with biologically inert colloid particles added. The colloid particles act as oncotic agents to retain fluid in the intravascular fluid compartment. The normal colloid oncotic pressure is 25; it is now possible to administer fluids which have colloid oncotic pressures of up to 70. In the absence of capillary leakage of colloid particles, these hyperoncotic solutions can expand the intravascular volume by up to 2–3 times their infused volume.

Albumin is derived from pooled human blood donations and is a 'biological' colloid.[9] Despite this, there are problems associated with albumin administration. Albumin is a blood product and carries with it the risks of infection transmission. Volume-for-volume, albumin is up to 10 times as expensive as other synthetic colloids.

Traditional blood transfusion practice has emphasised the importance of maintaining a near normal haemoglobin concentration in the acutely ill. However, the chosen target haemoglobin or haematocrit has been shown to be extremely variable in clinical practice.[10] Blood is an expensive product with limited availability. Transfusion also has short-term (anaphylaxis, infection) and possible longer term complications (immunosuppression).

THE CRYSTALLOID *VERSUS* COLLOID DEBATE

Proponents of colloid fluid therapy argue that administration of crystalloid alone results in a large fluid load (sometimes in great excess to the fluid volume which has been lost) to achieve the same haemodynamic status as with colloid.[5,8] This expansion of extracellular fluid may produce interstitial oedema in the tissues – most importantly in the lungs where it may impair gas exchange. Impaired gas exchange may counteract any gains in oxygen delivery through increased cardiac output by reducing arterial oxygen tension. Critically ill patients frequently experience hypo-albuminaemia and the colloid may act to improve the colloid oncotic pressure of the plasma towards normal. However, albumin is a poor indicator of colloid oncotic pressure in the critically ill, where a rise in acute phase proteins may attenuate the reduction in colloid oncotic pressure caused by hypo-albuminaemia.

Key point 1

- Despite a prolonged debate about the use of colloids versus crystalloids in resuscitation, it is likely that volume and speed of infusion are more important than choice of fluid.

Proponents of crystalloid therapy argue that any crystalloid which leaks into the extracellular space is rapidly evacuated by the lymphatic system. This is less true in the lungs which have a poorer lymphatic drainage. It has been argued that, in conditions of increased capillary leakage (*e.g.* sepsis), extravasation of colloid particles worsens and prolongs the tissue oedema which occurs.

The perfect colloid particle has yet to be devised. While crystalloid solutions are not associated with anaphylactic or anaphylactoid reactions, all synthetic colloids may induce an allergic reaction. Virtually all synthetic colloids may also impair coagulation.

Key point 2

- The routine use of albumin is not indicated in resuscitation and may be harmful in some groups.

Table 1 Summary of meta-analyses of crystalloid versus colloid randomised controlled trials

Study Year	Studies in the meta-analysis	Pooled patient numbers	Outcome
Alderson et al.[5] 2002	48 trials met inclusion criteria. 38 included data on mortality. 36 trials compared isotonic colloid and crystalloids, 12 trials incorporated hypertonic fluids	960 patients for isotonic colloids and crystalloids. Results also stratified for type of colloid (hetastarch – 7 trials with 197 patients; albumin – 18 trials with 641 patients; gelatin – 4 trials with 95 patients; dextran – 8 trials with 668 participants	Pooled relative risk showed no benefit for resuscitation with colloid over crystalloid. No significant advantages identified with each subgroup of colloid type
Choi et al.[11] 1999	Of 105 studies identified, 17 met the inclusion criteria. Studies were restricted to isotonic crystalloids versus colloids. Outcome measures were mortality, pulmonary oedema and length of stay.	814 patients in the studies identified as suitable	Pooled data did not identify any differences in outcome between crystalloid and colloid resuscitation. Possible survival advantage with crystalloid resuscitation in trauma patients on subgroup analysis. Clinically significant effects may not have been identified.
Schierhout & Roberts[12] 1998	37 randomised controlled trials identified, of which 26 incorporated isotonic colloids versus crystalloid and 11 incorporated hypertonic colloid/crystalloid solutions	Of the 26 eligible trials 19 reported mortality. These 19 trials had 1315 participants	No benefit displayed from colloid resuscitation. Authors concluded that colloid causes 4 extra deaths for every 100 patients resuscitated. Meta-analysis superseded by Cochrane Review of 2002 (see above)
Velanovich[33] 1989	8 studies identified. Non-randomised studies included	826 patients in 8 eligible trials	Pooled data suggested survival advantage with crystalloid, not statistically significant. Survival advantage prominent in trauma patients, though again not to statistical significance

EVIDENCE-BASED FLUID MANAGEMENT

A number of groups have used the technique of meta-analysis to examine critically the evidence in the crystalloid *versus* colloid, hypertonic crystalloid and albumin debates. The large number of clinical trials comparing colloid and crystalloid therapy in resuscitation has been subject to meta-analysis on a number of occasions (Table 1).[5,11,12] In general, resuscitation seems equally effective with either type of fluid provided sufficient volume is given.

Despite the proposed advantages of small volume hypertonic crystalloid resuscitation, a meta-analysis comparing isotonic to hypertonic crystalloid resuscitation in critically ill trauma, burns and surgical patients failed to show a definite advantage to hypertonic crystalloid.[14] In this meta-analysis, randomised controlled trials were identified which compared isotonic crystalloid resuscitation to hypertonic crystalloid resuscitation in patients with trauma burns or surgery. A total of 17 trials were identified with a total of 869 participants. Six trials were identified in surgical patients with a total of 271 participants. In these surgical patients, 1 trial related to intra-abdominal surgery, 2 examined coronary artery surgery, 2 looked at aortic reconstructive surgery, and 1 studied hemiarthroplasty, hysterectomy or radical prostatectomy. In this heterogeneous group of trials, the relative risk of death for surgical patients using hypertonic fluid resuscitation was 0.62, though the confidence intervals were wide (CI, 0.08–4.57).

Albumin has also been examined in a large meta-analysis which showed that the risk of death was higher in all patients given albumin resuscitation for hypovolaemia, burns and hypo-albuminaemia compared with crystalloid/no albumin.[13] In all, 35 randomised controlled trials were identified that met the study inclusion criteria. Mortality data were available in 31 of the trials. In 18 of the studies, albumin was used to resuscitate hypovolaemic patients. This gave 349 albumin-treated patients and 370 control patients. Mortality was 38/349 in the albumin-treated hypovolaemic patients and 26/370 in the control, a relative risk of 1.46 (CI, 0.97–2.22). For burns, three studies were identified giving a total of 81 albumin-treated patients and 82 controls. Mortality was 19/81 and 8/82, respectively, giving a relative risk of 2.4 (CI, 1.11–5.19) for mortality in albumin-treated burns patients. The third group of patients this meta-analysis identified was patients who were hypo-albuminaemic (there is an inverse correlation between albumin concentrations and survival from critical illness). Ten suitable studies were identified with 324 albumin-treated patients and 313 controls. Mortality in the two groups was 50/324 and 36/313 giving a relative risk for mortality with albumin treatment for hypo-albuminaemia of 1.38 (CI, 0.94–2.03).

It is unclear how relevant these conclusions are to abdominal surgery – the patient groups in the different randomised controlled trials were varied and included cardiopulmonary bypass, trauma, paediatric and septic patients as well as those undergoing abdominal surgery. Of the studies examined, only 5 are relevant to general surgical patients (with 121 albumin-treated patients and 141 controls) and 5 to vascular surgical patients.

Recent studies have challenged traditional blood transfusion practice. A Canadian multicentre study compared restricted transfusion (haemoglobin, 7.0–9.0 g/dl) with a liberal transfusion policy (haemoglobin, 10–12 g/dl) in critically ill patients.[15] Outcomes were improved in those receiving restricted transfusions. A further observational study on the critically ill found similar results with transfusion associated with poorer outcome even allowing for differences in illness severity and case mix.[16]

The applicability of these findings to the pre-operative situation is uncertain. No well-conducted, randomised, controlled trial of blood transfusion in abdominal surgery has been performed. Some studies report that patients with ischaemic heart disease do less well at lower haemoglobin levels.[17] Supra-normalisation studies in pre-operative patients also suggest that this group may benefit from higher O_2 delivery and hence higher haemoglobin levels.

Key point 3

- Relative anaemia is well tolerated in the critically ill and blood transfusion may worsen outcome.

MONITORING RESUSCITATION

Despite the development of a number of new monitoring modalities, there has been little real progress in improving clinically useful resuscitation end points in the last 20 years. A warm, well-perfused patient, with a normal mean arterial pressure and adequate urine output, still remains the gold standard in resuscitation. Non-invasive measurements of cardiac output and central venous oxygen tension monitoring continue to attract research interest. In one randomised control trial (RCT) in elderly patients with fractured neck of femur, fluid management using stroke volume end-points significantly improved postoperative outcome and reduced complication rates.[18]

Continuous recording of mixed venous oxygen saturation (SvO_2) has also been investigated as a target end-point in resuscitation. The measurement of true SvO_2 requires a pulmonary artery (PA) catheter to sample pulmonary capillary blood. Several groups have used more easily placed right arterial catheters to measure continuously a surrogate for the SvO_2 – the central venous oxygen saturation.[19] Variable findings have been reported, but a recent trial of early resuscitation in septic patients reported positive results.[20] This interesting RCT protocolised resuscitation in accident and emergency departments using central venous SO_2 as a target end-point. Protocolised patients with central venous O_2 measurements had a significantly better outcome than controls. It should be noted that the intervention group received more resuscitation fluid on average and were also more rapidly resuscitated. Both these factors may be important in explaining the improved outcome reported.

SUPRA-NORMALISATION

In the 1970s and 1980s, a North American group of surgeons and intensivists led by Shoemaker published a number of important papers on high-risk surgical patients.[21] Their findings can be summarised as follows:

1. The majority of patients who die after major surgery die with multi-organ failure. This is associated with inadequate oxygen delivery to the tissues.

2. Survivors of major surgery increase their cardiac index and oxygen delivery in the peri-operative period above baseline 'normal' valves. Non-survivors fail to increase O_2 delivery postoperatively.

3. Simple indices of circulatory status such as urine output, blood pressure and CVP do not correlate with outcome from high risk surgery, whereas cardiac index and oxygen delivery do correlate.

Key point 4

- Several studies report better outcome in both elective and non-elective 'high-risk' surgical patients who receive supra-normalisation protocols before operation.

These findings were confirmed and extended by many other groups. In particular, the increased surgical mortality in patients who are unable to increase their cardiac index has been observed by several groups.[22] The inference drawn from these studies was that patients who could not increase their cardiac output and oxygen delivery in response to surgery suffered from tissue hypoxia.

In a landmark study from 1988, Shoemaker and colleagues tested a hypothesis that enhancing cardiac output and oxygen delivery to the median levels observed in survivors would improve outcome in high-risk surgical patients.[23] Using fluid and inotropes as the interventions, they raised cardiac index to > 4.5 l/min/m^2 (measured using pulmonary artery flotation catheters). Surgical mortality was reduced from 33% (controls) to 4% (intervention group). This study has been criticised. The mortality in the control group was high; patients were allocated according to the clinical team which was on call at night and differences between the teams cannot be excluded.

A number of randomised, controlled studies have followed examining the effect of supra-normalisation in various groups (Table 2). In most studies, impressive results were achieved. However, only a small proportion relate to general surgery. In addition, some studies recruited both emergency and 'high-risk' elective patients without sufficient power for sub-group analysis. Even in studies focusing on elective surgery, the case-mix is very heterogeneous and most series contain both vascular, upper gastrointestinal and lower gastrointestinal cases. Major vascular cases are more likely to have significant cardiac co-morbidity and interventions aimed at raising cardiac output to above normal levels may have a different effect compared to a general surgical population.

Two studies have included significant numbers of abdominal surgical cases. Bennett's group randomised 107 patients into two groups before surgery.[24] Group 1 received standard peri-operative care while group 2 were admitted to a critical care area where a PA catheter was inserted and O_2 delivery augmented to a pre-set target using a combination of volume loading and inotropes. Outcome in the pre-optimised group was significantly improved (5.7% mortality) compared to the controls (22.2% mortality). Despite these results, some aspects of the study remain controversial. Mortality in the control

Table 2 Summary of randomised controlled trials of pre- and postoperative supra-normalisation

Study, Date	Patients	Methods	Outcomes
Lobo et al.[34] 2000	37 high-risk surgical patients (vascular and general); 18 controls and 19 in the intervention group	Patients in the treatment limb had supra-normal delivery of oxygen using a pulmonary artery catheter to guide therapy using fluids, inotropes vasodilators and vasopressors	33% mortality in the control group and 15.7% in the treatment group at 30 days. Study stopped early because of differences in mortality
Wilson et al.[3] 1999	138 patients undergoing major elective surgery at high risk of complications through the surgery or pre-existing conditions	Patients allocated to 1 of 3 groups – 2 had pre-operative optimisation using inotropes (adrenaline or dopexamine), invasive monitoring (with pulmonary artery catheter) and fluids. Control group received standard hospital perioperative care	3/92 pre-optimised patients died in hospital compared with 8/46 controls. Study was confounded by different use of critical care areas and normal ward care between the study and control groups
Sinclair et al.[18] 1997	40 patients presenting with fracture of the femoral neck. 20 patients allocated to the treatment group and 20 allocated to control group	During general anaesthesia, stroke volume was optimised using fluid boluses guided by an oesophageal Doppler ultrasound probe.	5% mortality in the treatment group versus 10% control mortality. Significant reductions (P < 0.05) in length of hospital stay in optimised group
Bishop et al.[35] 1995	115 major trauma patients (50 protocol and 65 control)	Protocol patients had a pulmonary artery catheter with goals of therapy equal to sur-vivor values of oxygen delivery & cardiac index	18% mortality in the treatment group and 37% mortality in the control group
Boyd et al.[24] 1993	107 patients (protocol 53, control 54) identified as having high risk. Heterogeneous surgical procedures of > 1.5 h duration	Both groups admitted pre-operatively to ITU for invasive monitoring (arterial and pulmonary artery). In addition, protocol group had oxygen delivery increased to target levels using inodilators and fluids	Control mortality 22.2% versus protocol mortality of 5.7%. Significant reduction in peri-operative morbidity in the protocol group
Shoemaker et al.[23] 1988	252 high-risk general surgical patients and 146 high-risk general surgical patients in separate series	Patients allocated to receive pre- or postoperative pulmonary artery catheterisation. In second series patients were allocated to receive no PA catheter (CVP only), PA catheter with normal goals, or PA catheter with supranormal goals of haemodynamic therapy	Series 1 – 21% of protocol patients and 38% of control patients died (statistically significant). In series 2, mortality rates were 23% (CVP), 33% series 2, mortality rates were 23% (CVP), 33% (PA control) and 4% (PA protocol). Difference between PA control and protocol group signifi-cant (P < 0.02), but borderline significance between PA protocol and CVP group

group appears high when compared to international figures, although UK data from NCEPOD suggest that control mortality was similar to national levels.[25]

This raises the important issue of best care. The study was performed before the recent UK critical care bed expansion. Not all control group patients initially received any form of critical care and this may have influenced their outcome. Other factors are also important in outcome following surgery, including the experience and seniority of the teams involved in the case. The impact of differences in teams was not investigated or controlled. Finally, both elective and emergency patients were included and, in some cases, supra-normalisation only occurred after surgery.

A second study was performed on elective, high-risk surgical patients in a large district general hospital in the UK.[3] Patients were randomised to three groups: standard care, pre-optimisation with adrenaline, and pre-optimisation with dopexamine. Outcome in both the pre-optimisation groups was better than standard care (standard mortality 17%, intervention mortality 3%) with significantly fewer major postoperative complications occurring in the dopexamine group.

Pre-optimisation may well be effective, but several issues are unresolved. These include the targets to be adopted, the method of monitoring and proper adjustments for patient location and clinical team experience. Finally, future trials should target more homogeneous groups of surgical patients (*e.g.* upper GI tract or elective aortic aneurysm replacement).

Supra-normalisation seems ineffective[26] or even harmful[27] in patients already admitted to critical care units. The role of the pulmonary artery catheter in the critically ill has also been challenged. One retrospective, observational study reported a worse outcome in patients who undergo PA catheterisation in critical care units.[28] Randomised control trials are currently being carried out to investigate further the risks *versus* benefits of PA catheters.

BETA-BLOCKADE

Supra-normalisation studies suggest that some high-risk patients undergoing major surgery would benefit from pre-operative augmentation of their cardiac index and oxygen delivery. However, an apparently conflicting management strategy has emerged – the use of β-blockade to prevent adverse cardiac events in the postoperative period following major surgery (Table 3).

The evidence base for this approach comes from two RCTs which looked at survival in patients who were β-blocked peri-operatively.[29,30] Mangano and co-workers demonstrated lower death rates in the postoperative period in patients undergoing vascular surgery who were given atenolol at induction of anaesthesia. This population had proven coronary artery disease or coronary artery disease risk factors. A further study by Poldermans and colleagues recruited high-risk patients with proven myocardial ischaemia on a stress echocardiogram (20% of those screened) and demonstrated significant reductions in mortality if those with proven ischaemia were β-blocked peri-operatively (17% *versus* 3.4%).[29] There were also reductions in significant non-fatal myocardial events (17% *versus* 0%). Other studies have shown reductions in myocardial ischaemic episodes using β-blockers, but major complications

Table 3 Summary of clinical trials of pre- and peri-operative β-blockade in high-risk, non-cardiac surgery

Study, Year	Patients	Methods	Outcomes
Mangano et al.[30] 1996	200 with proven coronary artery disease or risk factors for coronary artery disease undergoing non-cardiac surgery	Atenolol administered immediately pre-operatively until up to 7 days after surgery. Study criticised as patients who were already on β-blockers may have had them stopped if allocated to the placebo limb	No difference between atenolol treated and placebo group in hospital mortality. Overall mortality 55% lower and cardiovascular mortality 65% lower in the atenolol group 2 years post-surgery
Raby et al.[32] 1999	150 patients undergoing vascular surgery underwent pre-operative Holter monitoring; 26 of these had significant myocardial ischaemia by ST segment analysis. These 26 were allocated to β-blockade or control group	Esmolol or placebo infusion started immediately after surgery for 48 h	Fewer and shorter duration of ischaemic episodes in esmolol group, but mortality not statistically different between groups
Poldermans et al.[29] 1999	1351 patients having major vascular surgery. 846 found to have cardiac risk factors on screening. 173 of these had ischaemia on dobutamine stress echo-cardiography. 59 of these allocated to bisoprolol and 53 allocated to standard peri-operative care	Bisoprolol-treated patients received bisoprolol for 1 week before surgery and 30 days after surgery	17% of the control group died of cardiac causes during the peri-operative period compared to 3.4% of patients in the bisoprolol-treated group ($P = 0.02$). 17% of controls had non-fatal myo-cardial infarctions, compared to 0% of bisoprolol-treated patients ($P < 0.001\%$)
Urban et al.[31] 2000	109 patients having elective knee surgery under regional anaesthesia with proven or risk factors for ischaemic heart disease	Patients in treatment group received esmolol intravenously followed by metoprolol enterally after surgery until hospital discharge	Statistically significant greater incidence and duration of myocardial ischaemia in the control group postoperatively, but myocardial infarction and cardiac morbidity rates not significantly different between the groups

Key point 5

- Two large randomised controlled trials have demonstrated improved outcome in non-cardiac surgical patients with cardiac risk factors who are pre- or peri-operatively β-blocked.

Key point 6

- Organisational aspects of emergency surgical care, including timing, location of peri-operative care, team experience and seniority have important impacts on the survival of patients.

were not reduced significantly in the peri-operative period.[31,32] Despite the positive studies, the use of pre-operative β-blockade still remains controversial. The evidence for efficiency is only present in highly screened patients, mostly undergoing elective vascular surgery. A large empirical study of pre- and peri-operative β-blockade in unscreened high-risk surgical patients is needed.

CONCLUSIONS

In the last 20 years, several approaches to the resuscitation and optimisation of the high-risk surgical patient have been examined. Many of these trials have been heterogeneous in terms of patient entry and it is not possible to draw firm conclusions on abdominal surgical patients alone.

The colloid *versus* crystalloid debate may well have deflected attention away from the more important questions of resuscitation end-points, monitoring, speed, location and experience of clinical teams. Most trials demonstrate the beneficial effect of protocols in resuscitation. Supra-normalisation remains an attractive concept with a significant body of supporting evidence. However, the importance of the individual components (fluid loading, inotrope choice, case-mix, location of care) remains to be determined. Beta-blockade is also effective in improving outcome in some surgical patients with significant cardiac risk factors. Its broader applications to all high-risk patients remain controversial. As always, more large, multicentre, high-quality trials are needed.

Key points for clinical practice

- Despite a prolonged debate about the use of colloids *versus* crystalloids in resuscitation, it is likely that volume and speed of infusion are more important than choice of fluid.

- The routine use of albumin is not indicated in resuscitation and may be harmful in some groups.

Key points for clinical practice (continued)

- Relative anaemia is well tolerated in the critically ill and blood transfusion may worsen outcome.

- Several studies report better outcome in both elective and non-elective 'high-risk' surgical patients who receive supra-normalisation protocols before operation.

- Two large randomised controlled trials have demonstrated improved outcome in non-cardiac surgical patients with cardiac risk factors who are pre- or peri-operatively β-blocked.

- Organisational aspects of emergency surgical care, including timing, location of peri-operative care, team experience and seniority have important impacts on the survival of patients.

References

1. Grounds RM, Rhodes A, Bennett ED. Reducing surgical mortality and complications. In: Vincent J-L. (ed) *2001 Yearbook of Intensive Care and Emergency Medicine*. Berlin: Springer, 2001; 57–67.
2. Treasure T, Bennett D. Reducing the risk of major elective surgery. *BMJ* 1999; **318**: 1087–1088.
3. Wilson J, Woods I, Fawcett J *et al*. Reducing the risk of major elective surgery: randomised controlled trial of preoperative optimisation of oxygen delivery. *BMJ* 1999; **318**: 1099–1103.
4. Boyd O, Street M. Is perioperative intensive care therapy useful in patients with limited cardiovascular reserve? *Curr Opin Crit Care* 1999; **5**: 393–399.
5. Alderson P, Schierhout G, Roberts I, Bunn F. Colloids *versus* crystalloids for fluid resuscitation in critically ill patients. *Cochrane Database System Rev* 2000; CD000567.
6. Brown MD. Evidence-based emergency medicine. Hypertonic versus isotonic crystalloid for fluid resuscitation in critically ill patients. *Ann Emerg Med* 2002; **40**: 113–114.
7. Groeneveld AB. Albumin and artificial colloids in fluid management: where does the clinical evidence of their utility stand? *Crit Care* 2000; **4 (Suppl 2)**: S16–S20.
8. Waikar SS, Chertow GM. Crystalloids *versus* colloids for resuscitation in shock. *Curr Opin Nephrol Hypertens* 2000; **9**: 501–504.
9. Pulimood TB, Park GR. Debate: albumin administration should be avoided in the critically ill. *Crit Care* 2000; **4**: 151–155.
10. Hebert PC, Wells G, Marshall J *et al*. Transfusion requirements in critical care. A pilot study. Canadian Critical Care Trials Group. *JAMA* 1995; **273**: 1439–1444.
11. Choi PT, Yip G, Quinonez LG, Cook DJ. Crystalloids vs. colloids in fluid resuscitation: a systematic review. *Crit Care Med* 1999; **27**: 200–210.
12. Schierhout G, Roberts I. Fluid resuscitation with colloid or crystalloid solutions in critically ill patients: a systematic review of randomised trials. *BMJ* 1998; **316**: 961–964.
13. Alderson P, Bunn F, Lefebvre C *et al*. Human albumin solution for resuscitation and volume expansion in critically ill patients. *Cochrane Database System Rev* 2002; CD001208.
14. Bunn F, Roberts I, Tasker R, Akpa E. Hypertonic *versus* isotonic crystalloid for fluid resuscitation in critically ill patients. *Cochrane Database System Rev* 2002; CD002045.
15. Hebert PC, Wells G, Blajchman MA *et al*. A multicenter, randomized, controlled clinical trial of transfusion requirements in critical care. Transfusion Requirements in Critical Care Investigators, Canadian Critical Care Trials Group. *N Engl J Med* 1999; **340**: 409–417.

16. Vincent JL, Baron JF, Reinhart K *et al*. Anemia and blood transfusion in critically ill patients. *JAMA* 2002; **288**: 1499–1507.
17. Carson JL, Duff A, Poses RM *et al*. Effect of anaemia and cardiovascular disease on surgical mortality and morbidity. *Lancet* 1996; **348**: 1055–1060.
18. Sinclair S, James S, Singer M. Intra-operative intravascular volume optimisation and length of hospital stay after repair of proximal femoral fracture: randomised controlled trial. *BMJ* 1997; **315**: 909–912.
19. Rivers EP, Ander DS, Powell D. Central venous oxygen saturation monitoring in the critically ill patient. *Curr Opin Crit Care* 2001; **7**: 204–211.
20. Rivers E, Nguyen B, Havstad S *et al*. Early goal-directed therapy in the treatment of severe sepsis and septic shock. *N Engl J Med* 2001; **345**: 1368–1377.
21. Kern JW, Shoemaker WC. Meta-analysis of hemodynamic optimization in high-risk patients. *Crit Care Med* 2002; **30**: 1686–1692.
22. Savino JA, Del Guercio LR. Pre-operative assessment of high-risk surgical patients. *Surg Clin North Am* 1985; **65**: 763–791.
23. Shoemaker WC, Appel PL, Kram HB, Waxman K, Lee TS. Prospective trial of supranormal values of survivors as therapeutic goals in high-risk surgical patients. *Chest* 1988; **94**: 1176–1186.
24. Boyd O, Grounds RM, Bennett ED. A randomized clinical trial of the effect of deliberate peri-operative increase of oxygen delivery on mortality in high-risk surgical patients. *JAMA* 1993; **270**: 2699–2707.
25. Anon. *The Report of the National Confidential Enquiry into Perioperative Deaths 1996/1997*. London, NCEPOD, 1998.
26. Gattinoni L, Brazzi L, Pelosi P *et al*. A trial of goal-oriented hemodynamic therapy in critically ill patients. SvO$_2$ Collaborative Group. *N Engl J Med* 1995; **333**: 1025–1032.
27. Hayes MA, Timmins AC, Yau EH, Palazzo M, Hinds CJ, Watson D. Elevation of systemic oxygen delivery in the treatment of critically ill patients. *N Engl J Med* 1994; **330**: 1717–1722.
28. Connors AF, Speroff T, Dawson NV. The effectiveness of right heart catheterization in the initial care of critically ill patients. *JAMA* 2000; **27**: 889–897.
29. Poldermans D, Boersma E, Bax JJ *et al*. The effect of bisoprolol on perioperative mortality and myocardial infarction in high-risk patients undergoing vascular surgery. Dutch Echocardiographic Cardiac Risk Evaluation Applying Stress Echocardiography Study Group. *N Engl J Med* 1999; **341**: 1789–1794.
30. Mangano DT, Layug EL, Wallace A, Tateo I. Effect of atenolol on mortality and cardiovascular morbidity after noncardiac surgery. Multicenter Study of Perioperative Ischemia Research Group. *N Engl J Med* 1996; **335**: 1713–1720.
31. Urban MK, Markowitz SM, Gordon MA, Urquhart BL, Kligfield P. Postoperative prophylactic administration of beta-adrenergic blockers in patients at risk for myocardial ischemia. *Anesth Analg* 2000; **90**: 1257–1261.
32. Raby KE, Brull SJ, Timimi F *et al*. The effect of heart rate control on myocardial ischemia among high-risk patients after vascular surgery. *Anesth Analg* 1999; **88**: 477–482.
33. Velanovich V. Crystalloid *versus* colloid fluid resuscitation: a meta-analysis of mortality. *Surgery* 1989; **105**: 65–71.
34. Lobo SM, Salgado PF, Castillo VG *et al*. Effects of maximizing oxygen delivery on morbidity and mortality in high-risk surgical patients. *Crit Care Med* 2000; **28**: 3396–3404.
35. Bishop MH, Shoemaker WC, Appel PL *et al*. Prospective, randomized trial of survivor values of cardiac index, oxygen delivery, and oxygen consumption as resuscitation endpoints in severe trauma. *J Trauma* 1995; **38**: 780–787.

Timothy K. McCullough   Timothy G. Allen-Mersh

2

Recognition and significance of cancer cells in the circulation

Haematogenous metastasis requires detachment from the primary tumour, embolisation, arrest, implantation, proliferation and development of a surrounding stromal reaction.[1] Thus, the presence of metastases or micro-metastases can only be definitively established by histological identification of cancer cells with a tumour-related stromal support. Reliable identification and biopsy of such a micrometastatic site is frequently not possible, and current staging systems rely on surrogate variables (*e.g.* locoregional lymph node involvement within the excised tumour) that offer only a probability, rather than a certainty, of identifying residual disease.

Guidelines for treatment of colorectal cancer recommend that adjuvant chemotherapy should be given where there is histological evidence of lymph node involvement in the excised specimen.[2] However, 30% of node-negative colorectal patients relapse and die from metastases, and a similar proportion of node-positive patients are cured by surgical excision alone.[3] If colorectal cancer patients predicted by lymph node staging to be cured, but who are destined to develop recurrence could be identified, then the survival benefits of adjuvant treatment could also be offered to these patients. Similarly, if those patients with node-positive tumours who have been cured by surgery could be identified, then they could be spared the potential toxicity of adjuvant therapy, and the associated costs could be avoided. Many patients at low risk of developing recurrent disease opt for adjuvant chemotherapy because of this uncertainty. Detection of clinically occult residual cancer would allow the advantage of increased efficacy, with earlier adjuvant chemotherapy,[4] to be

Mr Timothy K. McCullough BSc MBBS MRCS, Research Fellow, Department of Surgery, Imperial College School of Science, Technology and Medicine, Chelsea and Westminster Hospital, 369 Fulham Road, London SW10 9NH, UK

Prof. Timothy G. Allen-Mersh BSc MD FRCS, Professor of Gastrointestinal Surgery, Imperial College School of Science, Technology and Medicine, Chelsea and Westminster Hospital, 369 Fulham Road, London SW10 9NH, UK (for correspondence)

Key point 1

- Earlier identification of residual disease leads to more effective treatment.

Key point 2

- There is an inherent inaccuracy in histological staging, which makes correct allocation of adjuvant therapy difficult.

---

gained in patients with proven residual disease without also treating patients who have been cured by tumour excision.

EXPERIMENTAL STUDIES OF TUMOUR CELLS IN THE CIRCULATION

Experimentally, Glaves[5] showed that the shedding of tumour cells into the circulation was sporadic, and Liotta et al.[6] demonstrated the greater ability of tumour cell clumps to produce metastases compared to single cells. Fidler[7] found that only 1% of radiolabelled melanoma cells survived for longer than 24 h after intravenous injection into mice, with most of the remaining cells localising within the lungs.

Proposed mechanisms for the clearing of circulating tumour cells (CTCs) from the circulation include mechanical trauma from turbulent blood flow, tumour cell deformation on passing through small vessels, shear forces, and host natural killer T-cells.[8] However, intravasation (gaining access to the circulation) and survival within the circulation may not be the main reason for metastatic inefficiency. Cameron et al.[9] developed an in vivo model to visualise metastasising cells. They found that the intravascular survival of injected melanoma cells was high, with most circulating cells able to extravasate (pass out of the circulation at a potential metastatic site), but that growth of an extravasated cell clump to form a metastasis was unlikely. Factors influencing whether these extravasated cells die, become dormant, or grow into metastases are poorly understood.

Thus, there is uncertainty about whether tumour cells in the circulation represent cancer dissemination, or are simply cells that have detached from the primary tumour and are destined to die without metastasising. The development of more sensitive techniques for detecting small numbers of CTCs has led to studies of the clinical significance of tumour cells in the blood.

Key point 3

- The study of circulating tumour cells has a long history, but new sensitive detection techniques have renewed interest in their significance.

CLINICAL DETECTION OF CIRCULATING TUMOUR CELLS

MORPHOMETRIC METHODS

Initially, clinical studies of cancer cells entering the circulation involved light microscopy, but inaccuracies based on uncertainty about morphometric identification of cancer cells led to scepticism of the results and to development of more specific detection methods. Light microscopy was used to identify tumour cell characteristics such as hyperchromatic nuclei, irregular chromatin pattern, abnormal mitoses and prominent nucleoli. Some normal blood precursors (*e.g.* megakaryocytes) gave false-positive results,[10] and it was also suggested that false positivity could result from epithelial cells being cored by percutaneous needle venesection.[10] Fluorescence-activated cell sorting (FACS) and immunocytochemistry have improved the accuracy of light microscopy in CTC detection. The technique relies on the binding of fluorescent ligands to the circulating cancer cell membranes, in proportion to the cell surface area. Different cell types can be sorted by the pattern of light scatter produced when they pass through a light beam. It has been applied to a variety of tumours, including gastric, breast and prostate cancers,[11–13] with *in vitro* sensitivities of up to 1 in 10^7 nucleated cells, where magnetic and immunocytochemical enrichment methods are used. This equates to one tumour cell in 20 ml of collected blood. *In vivo*, the sensitivity of FACS is reduced to about 1 tumour cell in 10^5 normal cells,[14] and some groups have questioned whether *in vitro* findings can currently be translated to clinical CTC detection.[15] As a result, the role of FACS in the clinical detection of circulating tumour cells remains uncertain, and most clinical CTC studies have relied on molecular detection techniques.

MOLECULAR DETECTION TECHNIQUES

Polymerase chain reaction (PCR)

The most sensitive methods for CTC identification are the polymerase chain reaction and reverse-transcription polymerase chain reaction (PCR and RT-PCR). The key insight was the process by which segments of DNA can be amplified *in vitro* by enzymatic replication to reach detectable concentrations.[16] The polymerase (Taq) – first derived from the bacterium *Thermus aquaticus* – promotes the high temperature (specific), high-yield, long-segment replication of genomic DNA by a factor of at least 10 million, and therefore permits DNA identification. In the case of cancers, this DNA may be a cancer-associated mutation or another cancer-specific sequence that amplifies only DNA arising from the target. Specific sense and anti-sense primers that bind to part of the upstream target sequence are used as the starting point for the polymerase, to begin copying the relevant part of the DNA strands. The cycling of the reaction-mixture temperature enables sequential denaturation (separation of the double-stranded template), annealing (binding of the primers to their targets), and extension (copying of the target sequence by Taq polymerase in 5' to 3' direction) such that after approximately 30 cycles, 10^9 cDNA copies can theoretically be made from a single initial target copy. In fact, due to the reaction kinetics and progressive inactivation of the enzyme, the number of copies generated is fewer. PCR requires consistent DNA abnormalities to detect

CTCs reliably, and has been used mainly in haematological malignancies that are frequently associated with specific DNA mutations.

RT-PCR

The absence of consistent DNA anomalies in most solid tumours has limited the use of PCR in CTC detection. RT-PCR is able to identify the transcripts of a given gene by detecting the messenger (m)RNA coding for the gene. Total RNA is extracted from the blood sample or other specimen, and undergoes reverse transcription to produce complimentary DNA (cDNA), which may then be amplified by PCR. In this way, tissue-specific mRNA can be detected within the specimen. If the selected mRNA/protein target is not expressed in the normal constituents of blood, but is identified within the blood, it may be concluded that it arises from cells of another tissue type not normally found in the circulation. A unique CTC marker has not been found, but it has been possible to use tissue, if not tumour. specific markers. Benign cells (*e.g.* of epithelial origin) are not thought to enter the circulation, and since free RNA has a very short half-life outside the cell, the presence of specific mRNA in blood suggests the presence of CTCs. An epithelium-specific marker can, therefore, be used for RT-PCR detection of CTCs from carcinomas.

RT-PCR has also been applied to the transcripts of specific mutations, such as k-ras and p53, not only in the blood, but also in lymph nodes for colorectal cancer and the urine for CTC of the bladder.[17,18] A significant finding has been that the p53 mutation found in CTCs from colorectal cancer patients matches that of the primary or metastatic tumour,[19,20] suggesting a clonal origin of CTCs from the relevant solid tumour. These mutations are unfortunately not ubiquitous among solid tumours, and the tissue-specific markers have proved more useful in CTC identification.

Key point 4

• The most sensitive methods are polymerase chain reaction-based, but polymerase chain reaction alone for circulating tumour cell detection is limited.

RT-PCR STUDIES IN SOLID TUMOURS

Breast cancer

Studies of CTC detection in breast cancer, have used targets, such as MUC-1, cytokeratin-19, carcinoembryonic antigen (CEA) and, most recently, mammaglobin mRNA, with varied success: CEA and CK-19 showed greater sensitivity than MUC-1, but CK-19 and MUC-1 showed greatest sensitivity[21] in predicting outcome. Mammaglobin has proved to be a specific marker, and also has a high *in vitro* sensitivity, but low numbers of cancer patients test positive in *in vivo* trials.[22] The practice of autologous blood stemcell re-infusion in patients undergoing chemotherapy has raised the question of contamination of the graft with breast cancer cells and RT-PCR may also have a role in identifying cancer cells in bone marrow products.[23]

Colorectal cancer

RT-PCR (mainly involving cytokeratin mRNA targets) has been used in the detection of colorectal cancer cells in resected lymph nodes, to improve on the sensitivity of existing histological staging. The cytokeratins make up a family whose members vary between tissue types. The usefulness of CK-8, CK-18 and CK-19 is limited by their presence in normal lymph nodes, endothelial tissue and fibroblasts.[24,25] CK-20 is not found in normal lymph nodes,[26] and has been used as a mRNA target for the detection of circulating and bone marrow colorectal cancer cells. CEA is expressed at elevated levels in almost all colorectal cancers,[27] and CEA mRNA has also been used as an RT-PCR target in colorectal cancer lymph node studies (Fig. 1). Other molecular markers (*e.g.* MUC-1) have been investigated,[28] with lesser success. It should be remembered that identification of lymph node involvement in the excised specimen is not direct evidence of residual disease. Perhaps for this reason, RT-PCR based attempts at lymph node staging have been associated with a high false positive rate in predicting residual disease.[29] Tumour cell detection in the blood (CTC) after treatment may be a more accurate predictor of recurrence.

Although RT-PCR is able to detect colorectal CTCs with an *in vitro* sensitivity of one tumour cell in 10^6 nucleated cells, its sensitivity *in vivo* is not clear. It has been suggested that the use of multiple mRNA targets and multiple blood samples may increase the sensitivity obtained with single mRNA targets.[20] Multiple mRNA targets address the heterogeneous expression between tumours, of proteins and their mRNAs. Multiple sampling increases the

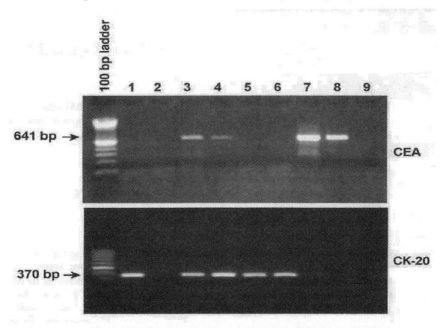

Fig. 1 Electrophoretic gel (agarose with ethidium bromide) that allows visualisation of PCR products when viewed under UV light. Top gel shows 641 bp fragment corresponding to CEA cDNA. Lanes 3, 4 and 8 are positive results from the blood of colon cancer patients and lane 7 is a positive control using colon cancer cell line HT29. Bottom gel shows 370 bp fragment corresponding to CK-20 cDNA. Lanes 1–3 and 5–8 are from colorectal cancer patients. Lanes 1, 3, 5 and 6 are positive. Lane 4 is a positive control using colon cancer cell line HT29.

probability of obtaining tumour cells in a venesection sample where there is sporadic tumour shedding into the blood and clumping. Estimates of false positivity vary, but are likely to be as high as 10–15%, as a result of sample contamination by venesection-cored skin cells expressing the target mRNA, illegitimate transcription during RT, or genomic contamination in PCR preparation. The use of pre-flushed venesection cannulae reduces skin cell contamination of percutaneous venesected blood samples.[30]

As with lymph node studies, the markers most used for CTC detection have been CEA and CK-20, although guanylyl cyclase C may be a more specific marker.[31]

Studies thus far have shown that CTCs are a consistent finding in invasive colorectal carcinoma, with little correlation to histological stage, and that clearance of the cells from the circulation after resection may be of more prognostic significance. In patients tested at 24 h after complete colorectal cancer resection, CTC prevalence fell in earlier stage (Dukes' A and B) but not in more advanced stage (Dukes' C) tumours.[32] CTC detection at 24 h after primary tumour resection seems to have a similar accuracy to lymph node staging in predicting colorectal cancer recurrence. The combination of CTC and lymph node status is capable of identifying over 90% of patients destined to develop recurrence.[33]

Lung cancer

The role of lung cancer CTC detection has mainly been to evaluate response to chemotherapy. The principal targets used in lung cancer have been CEA, CK-19, and squamous cell antigen mRNA. Studies suggest sensitivities between 50% *in vivo*[34] and 100% *in vitro*[35] in cancer cell detection in blood, but report poor specificity, especially for CK-19,[34] which was detectable in no-cancer control blood samples. There has been little work on predicting lung cancer recurrence using circulating tumour cell detection

Malignant melanoma

Tyrosinase mRNA has been a target used in detection of circulating malignant melanoma cells for over a decade;[36] although other targets (*e.g.* MART-1 mRNA) have also been used, there is still controversy about whether tyrosinase mRNA is of prognostic value in the monitoring of melanoma patients. Variation in both sensitivity and specificity in detecting circulating melanoma cells is reported from studies involving patients with all stages of disease. One explanation is that many different experimental protocols have been used and there has been little standardisation between studies.[37,38] Gogas et al.[39] found that of CTC-positive patients undergoing adjuvant interferon therapy after resection of stage IIb or III melanoma, those who tested positive in the follow-up period had a higher chance of relapse than those who became negative after resection. Other groups suggest that RT-PCR on blood using the tyrosinase mRNA target may be useful in monitoring early stage, but not late stage, tumours.[40] Most studies examining outcome in melanoma have been small and with limited longer-term follow-up; there is no current consensus on the role of RT-PCR in melanoma.

> **Key point 6**
>
> • Current molecular detection methods need standardising, and need to be more robust for introduction into clinical usage.

Prostate cancer

Evidence from several studies suggests that CTC identification using a prostate-specific antigen (PSA) mRNA target, correlates with adverse tumour stage and may have a role in pre- and postoperative assessment.[41] However, results of studies detecting PSA mRNA in the blood of prostate cancer patients have suggested varied sensitivities[42,43] in predicting outcome, and differences in the protocols used in CTC identification may account for this.

> **Key point 7**
>
> • The prognostic significance of circulating tumour cell detection is becoming apparent.

THE FUTURE

Although RT-PCR currently remains the gold standard for the detection of CTCs, technical difficulties persist, and it is not yet clear whether the test is robust, reproducible and useful in clinical practice. Portability of blood samples for RT-PCR will require an effective means of RNA preservation, without which the shelf-life of a fresh sample is thought to be about 30 min.[44] Newer molecular techniques are being evaluated, for example nucleic acid sequence-based amplification (NASBA), which may eliminate the problem of genomic DNA contamination and the difficulties posed by primer design.[45] These methods remain at an early stage of development in their potential application to CTC detection.

Although standardisation of the current varied RT-PCR protocols would allow comparisons between studies, techniques for CTC detection are still being optimised, and there may be difficulties in obtaining consensus about protocols. In 1975, Salsbury predicted that CTC detection would be of no prognostic value.[10] He was probably right about detection before treatment where CTCs seem to be almost ubiquitous in the presence of invasive cancer, but emerging results suggest that CTC detection may have an important role in predicting recurrence after apparently curative treatment. The availability of cancer cells within the circulation in patients with occult residual disease will also provide a source for tumour genotyping, allowing more rational allocation of treatments.

Key points for clinical practice

- .Earlier identification of residual disease leads to more effective treatment.

- .There is an inherent inaccuracy in histological staging, which makes correct allocation of adjuvant therapy difficult.

- .The study of circulating tumour cells has a long history, but new sensitive detection techniques have renewed interest in their significance.

- .The most sensitive methods are polymerase chain reaction-based, but polymerase chain reaction alone for CTC detection is limited.

- .Reverse transcriptase-polymerase chain reaction is the most widely used molecular detection technique for circulating tumour cells.

- .Current molecular detection methods need standardising, and need to be more robust for introduction into clinical usage.

- .The prognostic significance of circulating tumour cell detection is becoming apparent.

References

1. Hermanek P, Hutter RV, Sobin LH, Wittekind C, International Union Against Cancer. Classification of isolated tumor cells and micrometastasis. *Cancer* 1999; **86**: 2668–2673.
2. Benson 3rd AB, Choti MA, Cohen AM *et al*. NCCN Practice guidelines for colorectal cancer. *Oncology (Huntingt)* 2000; **14**: 203–212.
3. Allum WH, Slaney G, McConkey CC, Powell J. Cancer of the colon and rectum in the West Midlands, 1957–1981. *Br J Surg* 1994; **81**: 1060–1063.
4. Nordic Gastrointestinal Tumor Adjuvant Therapy Group. Expectancy or primary chemotherapy in patients with advanced asymptomatic colorectal cancer: a randomized trial. *J Clin Oncol* 1992; **10**: 904–911.
5. Glaves D. Correlation between circulating cancer cells and incidence of metastases. *Br J Cancer* 1983; **48**: 665–673.
6. Liotta LA, Saidel MG, Kleinerman J. The significance of hematogenous tumor cell clumps in the metastatic process. *Cancer Res* 1976; **36**: 889–894.
7. Fidler IJ. Metastasis: quantitative analysis of distribution and fate of tumor emboli labeled with ^{125}I-5-iodo-2'-deoxyuridine. *J Natl Cancer Inst* 1970; **45**: 773–782.
8. Weiss L, Nannmark U, Johansson BR, Bagge U. Lethal deformation of cancer cells in the microcirculation: a potential rate regulator of hematogenous metastasis. *Int J Cancer* 1992; **50**: 103–107.
9. Cameron MD, Schmidt EE, Kerkvliet N *et al*. Temporal progression of metastasis in lung: cell survival, dormancy, and location dependence of metastatic inefficiency. *Cancer Res* 2000; **60**: 2541–2546.
10. Salsbury AJ. The significance of the circulating cancer cell. *Cancer Treat Rev* 1975; **2**: 55–72.

11. Pituch-Noworolska A, Wieckiewicz J, Krzeszowiak A *et al*. Evaluation of circulating tumour cells expressing CD44 variants in the blood of gastric cancer patients by flow cytometry. *Anticancer Res* 1998; **18**: 3747–3752.

12. Beitsch PD, Clifford E. Detection of carcinoma cells in the blood of breast cancer patients. *Am J Surg* 2000; **180**: 446–448; discussion 448–449.

13. Fadlon EJ, Rees RC, McIntyre C, Sharrard RM, Lawry J, Hamdy FC. Detection of circulating prostate-specific antigen-positive cells in patients with prostate cancer by flow cytometry and reverse transcription polymerase chain reaction. *Br J Cancer* 1996; **74**: 400–405.

14. Molino A, Colombatti M, Bonetti F *et al*. A comparative analysis of three different techniques for the detection of breast cancer cells in bone marrow. *Cancer* 1991; **67**: 1033–1036.

15. Tsavellas G, Huang A, McCullough T, Patel H, Araia R, Allen-Mersh TG. Flow cytometry correlates with RT-PCR for detection of spiked but not circulating colorectal cancer cells. *Clin Exp Metastasis* 2002; **19**: 495–502.

16. Saiki RK, Gelfand DH, Stoffel S *et al*. Primer-directed enzymatic amplification of DNA with a thermostable DNA polymerase. *Science* 1988; **239**: 487–491.

17. Hayashi N, Ito I, Yanagisawa A *et al*. Genetic diagnosis of lymph-node metastasis in colorectal cancer. *Lancet* 1995; **345**: 1257–1259.

18. Sidransky D, Von Eschenbach A, Tsai YC *et al*. Identification of p53 gene mutations in bladder cancers and urine samples. *Science* 1991; **252**: 706–709.

19. Khan ZA, Jonas SK, Le-Marer N *et al*. p53 mutations in primary and metastatic tumors and circulating tumor cells from colorectal carcinoma patients. *Clin Cancer Res* 2000; **6**: 3499–3504.

20. Wharton RQ, Jonas SK, Glover C *et al*. Increased detection of circulating tumor cells in the blood of colorectal carcinoma patients using two reverse transcription-PCR assays and multiple blood samples. *Clin Cancer Res* 1999; **5**: 4158–4163.

21. Berois N, Varangot M, Aizen B *et al*. Molecular detection of cancer cells in bone marrow and peripheral blood of patients with operable breast cancer. Comparison of CK19, MUC1 and CEA using RT-PCR. *Eur J Cancer* 2000; **36**: 717–723.

22. Silva AL, Tome MJ, Correia AE, Passos-Coelho JL. Human mammaglobin RT-PCR assay for detection of occult breast cancer cells in hematopoietic products. *Ann Oncol* 2002; **13**: 422–429.

23. Kruger WH, Stockschlader M, Hennings S *et al*. Detection of cancer cells in peripheral blood stem cells of women with breast cancer by RT-PCR and cell culture. *Bone Marrow Transplant* 1996; **18 (Suppl 1)**: S18–S20.

24. Traweek ST, Liu J, Battifora H. Keratin gene expression in non-epithelial tissues. Detection with polymerase chain reaction. *Am J Pathol* 1993; **142**: 1111–1118.

25. Gunn J, McCall JL, Yun K, Wright PA. Detection of micrometastases in colorectal cancer patients by K19 and K20 reverse-transcription polymerase chain reaction. *Lab Invest* 1996; **75**: 611–616.

26. Dorudi S, Kinrade E, Marshall NC, Feakins R, Williams NS, Bustin SA. Genetic detection of lymph node micrometastases in patients with colorectal cancer. *Br J Surg* 1998; **85**: 98–100.

27. Shuster J, Thomson DM, Fuks A, Gold P. Immunologic approaches to diagnosis of malignancy. *Prog Exp Tumor Res* 1980; **25**: 89–139.

28. Hardingham JE, Hewett PJ, Sage RE *et al*. Molecular detection of blood-borne epithelial cells in colorectal cancer patients and in patients with benign bowel disease. *Int J Cancer* 2000; **89**: 8–13.

29. Mori M, Mimori K, Ueo H *et al*. Clinical significance of molecular detection of carcinoma cells in lymph nodes and peripheral blood by reverse transcription-polymerase chain reaction in patients with gastrointestinal or breast carcinomas. *J Clin Oncol* 1998; **16**: 128–132.

30. Wharton RQ, Patel H, Jonas SK, Glover C, Weston M, Allen-Mersh TG. Venesection needle coring increases positive results with RT-PCR for detection of circulating cells expressing CEA mRNA. *Clin Exp Metastasis* 2000; **18**: 291–294.

31. Bustin SA, Gyselman VG, Williams NS, Dorudi S. Detection of cytokeratins 19/20 and guanylyl cyclase C in peripheral blood of colorectal cancer patients. *Br J Cancer* 1999; **79**: 1813–1820.

32. Patel H, Le Marer N, Wharton RQ *et al*. Clearance of circulating tumor cells after excision of primary colorectal cancer. *Ann Surg* 2002; **235**: 226–231.

33. McCullough TK, Evans AJ, Hanna AJ, Wharton RQ, Patel H, Allen-Mersh TG. Detection of circulating tumour cells at 24 h after primary resection predicts colorectal cancer recurrence. *Br J Surg* 2002; **89**: 68.

34. Krismann M, Todt B, Schroder J *et al*. Low specificity of cytokeratin 19 reverse transcriptase-polymerase chain reaction analyses for detection of hematogenous lung cancer dissemination. *J Clin Oncol* 1995; **13**: 2769–2775.

35. Dingemans AM, Brakenhoff RH, Postmus PE, Giaccone G. Detection of cytokeratin-19 transcripts by reverse transcriptase-polymerase chain reaction in lung cancer cell lines and blood of lung cancer patients. *Lab Invest* 1997; **77**: 213–220.

36. Smith B, Selby P, Southgate J, Pittman K, Bradley C, Blair GE. Detection of melanoma cells in peripheral blood by means of reverse transcriptase and polymerase chain reaction. *Lancet* 1991; **338**: 1227–1229.

37. Seiter S, Rappl G, Tilgen W, Ugurel S, Reinhold U. Facts and pitfalls in the detection of tyrosinase mRNA in the blood of melanoma patients by RT-PCR. *Recent Results Cancer Res* 2001; **158**: 105–112.

38. Keilholz U, Willhauck M, Rimoldi D *et al*. Reliability of reverse transcription-polymerase chain reaction (RT-PCR)-based assays for the detection of circulating tumour cells: a quality-assurance initiative of the EORTC Melanoma Cooperative Group. *Eur J Cancer* 1998; **34**: 750–753.

39. Gogas H, Kefala G, Bafaloukos D *et al*. Prognostic significance of the sequential detection of circulating melanoma cells by RT-PCR in high-risk melanoma patients receiving adjuvant interferon. *Br J Cancer* 2002; **87**: 181–186.

40. Waldmann V, Wacker J, Deichmann M, Jackel A, Bock M, Naher H. Prognosis of metastatic melanoma: no correlation of tyrosinase mRNA in bone marrow and survival time. *Recent Results Cancer Res* 2001; **158**: 118–125.

41. Gomella LG, Raj GV, Moreno JG. Reverse transcriptase polymerase chain reaction for prostate specific antigen in the management of prostate cancer. *J Urol* 1997; **158**: 326–337.

42. de la Taille A, Olsson CA, Katz AE. Molecular staging of prostate cancer: dream or reality? *Oncology (Huntingt)* 1999; **13**: 187–194; discussion 194–198, 204–205.

43. Ghossein RA, Scher HI, Gerald WL *et al*. Detection of circulating tumor cells in patients with localized and metastatic prostatic carcinoma: clinical implications. *J Clin Oncol* 1995; **13**: 1195–1200.

44. Tsui NB, Ng EK, Lo YM. Stability of endogenous and added RNA in blood specimens, serum, and plasma. *Clin Chem* 2002; **48**: 1647–1653.

45. Burchill SA, Perebolte L, Johnston C, Top B, Selby P. Comparison of the RNA-amplification based methods RT-PCR and NASBA for the detection of circulating tumour cells. *Br J Cancer* 2002; **86**: 102–109.

Simon R. Bramhall

3

The matrix metalloproteinases: their potential clinical role

The extracellular matrix (ECM) is important in cell and tissue support, and in forming different tissue compartments. The matrix also provides a surface for molecular sieving and cellular regulation. Extracellular barriers are formed by the matrix (Table 1), comprising the basement membrane and interstitial stroma, and the subendothelial basement membrane. The principal component of the basement membrane is type IV collagen providing the scaffold upon which the other major components (laminin and heparan sulphate proteoglycan) and the minor components of the matrix are assembled. Under

Table 1 The extracellular matrix

	Function	Composition
Basement Membrane	Boundary between parenchyma and stroma	Type IV collagen Laminin Fibronectin Type V collagen Heparan sulphate proteoglycan

Interstitial stroma	Separates blood vessels and lymphatics from organ parenchyma	Type IV collagen
		Elastin
		Anchoring fibres and fibrils
		Ground substance
		    Type I collagen
		    Type III collagen
		    Type V collagen
		    Fibronectin
		    Elastin
		    Proteoglycans

Mr Simon R Bramhall MD FRCS, Consultant Hepatobiliary and Transplant Surgeon, Liver Unit, The Queen Elizabeth Hospital, Edgbaston, Birmingham B15 2TH, UK

Key point 1

- A complex series of regulatory enzymes control extracellular matrix integrity that may be disrupted by cell/basement membrane attachment, excess secretion of proteolytic enzymes or a reduction in the secretion of inhibitors.

normal conditions, the ECM is an insoluble structure that cannot be breached by cells. However, focal permeability may occur during healing, remodelling, tissue inflammation and neoplastic development. Within the human genome, over 500 genes have been identified that encode proteases or protease-like proteins.[1] A complex series of regulatory enzymes control ECM integrity and this may be disrupted by: (i) cell/basement membrane attachment via cell surface receptors; (ii) excess cellular secretion of proteolytic enzymes or a reduction in the secretion of inhibitors; and (iii) tumour cell migration into the region modified by proteolysis.

The defining characteristic of tumours is their ability to invade tissues and generate metastases. Invasion is defined as the process of movement, penetration or infiltration of cells into adjacent tissues. Tumour cell invasion has to occur at three sites for the successful establishment of metastases: (i) the immediate tumour-host interface; (ii) the local vascular or lymphatic endothelium; and (iii) the endothelium at the site of the metastases. The degradation of ECM is an essential step in the processes of invasion and metastasis. ECM degradation is, however, not limited to malignant cells, and ECM degradation is also characteristic of a number of 'benign' conditions including the arthropathies, vascular aneurysms and atherosclerosis.

In scirrhous tumours, there is an intense stromal reaction, which is a direct result of the malignant epithelial cells themselves. For example, loss of basement membrane integrity in breast and colorectal cancers has been shown to be associated with an increased risk of metastasis and poor prognosis. Loss of continuity of type IV collagen in the basement membrane and absence of basement membrane proteoglycans are common features of pancreatic cancer. These findings indicate that proteolytic degradation is likely to be an important aspect of the invasive phenotype.

MATRIX METALLOPROTEINASES

The matrix metalloproteinases (MMPs) are a family of 24 proteolytic enzymes that share common characteristics (Table 2).

1. Each degrades at least one component of the ECM, basement membrane proteins and bioactive mediators.

2. All contain a zinc ion.

3. All are secreted as a pro-enzyme, which in each case is activated by cleavage of defined peptide sequences.

4. All share sequence homologies.

Table 2 Nomenclature of the human matrix metalloproteinases

Domain organisation	Group	Names		
Archetypal MMPs	Collagenases	MMP1	Type I collagenase	Interstitial collagenase
		MMP8	Collagenase 2	PMN collagenase
		MMP13	Collagenase 3	
	Stromelysins	MMP3	Stromelysin	Transin
		MMP10	Stromelysin 2	Transin 2
	Other MMPs	MMP12	Metalloelastase	
		MMP19		
		MMP20	Enamelysin	
		MMP27	MMP22	C-MMP
Gelatinases		MMP2	72 kDa type IV collagenase	Gelatinase A
		MMP9	92 kDa type IV collagenase	Gelatinase B
Matrilysins		MMP7	**PU**tative **M**atrix metallo**P**roteinase (PUMP1)	Matrilysin
		MMP26		Matrilysin 2
Convertase-activatable MMPs	Secreted	MMP11	Stromelysin 3	
		MMP21	X-MMP	
		MMP28	Epilysin	
	Membrane associated	MMP14	MT1-MMP	Membrane-type matrix metallo-proteinase 1
		MMP15	MT2-MMP	
		MMP16	MT3-MMP	
		MMP24	MT5-MMP	
		MMP17	MT4-MMP	
		MMP25	MT6-MMP	
		MMP23A		
		MMP23B		

5. All are inhibited by specific tissue inhibitors of the metalloproteinases (TIMPs; Table 3).

6. All are involved in normal re-modelling processes, such as embryonic development, post partum involution of the uterus, bone and growth plate remodelling, ovulation and wound healing.

7. They also play a major role in pathological processes, including rheumatoid arthritis, periodontitis, vascular disease as well as tumour invasion and metastasis.

Key point 2

- The matrix metalloproteinases are a family of 24 proteolytic enzymes that share common characteristics.

Table 3 Status in development of MMPIs

MMPI	Company	Mechanism	Tumour	Status
Batimastat (BB94)	BBiotech	Broad spectrum	Advanced solid	Discontinued PI
Marimastat (BB2516)	BBiotech	Broad spectrum	Pancreatic, gastro-oesophageal	Awaiting mature data from adjuvant study
Tanomastat (BAY 12-9566)	Bayer	MMP2,3,9	SCLC, NSCLC, pancreas, ovary	Discontinued PIII
Prinomastat (AG3340)	Agouron	MMP2,3,9,14	NSCLC, prostate	Discontinued PIII
MMI270 CGS27023A	Novartis	Broad spectrum	Advanced solid	Awaited
Neovastat (AE-941)	Aeterna		Breast, prostate, NSCLC, renal	Awaited
BMS275291	Bristol Myers Squibb	MMP1,2,8,9,14	Advanced solid	Awaited
Metastat (COL-3)	CollaGenex	MMP2	Advanced solid	Discontinued PI

SCLC, small cell lung cancer; NSCLC, non-small cell lung cancer, PI, phase I trial; PIII, phase III trial.

The range of targets for MMPs is more complex than initially imagined and, in addition to their classical connective tissue re-modelling functions, they are known to regulate precisely the function of bioactive molecules by proteolytic processing. MMPs mediate cell-surface receptor cleavage and release, cytokine activation and inactivation and release of apoptotic ligands.[2] Many of these cellular processes regulated by MMPs will promote tumour growth (proliferation, adhesion, dispersion, migration, differentiation, angiogenesis, apoptosis and host defence evasion), but some may also suppress normal tissue function and host defence mechanisms. The overall effect of MMP suppression is, therefore, not entirely straightforward. Recent observations have revealed that MMPs may play a fundamental role in early stage disease despite the classical belief that their role is in disease progression and malignant metastasis.[2,3] More recently, two large metalloproteinase-related families with the ability to degrade ECM have been described – the ADAMs and the ADAMTSs.[4,5] MMP inhibition may cross-inhibit the ADAMs and the

Key point 3

• Matrix metalloproteinases mediate basement membrane/extracellular matrix degradation in the early stages of malignant transformation promoting the production of a pericellular environment that produces genetic instability and later promotes metastasis.

ADAMTSs and this might account for the side-effects seen with long-term MMP inhibition.[6]

STRUCTURE

The MMPs contain several distinct conserved domains. The first is the leader sequence that is cleaved during activation of the enzyme and contains the highly conserved sequence **PRCGVPNPD**. The catalytic domain is the zinc-binding area or metal ion binding domain (MBD) and incorporates a signal peptide, an N-terminal propeptide, and a haemopexin carboxy-terminal domain determines substrate specificity interactions with cell-surface receptors and TIMPs.[7] The two matrilysins lack the haemopexin domain, but are otherwise similar in sequence, the six MT-MMPs are inserted into the plasma membrane by a transmembrane segment or a glycosylphosphatidylinositol anchor, and MMP2 and MMP9 have three fibronectin modules that function as a collagen-binding domain.[8] Several MMPs including all six of the MT-MMPs, and MMP23A and MMP23B have an insert in the propeptide that can be cleaved by furin-like proprotein convertase proteases.

REGULATION OF SECRETION

MMP activity is principally regulated at three levels – transcription, pro-enzyme activation, and inhibition. Additional fine-tuning of MMP activity can occur as a result of several other processes.[9] These mechanisms operate to ensure that proteolytic activity is delivered to those sites where it is necessary but, in disease states (such as cancer) these mechanisms are circumvented to allow the uncontrolled proteolytic activity that leads to a specific phenotypic effect (Fig. 1).

MMPs are independently regulated at a transcriptional level in a number of complex ways. Under physiological conditions, MMP expression is quiescent but can be induced with the expression of a number of signals, typically from the stroma, infiltrating host defence cells or in malignancy by the epithelial cells. The same MMP can be transcriptionally induced or repressed by different agents depending on the tumour type. The genes for the MMP family do, however, share a number of common features including similarities in the promoter sequences.

Interleukin-1 (IL-1) has been shown to modulate transcription of the MMP genes by binding to the PEA3 transcription factor and initiating transcription. IL-1 induces c-*fos*, c-*myc* and c-*jun* expression in human skin fibroblasts, and together with tumour necrosis factor-α (TNF-α) can trigger transcription leading to increased MMP expression; this effect can be augmented by transforming growth factor-β (TGF-β). TGF-β can function as both a positive and negative regulator of MMP gene transcription in both normal and tumour cells.[10] The overall effect on proteolytic activity by TGF-β is further complicated by its effect on naturally occurring MMP inhibitors and the addition of TGF-β to a fibrosarcoma cell line increased the expression of MMP2, MMP9 and TIMP1, but the overall effect was a reduction in the invasive capacity of the cells. *In vitro* work has also suggested that the effects of TGF-β may be augmented by TNF-α or IL-1, leading to the view that TGF-

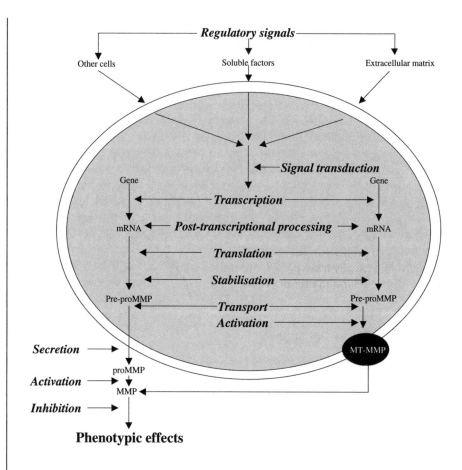

Fig. 1 The levels of MMP regulation (bold italic text) that could be targeted therapeutically.

β may increase the stability of mRNA for the MMPs whilst TNF-α or IL-1 act via the transcription pathway to increase synthesis of the enzymes.

The signal transduction pathways that mediate transcriptional activation are diverse, but the majority converge on the AP-1 transcription factor. The AP-1 binding sites/TPA responsive elements (AP-1, transcription activator protein; TPA, 12-O-tetradecanoylphorbol-13-acetate, a phorbol ester) is a DNA-binding complex formed from the products of two proto-oncogenes *c-fos* and *c-jun*, whose function is enhanced by the tumour promoting TPA. Several other nuclear factors influence MMP expression including: (i) the Ets oncoproteins that, along with IL-1, bind to the PEA3 transcription factor immediately upstream of the AP-1 binding site initiating transcription; (ii) NF-κB that induces selective MMPs; (iii) STATs that mediate the effects of interferons; (iv) Tcf4; (v) CIZ; (vi) p53; and (vii) Cbfa1. TGF-β inhibitory element (TIE) and AG-rich element (AGRE) have also been identified in the promoters of several MMP genes and can act as negative regulatory elements.[11]

Variability in MMP expression can also occur with the presence of single nucleotide polymorphisms in MMP promoters and specific MMP1 and MMP3 alleles have been associated with increased susceptibility to certain types of malignancy.[12]

Activation

MMPs are synthesised as inactive zymogens and require activation for function. An unpaired cysteine residue in the prodomain of MMPs forms a cysteine-switch. Following initial cleavage, the prodomain partially unfolds and exposes additional sites for further cleavage by other activating enzymes including other members of the MMP family. Binding to a ligand or substrate may also lead to a disengagement of the propeptide causing activation.[13] Several MMPs have important roles as activators of other pro-MMPs but are themselves activated by other classes of proteases. In most cases, therefore, the activation of MMPs requires the presence of proteases from other classes acting either directly or indirectly in a proteolytic cascade.

Activation usually takes place in the immediate pericellular space, but binding to cell-surface bound matrix molecules may protect against activation. The pro-MMP2 activation mechanism mediated by the MT-MMPs involves the formation of a multi-protein cell-surface molecule involving MT-MMP and TIMP2 binding pro-MMP2 at the haemopexin domain and also involving integrins as adhesion molecules securing the complex.[14] The MT-MMPs, MMP11, MMP23 and MMP28 are activated intracellularly by furin-like proprotein convertases.[15]

The MMP-activating enzyme systems can be de-regulated during pathological processes and, during tumour progression, distinct systems of activating enzymes may be over-expressed as part of the localisation of degradative processes to the cell surface.[16]

Endogenous MMP inhibition

The activity of the MMPs on the ECM is dependent on the balance between the enzymes and their inhibitors – the TIMPs. Four major mammalian TIMPs have been described (TIMP1–4), these bind non-covalently to the active MMPs in a 1:1 stoichiometric manner and the close ratio of TIMPs to MMPs which is required to neutralise enzymatic activity means that small changes in the levels of either leads to biologically significant changes in net proteolytic activity. Reduced levels of TIMPs generally correlate with an increase in malignant potential or progression.

Several recently described proteins are also capable of inhibiting MMPs or contain homologous TIMP inhibitory domains, but their targets and relevance in pathological processes remains unclear.

Key point 4

- Elastin loss is a manifestation of excessive elastolysis, which causes recruitment of inflammatory cells and consequently over-production of cellular proteases. The connective tissue destruction in aneurysms is mediated by the matrix metalloproteinases.

ROLE IN TUMOUR INVASION

The classical belief that MMPs were involved in tumour invasion and metastasis has had to be modified with recent findings.[2,3] It is now believed that MMPs mediate basement membrane and ECM degradation in the early stages of malignant transformation promoting the production of a pericellular environment that produces genetic instability and, later in the process, promotes metastasis.[17] MMPs promote growth initiation and then sustain growth in both primary tumours and metastases by: (i) activating/inactivating growth factors/growth factor binding proteins; (ii) releasing mitogenic factors from the ECM; (iii) processing adhesion molecules; and (iv) cleavage of the pro-apoptotic Fas ligand.[18] MMPs may also help to circumvent natural host immunity by destroying chemokine gradients that attract immune cells.[19] They also have profound effects on angiogenesis by mobilising or activating pro-angiogenic factors like bFGF, VEGF or TGF-β and negatively by generating angiogenesis inhibitors such as angiostatin and endostatin from larger precursor proteins.[2,20]

Despite the more recent conflicting evidence, MMP activity has been correlated with malignant potential in a number of older studies. MMP9 secretion by cancer cell lines has been correlated with increased metastatic potential, collagenase production has been correlated with tumour grade and stromal, vascular and lymphatic invasion and stromelysin expression has been shown to correlate with tumour progression. Increased collagenolytic activity compared to normal tissue has been demonstrated in endometrial, ovarian, prostate, colorectal, gastric, breast and lung carcinoma, while excess activity of the stromelysins has been recorded in squamous cell carcinomas. Extensive *in vitro* data suggest that expression of mRNA encoding for MMP2 and TIMP2 is epithelial cell in origin, but *in situ* hybridisation studies have localised the mRNA expression of MMP2 and TIMP2 principally to the tumour stroma in human skin and colorectal neoplasia. MMP2 protein has been found predominantly in the malignant epithelial cells of both breast and colorectal cancer using immuno-histochemical methods, MMP9 has been demonstrated in squamous cell carcinoma cells but not in basal cell carcinomas or normal skin, MMP11 is expressed almost exclusively in the stroma of malignant breast tumours, and MMP1 is principally a product of fibroblasts which is up-regulated in the stroma of tumours. These findings suggest the importance of tumour/stromal cell interactions in the production of degradative enzymes, and also the existence of specific differences in MMP production between tumour types.

ROLE IN VASCULAR DISEASE

The cause of aneurysmal degeneration is largely unknown, but it is recognised that abdominal aortic aneurysms have chronic transmural inflammation and

---

Key point 5

- Most approaches aimed at reducing matrix metalloproteinase activity are experimental and few have reached the clinical arena.

destruction of connective tissue proteins within the outer aortic wall. Initiation and expansion of aneurysms is attributed to loss of elastin, normally responsible for the resilience of the aorta, whereas loss of fibrillar collagens (types I and III), the major source of tensile strength, are believed to ultimately result in rupture. Several studies have shown evidence of increased collagen breakdown and increased synthesis, consistent with increased turnover. Elastin has an extremely long half-life (40–70 years) and loss is almost certainly a manifestation of excessive elastolysis rather than reduced synthesis. This is supported by experimental models in which aneurysm formation can be induced by infusion of elastase, which causes recruitment of inflammatory cells and consequently overproduction of cellular proteases. Several recent studies indicate that the connective tissue destruction in aneurysms is mediated by the MMPs. MMP2 and MMP9 are the most prominent elastolytic proteins secreted by human aneurysm tissue and in organ culture. TIMPs are also overproduced in human aneurysms although their role in pathogenesis remains unclear. MMPs have also been reported to be overexpressed in the thoracic aortic aneurysms associated with Marfan's syndrome and plasma levels of MMP9 have been shown to be higher in patients with abdominal aortic aneurysms than in healthy volunteers. Organ culture studies suggest that diseased aortic tissue is the source of MMP9.[21] These elevated circulating levels of MMPs decrease after surgical repair.[22]

Recently, several agents derived from tetracycline-type antibiotics have been shown to prevent aneurysm formation or retard growth in experimental models. Their mechanism of action is not thought to be related to their antibiotic properties.[23]

POTENTIAL STRATEGIES FOR MMP INHIBITION

Most approaches aimed at reducing MMP activity are experimental and few have reached the clinical arena. Several approaches to inhibit MMP gene expression have been reported and involve blocking extracellular factors, signal transduction pathways, or activating nuclear factors.

MMP transcripts have been targeted using ribozymes and anti-sense constructs, and these methods have been shown to reduce MMP production in cancer cells and TIMP1 expression in normal cells. The ability to translate the *in vitro* inhibition of extracellular factors that reduce MMP expression to the clinical arena is fraught with difficulties because of the diversity of agents involved and the opposing actions of several different factors on MMP production. Interferon-γ (IFN-γ), IFN-β and IFN-α, however, have all have been shown to inhibit the transcription of MMPs and could have a potential therapeutic role.[24] Another group of cytokines have been shown to up-regulate MMP expression and blocking their function could be a further therapeutic strategy. TNF-α monoclonal blocking antibodies have been shown to be effective in the treatment of rheumatoid arthritis and could, at least in part, be functioning by blocking TNF-α-induced MMP production.[25] Further potential cytokine targets include IL-1, epidermal growth factor receptors and TGF-β.[26,27]

Several experimental strategies have been used *in vitro* to block signal transduction. A medicinal alkaloid called Halofuginone can interfere with TGF-β signalling and, in doing so, block MMP2 expression.[28] Selective inhibition of the p38 MAPK pathway, the Ras responsive element and the Ras farnesyl transferase pathway can also abolish or reduce the expression of several MMPs and reduce *in vitro* MMP-induced invasion.[29]

Targeting nuclear factors responsible for MMP gene regulation can also modify MMP expression. The general nuclear factors AP-1 and NF-κB if blocked might effect MMP gene expression or more specific factors such as Cbfa1, that selectively modify MMP expression, could be targeted. Many extracellular signalling pathways converge via the AP-1 binding site and several natural products have been reported to inhibit AP-1 binding activity and, therefore, AP-1-induced transcription.[30,31] The NF-κB transcription pathway can also be targeted to inhibit MMP production.[32,33]

Post-transcriptional MMP regulation usually involves the blocking of pro-MMP activation. Plasmin inhibitors can prevent the cleavage of pro-MMPs, but the obvious target is the MMP activating MT-MMPs. Anti-MT1-MMP monoclonal antibodies have been shown to inhibit proteolytic activity and impair endothelial cell migration.[34] Selective furin inhibition has been shown to prevent the activation of MT1-MMP and reduce pro-MMP2 processing which, in turn, prevented tumour growth and invasion.[35,36] The anti-angiogenic factor thrombospondin-1 inhibits pro-MMP2 and pro-MMP9 activation and endostatin inhibits processing and activation of pro-MMP2 by MT1-MMP.[37–39] The feasibility of targeting post-transcriptional MMP regulation with therapeutic intent has been supported by the observation that HIV aspartyl protease inhibitors promote the regression of Kaposi sarcoma in AIDS patients.[40] HIV aspartyl protease inhibitors also modulate the activity of several host proteases and also block pro-MMP2 activation.[41]

THERAPEUTIC ROLE OF MMPIS

The first therapeutic application of MMPI strategies involved TIMPs. Exogenous human recombinant TIMP1 reduced *in vitro* invasion and metastatic lung colonisation by human tumour xenografts. TIMP2 inhibited the invasion of smooth muscle cell monolayers by HT1080 cells and *ras*-transformed rat embryo fibroblasts and prevented collagen degradation and invasion by tumour cell lines *in vitro*. TIMP1 transgenic mice were also shown to have varying effects on tumour growth. Protein-based therapies are difficult to deliver in a clinical setting because of poor pharmacokinetics and, in addition, the TIMPs have been shown to have tumour-promoting activity.

Because of the importance of MMPs in tumour invasion and metastasis, low molecular weight inhibitors of the MMPs have been developed for clinical application. The first synthetic compound to enter clinical trials in patients with cancer was a broad-spectrum MMPI called batimastat, developed by British Biotech Pharmaceuticals Limited (Oxford, UK). Batimastat has inhibitory activity against all the MMPs in low nanomolar concentrations, but appears to be specific for the MMPs. Batimastat reduced the tumour burden in nude mice given human ovarian carcinoma xenografts and increased their survival up to 6-fold compared to controls. The major drawback of batimastat was its low solubility and further development by British Biotech led to an analogue with greater solubility, marimastat. An initial non-randomised dose finding study in 113 patients with pancreatic cancer followed. The majority of

> **Key point 6**
>
> • The study of marimastat in gastro-oesphageal cancer provided the first demonstration of a therapeutic benefit for an matrix metalloproteinase inhibitor in cancer patients.

patients completed the 28-day study and the principal side-effect was arthralgia. In evaluable patients, 30% showed no increase or fall in CA19-9 levels and 49% had radiological stable disease. The median survival was 245 days for those with a stable or falling CA19-9 level and 128 days in those with rising CA19-9. Following this investigation, marimastat has been studied in a number of tumour types and three randomised studies have been published.

A total of 414 patients with unresectable pancreatic cancer were randomized to receive marimastat 5, 10 or 25 mg b.i.d. or gemcitabine. There was no significant difference in survival between 5 mg, 10 mg or 25 mg b.i.d. marimastat and gemcitabine. Median survival times were 111, 105, 125 and 167 days and 1-year survival was 14%, 14%, 20% and 19%, respectively. In a Cox's proportional hazard model, there was no significant difference in survival between patients treated with marimastat 25 mg b.i.d. and gemcitabine, but there was between patients treated with gemcitabine and marimastat 10 mg and 5 mg b.i.d. ($P < 0.003$).[42] Following this study, a further 239 patients with unresectable pancreatic cancer were randomized to receive gemcitabine in combination with either marimastat or placebo. There was no significant difference in survival between gemcitabine and marimastat and gemcitabine and placebo. Median survival times were 165.5 and 164 days and 1-year survival was 18% and 17%, respectively. There were no significant differences in overall response rates, progression-free survival or time-to-treatment failure between the treatment arms (Fig. 2).[43] Running concurrently with the studies

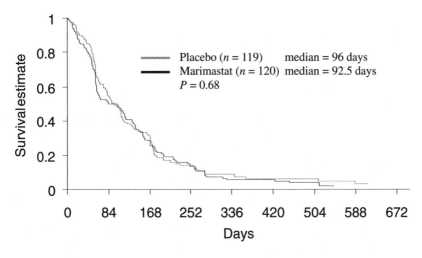

Fig. 2 Overall progression-free survival in the gemcitabine + marimastat *versus* gemcitabine + placebo study in advanced pancreatic cancer.[43]

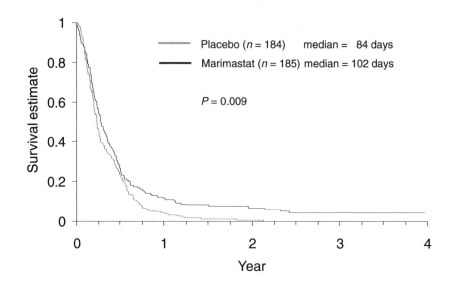

Fig. 3 Overall progression-free survival in the marimastat *versus* placebo study in advanced gastro-oesophageal cancer.[44]

in pancreatic cancer, 369 patients with non-resectable gastric and gastro-oesophageal adenocarcinoma, who had received no more than a single regimen of 5-fluorouracil-based chemotherapy, were randomised to receive either marimastat (10 mg b.i.d.) or placebo. At study completion, there was a modest difference in survival in favour of marimastat ($P = 0.07$). This survival benefit was maintained over a further 2 years of follow-up ($P < 0.03$). The median survival was 138 days for placebo and 160 days for marimastat, with 2-year survival of 3% and 9%, respectively. A significant survival benefit was identified at study completion in the pre-defined sub-group of 123 patients who had received prior chemotherapy ($P < 0.05$). This benefit increased with 2 years' additional follow-up ($P = 0.006$), with 2-year survival of 5% and 18%, respectively. Progression-free survival was also significantly longer for patients receiving marimastat compared to placebo ($P = 0.009$; Fig. 3).[44] In each of these studies, marimastat was well tolerated. In the study comparing marimastat with gemcitabine in pancreatic cancer, those patients with early stage disease and treated with marimastat did equally as well as those treated with gemcitabine (Fig. 4). In the study of marimastat *versus* placebo in gastro-oesophageal cancer, the improvement in survival was also more marked in those patients with low volume disease, but neither of these sub-groups were pre-defined.

The 20% 1-year survival of 25 mg marimastat was similar to that with gemcitabine and, together with its good tolerance and oral administration, warranted further investigation in pancreatic cancer, but combination of marimastat with gemcitabine was disappointing although the numbers in this study were perhaps too small. The study in gastro-oesophageal cancer provided one of the first demonstrations of a therapeutic benefit for an MMP inhibitor in cancer patients. The greatest benefit was observed in patients who had previously received chemotherapy although this finding remains unexplained. These randomised data were also supported by a phase II study of marimastat

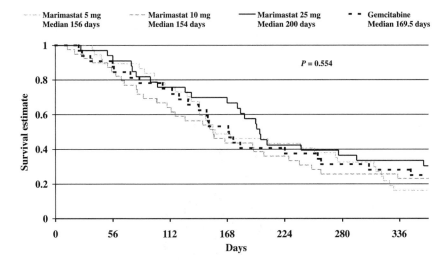

Fig. 4 Progression-free survival in patients with stage I/II/III pancreatic cancer treated with one of three doses of marimastat or gemcitabine.[42]

Key point 7

• Matrix metalloproteinases are most important in the early stages of tumourigenesis and their role is probably diminished following metastases.

---

in combination with Temozolomide in patients with glioblastoma multiforme in which the combination improved the outcome in these patients.[45]

British Biotech's development and subsequent broad patent protection on peptide-based hydroxamate inhibitors prompted the development of new chemical approaches in inhibitor design that led to more selective inhibitors. Several of these have entered trials in a variety of tumour types, but publication of data from these studies is still awaited or the studies have been suspended (Table 3).

The lack of efficacy of MMPIs studied in cancer is not surprising.[3] It is now established that MMPs are most important in the early stages of tumourigenesis and their role is probably diminished following metastases.

Key point 8

• Treatment of cancer by low molecular weight matrix metallo-proteinase inhibitors is novel with considerable potential, but the currently available matrix metalloproteinase inhibitors are too crude for wide-spread applicability.

Key point 9

- Current data demonstrate proof-of-principle that matrix metallo-proteinase inhibition has a role to play in the treatment of malignancy and possibly in the treatment of aneurysmal disease.

The difficulty in designing trials for new agents that act early in tumourigenesis is, of course, that most agents need a track record in advanced disease before being applied to early disease; however, this barrier needs to be overcome if this class of agents is to achieve its potential. In addition, the lack of success may also be because most of the MMPIs to reach clinical trials target a wide range of MMPs even those that may actually be beneficial.[3] The *in vivo* consequence of MMP inhibition might also be unpredictable with recent reports of synthetic MMPIs leading to a paradoxical increase in MMP production.[46,47] The MMPs also only form one class of proteolytic enzymes and to achieve disease amelioration by proteolytic inhibition may require blocking several groups of proteolytic enzymes.

CONCLUSIONS

The MMP enzyme system appears to play an important role in cancer invasion and metastasis, and has more recently been implicated in the growth of vascular aneurysms.

To target MMPs for therapeutic intervention effectively is a challenge, but the multiple mechanisms of MMP regulation offer exciting opportunities. The transfer of molecular technologies into the clinical arena will require the development of new study end points and surrogate markers for assessing efficacy and new imaging techniques that will allow the *in vivo* analysis of MMP inhibition.[3,48,49]

Treatment of cancer by low molecular weight MMPIs is a novel approach with considerable potential for use in the adjuvant and palliative settings, but the currently available MMP inhibitors are too crude a tool for wide-spread clinical applicability; however, they do demonstrate proof-of-principle that MMP inhibition has a role to play in the treatment of malignancy and possibly in the palliative treatment of aneurysmal disease.

Key points for clinical practice

- A complex series of regulatory enzymes control extracellular matrix integrity that may be disrupted by cell/basement membrane attachment, excess secretion of proteolytic enzymes or a reduction in the secretion of inhibitors.

- The matrix metalloproteinases are a family of 24 proteolytic enzymes that share common characteristics.

Key points for clinical practice (continued)

- Matrix metalloproteinases mediate basement membrane/extracellular matrix degradation in the early stages of malignant transformation promoting the production of a pericellular environment that produces genetic instability and later promotes metastasis.

- Elastin loss is a manifestation of excessive elastolysis, which causes recruitment of inflammatory cells and consequently overproduction of cellular proteases. The connective tissue destruction in aneurysms is mediated by the matrix metalloproteinases.

- Most approaches aimed at reducing matrix metalloproteinase activity are experimental and few have reached the clinical arena.

- The study of marimastat in gastro-oesphageal cancer provided the first demonstration of a therapeutic benefit for an matrix metalloproteinase inhibitor in cancer patients.

- Matrix metalloproteinases are most important in the early stages of tumourigenesis and their role is probably diminished following metastases.

- Treatment of cancer by low molecular weight matrix metalloproteinase inhibitors is novel with considerable potential, but the currently available matrix metalloproteinase inhibitors are too crude for wide-spread applicability.

- Current data demonstrate proof-of-principle that matrix metalloproteinase inhibition has a role to play in the treatment of malignancy and possibly in the treatment of aneurysmal disease.

References

1. Lopez-Otin C, Overall CM. Protease degradomics: a new challenge for proteomics. *Nat Rev Mol Cell Biol* 2002; **3**: 509–519.
2. Egeblad M, Werb Z. New functions for the matrix metalloproteinases in cancer progression. *Nat Rev Cancer* 2002; **2**: 161–174.
3. Coussens LM, Fingleton B, Matrisian LM. Matrix metalloproteinase inhibitors and cancer: trials and tribulations. *Science* 2002; **295**: 2387–2392.
4. Blobel CP. Functional and biochemical characterization of ADAMs and their predicted role in protein ectodomain shedding. *Inflamm Res* 2002; **51**: 83–84.
5. Cal S, Obaya AJ, Llamazares M *et al*. Cloning, expression analysis, and structural characterization of seven novel human ADAMTSs, a family of metalloproteinases with disintegrin and thrombospondin-1 domains. *Gene* 2002; **283**: 49–62.
6. Naglich JG, Jure-Kunkel M, Gupta E *et al*. Inhibition of angiogenesis and metastasis in two murine models by the matrix metalloproteinase inhibitor, BMS-275291. *Cancer Res* 2001; **61**: 8480–8485.
7. Overall CM. Molecular determinants of metalloproteinase substrate specificity: matrix metalloproteinase substrate binding domains, modules, and exosites. *Mol Biotechnol* 2002; **22**: 51–86.

8. Uria JA, Lopez-Otin C. Matrilysin-2, a new matrix metalloproteinase expressed in human tumors and showing the minimal domain organization required for secretion, latency, and activity. *Cancer Res* 2000; **60**: 4745–4751.

9. Overall CM, Lopez-Otin C. Strategies for MMP inhibition in cancer: innovations for the post-trial era. *Nat Rev Cancer* 2002; **2**: 657–672.

10. Jimenez MJ, Balbin M, Alvarez J *et al*. A regulatory cascade involving retinoic acid, Cbfa1, and matrix metalloproteinases is coupled to the development of a process of perichondrial invasion and osteogenic differentiation during bone formation. *J Cell Biol* 2001; **155**: 1333–1344.

11. Benderdour M, Tardif G, Pelletier JP *et al*. A novel negative regulatory element in the human collagenase-3 proximal promoter region. *Biochem Biophys Res Commun* 2002; **291**: 1151–1159.

12. Biondi ML, Turri O, Leviti S *et al*. MMP1 and MMP3 polymorphisms in promoter regions and cancer. *Clin Chem* 2000; **46**: 2023–2024.

13. Bannikov GA, Karelina TV, Collier IE, Marmer BL, Goldberg GI. Substrate binding of gelatinase B induces its enzymatic activity in the presence of intact propeptide. *J Biol Chem* 2002; **277**: 16022–16027.

14. Overall CM, King AE, Sam DK *et al*. Identification of the tissue inhibitor of metalloproteinases-2 (TIMP-2) binding site on the hemopexin carboxyl domain of human gelatinase A by site-directed mutagenesis. The hierarchical role in binding TIMP-2 of the unique cationic clusters of hemopexin modules III and IV. *J Biol Chem* 1999; **274**: 4421–4429.

15. Pei D, Kang T, Qi H. Cysteine array matrix metalloproteinase (CA-MMP)/MMP-23 is a type II transmembrane matrix metalloproteinase regulated by a single cleavage for both secretion and activation. *J Biol Chem* 2000; **275**: 33988–33997.

16. Velasco G, Cal S, Merlos-Suarez A *et al*. Human MT6-matrix metalloproteinase: identification, progelatinase A activation, and expression in brain tumors. *Cancer Res* 2000; **60**: 877–882.

17. Sternlicht MD, Lochter A, Sympson CJ *et al*. The stromal proteinase MMP3/stromelysin-1 promotes mammary carcinogenesis. *Cell* 1999; **98**: 137–146.

18. Noe V, Fingleton B, Jacobs K *et al*. Release of an invasion promoter E-cadherin fragment by matrilysin and stromelysin-1. *J Cell Sci* 2001; **114**: 111–118.

19. McQuibban GA, Gong JH, Tam EM *et al*. Inflammation dampened by gelatinase A cleavage of monocyte chemoattractant protein-3. *Science* 2000; **289**: 1202–1206.

20. Cornelius LA, Nehring LC, Harding E *et al*. Matrix metalloproteinases generate angiostatin: effects on neovascularization. *J Immunol* 1998; **161**: 6845–6852.

21. McMillan WD, Pearce WH. Increased plasma levels of metalloproteinase-9 are associated with abdominal aortic aneurysms. *J Vasc Surg* 1999; **29**: 122–127; discussion 127–129.

22. Sangiorgi G, D'Averio R, Mauriello A *et al*. Plasma levels of metalloproteinases-3 and -9 as markers of successful abdominal aortic aneurysm exclusion after endovascular graft treatment. *Circulation* 2001; **104**: I288–I295.

23. Thompson RW, Baxter BT. MMP inhibition in abdominal aortic aneurysms. Rationale for a prospective randomized clinical trial. *Ann NY Acad Sci* 1999; **878**: 159–178.

24. Ma Z, Qin H, Benveniste EN. Transcriptional suppression of matrix metalloproteinase-9 gene expression by IFN-gamma and IFN-beta: critical role of STAT-1alpha. *J Immunol* 2001; **167**: 5150–5159.

25. Mengshol JA, Mix KS, Brinckerhoff CE. Matrix metalloproteinases as therapeutic targets in arthritic diseases: bull's-eye or missing the mark? *Arthritis Rheum* 2002; **46**: 13–20.

26. Lal A, Glazer CA, Martinson HM *et al*. Mutant epidermal growth factor receptor up-regulates molecular effectors of tumor invasion. *Cancer Res* 2002; **62**: 3335–3339.

27. Muraoka RS, Dumont N, Ritter CA *et al*. Blockade of TGF-beta inhibits mammary tumor cell viability, migration, and metastases. *J Clin Invest* 2002; **109**: 1551–1559.

28. McGaha TL, Phelps RG, Spiera H, Bona C. Halofuginone, an inhibitor of type-I collagen synthesis and skin sclerosis, blocks transforming-growth-factor-beta-mediated Smad3 activation in fibroblasts. *J Invest Dermatol* 2002; **118**: 461–470.

29. Zhang Y, Thant AA, Machida K *et al*. Hyaluronan-CD44s signaling regulates matrix metalloproteinase-2 secretion in a human lung carcinoma cell line QG90. *Cancer Res* 2002; **62**: 3962–3965.

30. Sato T, Koike L, Miyata Y *et al.* Inhibition of activator protein-1 binding activity and phosphatidylinositol 3-kinase pathway by nobiletin, a polymethoxy flavonoid, results in augmentation of tissue inhibitor of metalloproteinases-1 production and suppression of production of matrix metalloproteinases-1 and -9 in human fibrosarcoma HT-1080 cells. *Cancer Res* 2002; **62**: 1025–1029.

31. Mohan R, Sivak J, Ashton P *et al.* Curcuminoids inhibit the angiogenic response stimulated by fibroblast growth factor-2, including expression of matrix metalloproteinase gelatinase B. *J Biol Chem* 2000; **275**: 10405–10412.

32. Mix KS, Mengshol JA, Benbow U *et al.* A synthetic triterpenoid selectively inhibits the induction of matrix metalloproteinases 1 and 13 by inflammatory cytokines. *Arthritis Rheum* 2001; **44**: 1096–1104.

33. Pan MR, Chuang LY, Hung WC. Non-steroidal anti-inflammatory drugs inhibit matrix metalloproteinase-2 expression via repression of transcription in lung cancer cells. *FEBS Lett* 2001; **508**: 365–368.

34. Galvez BG, Matias-Roman S, Albar JP, Sanchez-Madrid F, Arroyo AG. Membrane type 1-matrix metalloproteinase is activated during migration of human endothelial cells and modulates endothelial motility and matrix remodeling. *J Biol Chem* 2001; **276**: 37491–37500.

35. Bassi DE, Lopez De Cicco R, Mahloogi H *et al.* Furin inhibition results in absent or decreased invasiveness and tumorigenicity of human cancer cells. *Proc Natl Acad Sci USA* 2001; **98**: 10326–10331.

36. Khatib AM, Siegfried G, Chretien M, Metrakos P, Seidah NG. Proprotein convertases in tumor progression and malignancy: novel targets in cancer therapy. *Am J Pathol* 2002; **160**: 1921–1935.

37. Bein K, Simons M. Thrombospondin type 1 repeats interact with matrix metalloproteinase 2. Regulation of metalloproteinase activity. *J Biol Chem* 2000; **275**: 32167–32173.

38. Rodriguez-Manzaneque JC, Lane TF, Ortega MA *et al.* Thrombospondin-1 suppresses spontaneous tumor growth and inhibits activation of matrix metalloproteinase-9 and mobilization of vascular endothelial growth factor. *Proc Natl Acad Sci USA* 2001; **98**: 12485–12490.

39. Kim YM, Jang JW, Lee OH *et al.* Endostatin inhibits endothelial and tumor cellular invasion by blocking the activation and catalytic activity of matrix metalloproteinase. *Cancer Res* 2000; **60**: 5410–5413.

40. Sgadari C, Barillari G, Toschi E *et al.* HIV protease inhibitors are potent anti-angiogenic molecules and promote regression of Kaposi sarcoma. *Nat Med* 2002; **8**: 225–232.

41. Liang JS, Distler O, Cooper DA *et al.* HIV protease inhibitors protect apolipoprotein B from degradation by the proteasome: a potential mechanism for protease inhibitor-induced hyperlipidemia. *Nat Med* 2001; **7**: 1327–1331.

42. Bramhall SR, Rosemurgy A, Brown PD, Bowry C, Buckels JAC. Marimastat as first line therapy for patients with unresectable pancreatic cancer – a randomized trial. *J Clin Oncol* 2001; **19**: 3447–3455.

43. Bramhall SR, Schulz J, Nemunaitis J *et al.* A double-blind placebo-controlled, randomised study comparing gemcitabine and marimastat with gemcitabine and placebo as first line therapy in patients with advanced pancreatic cancer. *Br J Cancer* 2002; **87**: 161–167.

44. Bramhall SR, Hallissey MT, Whiting J *et al.* Marimastat as maintenance therapy for patients with advanced gastric cancer: a randomised trial. *Br J Cancer* 2002; **86**: 1864–1870.

45. Groves MD, Puduvalli VK, Hess KR *et al.* Phase II trial of temozolomide plus the matrix metalloproteinase inhibitor, marimastat, in recurrent and progressive glioblastoma multiforme. *J Clin Oncol* 2002; **20**: 1383–1388.

46. Kruger A, Soeltl R, Sopov I *et al.* Hydroxamate-type matrix metalloproteinase inhibitor batimastat promotes liver metastasis. *Cancer Res* 2001; **61**: 1272–1275.

47. Maquoi E, Munaut C, Colige A *et al.* Stimulation of matrix metalloproteinase-9 expression in human fibrosarcoma cells by synthetic matrix metalloproteinase inhibitors. *Exp Cell Res* 2002; **275**: 110–121.

48. Weissleder R. Scaling down imaging: molecular mapping of cancer in mice. *Nat Rev Cancer* 2002; **2**: 11–18.

49. Schatzkin A, Gail M. The promise and peril of surrogate end points in cancer research. *Nat Rev Cancer* 2002; **2**: 19–27.

Carolynne Vaizey

4

Physiological concepts in the treatment of faecal incontinence including sacral nerve stimulation

The once taboo subject of faecal incontinence is now becoming accepted as a common cause of major disability. Studies have shown that daily or weekly episodes of faecal incontinence affect about 2% of the adult population.[1] However, urinary incontinence still commands a significantly higher public profile, and many of the newer treatments for faecal incontinence have been inspired by those developed by urologists.

Key point 1

- There is a surprisingly high incidence of faecal incontinence, and it is not just a disability of the elderly.

The maintenance of faecal continence is a product of stool consistency, colorectal activity and the harmonious functioning of the external and the internal anal sphincters.[2] The external sphincter, a skeletal-type voluntary muscle, works as the 'emergency brakes' providing the ability to defer defecation and preventing urge incontinence. Like other skeletal muscles, it is fatiguable, capable of producing only short-lived increases in anal canal pressure usually in response to rises in intrarectal or intra-abdominal pressure. The internal sphincter, a smooth and therefore involuntary muscle, maintains closure of the anal canal, preventing leakage of stool or passive incontinence. It is maintained in near maximal contraction, but relaxes in response to rectal distension.

The introduction of endo-anal sonography in the late 1980s provided incomparable images of the anal sphincter mechanism and radically altered thinking about the aetiology of faecal incontinence. The previously held view

---

Ms Carolynne Vaizey MD FRCS FCS(SA), Consultant Colorectal Surgeon, The Middlesex Hospital, Mortimer Street, London W1T 3AA, UK

Key point 2

- The biggest advance in incontinence has been endo-anal ultrasonography which allows for improved selection for surgery.

Key point 3

- Most cases of incontinence are due to defective or atrophic anal sphincter muscles.

that pudendal nerve damage was the underlying cause in most patients[3] was quickly shattered. Sphincter defects or atrophy are now known to account for the majority of cases of incontinence. Of women with faecal incontinence and obstetric damage as the only risk factor, 90% were found to have sphincter muscle damage on endo-anal ultrasonography.[4] The first report of internal sphincter muscle atrophy was published in 1997.[5] As the external anal sphincter muscle is less distinct on ultrasonography than the hypo-echoic internal sphincter, endocoil magnetic resonance imaging (MRI) has been used to assess the external sphincter.[6] The literature is divided on the question as to whether prolonged pudendal nerve latencies affect the outcome of a sphincter repair. However, Briel's group has shown a clear affect of external sphincter atrophy on continence after sphincteroplasty.[7] MRI, with or without the use of an endo-anal coil, is not an economically practical substitute for endo-anal ultrasonography, but can provide superior images of the external sphincter in equivocal cases.[8]

Table 1 The St Mark's Score[9]

	Never	Rarely	Sometimes	Weekly	Daily
Incontinence for solid stool	0	1	2	3	4
Incontinence for liquid stool	0	1	2	3	4
Incontinence for gas	0	1	2	3	4
Alteration in life-style	0	1	2	3	4

	No	Yes
Need to wear a pad or plug	0	2
Taking constipating medicines	0	2
Lack of ability to defer defecation for 15 min	0	4

Never	no episodes in the past 4 weeks
Rarely	1 episode in the past 4 weeks
Sometimes	> 1 episode in the past 4 weeks but < 1 a week
Weekly	1 or more episodes a week but < 1 a day
Daily	1 or more episodes a day

Add one score from each row
Minimum score =   0 = perfect continence
Maximum score = 24 = totally incontinent.

As there are no reliable medications to counteract increased colonic activity or 'irritable bowel syndrome', treatments classically focus on firming the stools or on improving the sphincter mechanism. The treatment of faecal incontinence has been a rapidly changing field over the past decade with many newer therapies dying a slow death under the scrutiny of long-term follow-up. Results of surgery were poorly standardised prior to the introduction of validated continence scoring systems in the latter part of the 1990s. Prior to this, reports were generally of the operating surgeon's short-term subjective assessment of symptom improvement, with no regard to the need for anti-diarrhoeal medications and no assessment of quality-of-life. The scoring system which correlates best with in-depth clinical symptom assessment is the St Mark's Score which is a modification of the Wexner continence score (Table 1).[9] This system, together with a bowel diary and a disease-specific quality-of-life instrument, has revolutionised postoperative patient assessments.

CURRENT CONSERVATIVE THERAPIES

Loperamide or other stool-firming agents should be used as the first line of therapy for patients with faecal incontinence who do not suffer from concomitant difficulty with defecation. Ideally, it is used initially in very small, carefully titrated doses, often in the form of a paediatric syrup at first to avoid causing any discomfort or constipation. Biofeedback therapy, based around an exercise programme with visual computerised feedback to the patient is now an established conservative therapy. It is particularly successful for patients who have intact but weakened sphincter muscles.[10] The anal plug (Conveen, Coloplast Ltd, UK) is a somewhat conical, tampon-like device which can be useful in the prevention of faecal leakage. However, it is not comfortable for many patients and some find it aesthetically unacceptable.

Key point 4

- Conservative options should be used before consideration for surgery

---

SIMPLE PROCEDURES AND REPAIRS

In the 1970s, Parks developed the overlapping sphincter repair technique for the defective anal sphincter and the post-anal repair for idiopathic or 'neurogenic incontinence' in the absence of a reparable defect. The overlapping repair was shown to improve continence in 60–90% of patients in the short-term, but this is now known to drop to about 50% after an interval of 5 years.[11] Post-anal repair was said to provide short-term benefit in up to 83% of patients, but improvement persisted in as few as 28% of patients in the longer term with only 21% fully continent. In response to these long-term results and the change of emphasis away from neurogenic injury, this latter operation has fallen into disrepute. Although the overlapping repair is still used for external anal sphincter muscle defects, there is now a more cautious patient-selection process which usually follows an initial trial of conservative therapies. Repeat overlapping repair is also an option for selected patients with a persistent sphincter defect but an intrinsically functional external sphincter.[12]

Key point 5

- Prevention is better than cure particularly in view of the disappointing long-term results of most therapies.

The most common cause of a reparable defect in the anal sphincter muscles is obstetric trauma; in the absence of sepsis, single post-surgical or traumatic injuries to the external sphincter or to both sphincters can usually be treated in the same manner. Defects in the internal anal sphincter muscle, such as those seen after an over-enthusiastic lateral sphincterotomy, are not amenable to simple surgical repair.[13] This is not entirely surprising for a smooth muscle, about 2 mm in thickness, which is in a state of constant contraction.

With the posterior repair falling into disrepute, the options for patients without a reparable defect who fail conservative therapies are limited. There was initial enthusiasm over topical treatment with the pharmacological agent phenylephrine when it was shown to enhance the function of the normal internal anal sphincter muscle.[14] However, its effect on the weakened sphincter has not lived up to expectations. The use of bulking agents to promote closure of the lax anal canal has been slow to develop. An initial report of the use of collagen injections for internal sphincter insufficiency[15] showed acceptable early results, but no long-term results were published. PTP implants (Uroplasty Ltd, Reading, UK), which are silicone based and, therefore, non-absorbable, are now licensed for use in faecal incontinence. Previously known as Bioplastique in pilot studies, the injections consist of textured polydimethylsiloxane particles suspended in a bio-excretable carrier hydrogel of polyvinylpyrrolidone (povidone, PVP). An initial pilot study showed mixed results, but a subsequent trial using a refined technique has been more promising.[16]

SACRAL NERVE STIMULATION

An alternative approach to the treatment of faecal incontinence is sacral nerve stimulation. Continuous stimulation of the sacral nerves has been used in the treatment of patients with bladder dysfunction since 1981. The first report describing its use for faecal incontinence[17] appeared to show good results for patients with a weak, but intact, external sphincter. The implication was that its main action was to enhance external sphincter function. Patients underwent a short trial of stimulation using percutaneous electrodes, usually placed through the S3 foramen, and an external stimulator. If there was symptomatic improvement over several days, the patients proceeded to implantation of a permanent electrode and a stimulator, identical to that used for dynamic graciloplasty. The permanent implantation of the electrode was performed through an incision over the sacrum. Connecting leads were tunnelled to the

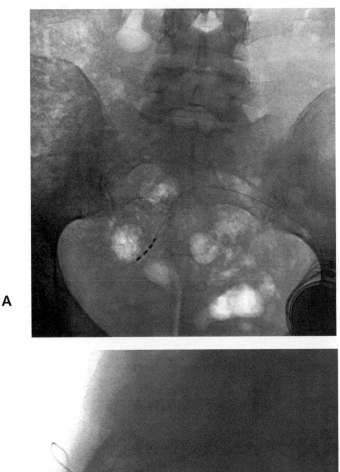

A

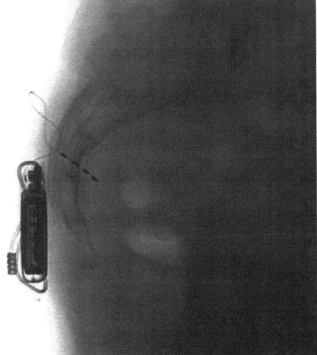

B

Fig. 1 Anteroposterior (A) and lateral (B) X-ray views of an implanted sacral nerve permanent electrode and stimulator. The upper traces show rectal activity and the lower traces anal activity. Stimulation appears to reduce rectal contractile activity and to cause qualitative changes in anal contractile activity with induction of slow wave activity and a reduction in transient relaxations.

stimulator, which was implanted in the anterior abdominal wall. The operation has since been modified with the stimulator now usually implanted into the buttock and the electrode implanted percutaneously (Fig. 1).

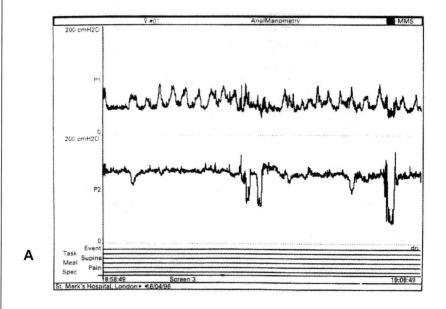

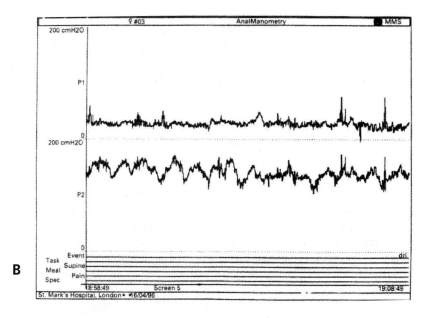

Fig. 2 Ten-minute traces from 24-h ambulatory studies of a patient before and with sacral nerve stimulation. These show evidence of the effects of the stimulation on the anorectum. (A) Before stimulation; P1 = rectal trace, P2 = anal trace. (B) With stimulation; P1 = rectal trace, P2 = anal trace. Stimulation appears to produce a general decrease in rectal activity and to eliminate the spontaneous decreases in anal resting pressure. Additionally, there is induction of internal anal sphincter slow wave activity with stimulation.

After 26 years of experience with this technique in urological cases, the mechanism of action of the stimulation has not been fully defined although it appears to alter sacral nerve reflexes, rather than directly change motor function. A detailed physiological study on patients with faecal incontinence failed to show a major effect on the external sphincter but did show an effect on rectal capacity and on rectal activity. Additionally, there was a qualitative, rather than a quantitative, effect on the internal sphincter muscle with the induction of slow wave activity and a decrease in the number of spontaneous falls in pressure (Fig. 2).[18] For the sceptics, a double-blind cross-over trial on patients with faecal incontinence[19] provided unique evidence that it has more than a placebo effect. Larger studies have now duplicated the initial excellent results,[20,21] and the effect has been shown to last at a median follow-up of 2 years (range, 3–60 months).[22]

NEOSPHINCTERS

Disruption of the anal sphincters not amenable to simple repair can range from a single defect in the internal sphincter to total disruption of the sphincter mechanism with little or no residual muscle. Internal sphincter defects are frequently due to common surgical procedures. Extensive external and internal anal sphincter damage can result from obstetric, surgical or other trauma, or follow previous unsuccessful surgery aimed at sphincter repair.

New treatments have been devised for patients with extensive or irreparable sphincter damage who suffer from severe incontinence. They may also have application for patients with profoundly weak, but intact, sphincters or those with congenital defects. These treatments involve radical surgery such as a replacement of the sphincter muscle with an electronically stimulated striated muscle or the more simple implantation of an artificial sphincter device. Caution should be exercised in the congenital group, however, as there are often associated hindgut abnormalities. An example of this would be the commonly seen rectal sensory deficit in patients born with an imperforate anus.

DYNAMIC GRACILOPLASTY

The use of skeletal muscle wrapped around the anus to improve continence was first described by Pickrell in 1952 using the gracilis muscle. The procedure was reliant to some extent on the muscle being so tightly wrapped as to cause a degree of obstruction. The results were poor and the operation fell into disrepute. Other muscles such as gluteus maximus and obturator internus were also trialed as anal canal 'wraps'. The gluteus muscles should be easier to use in the maintenance of continence than gracilis muscle as they are natural synergists of the anal sphincter, but results were poor and the resultant functional deficit worse than that following a graciloplasty.

The use of muscle wraps was revived with the discovery that chronic stimulation of a skeletal muscle can convert fast twitch, fatiguable muscle into slow twitch, muscle capable of continuous contraction. With chronic stimulation, there is an increase in the number of capillaries, an increase in aerobic-oxidative capacity and a decrease in muscle fibre diameter; the actual number of muscle fibres remaining unchanged.[23] The first chronically stimulated graciloplasty was performed in 1986 by Baeten in Maastricht.

The operative procedure involves two components that can be performed at one operation. The gracilis muscle is first mobilised and then wrapped, scarf-like, around the anus to be inserted onto the opposite ischial tuberosity or tethered to the skin. Implantation of the stimulator, electrode and connecting leads is the next phase. The electrode may be in the form of a cuff placed directly around the nerve, located at the top of the thigh, or a wire placed adjacent to the nerve branches. Connecting leads tunnel up to a pocket on the anterior abdominal wall created for the stimulator. A programme of incremental muscle stimulation usually spans a period of weeks before the muscle is fully trained to achieve a state of continuous contraction.[24] For defecation, the patient must switch off the stimulator to allow the muscle to relax and this is achieved using a hand-held patient programmer which communicates with the stimulator by telemetry.

Baeten's work, combined with that of Williams in London, lead to a temporary revival of this technique under the new name of the 'dynamic graciloplasty'.[25,26] However, the complication and re-operation rates are high,[27] and many are very hesitant to take on this relatively complex surgery. The most common complications encountered are technical problems with the muscle wrap and with the muscle stimulation, infection and difficulty with defecation.[28] Major contra-indications to the dynamic graciloplasty include pre-existing peri-anal sepsis, thereby excluding patients with Crohn's disease, and neurological disorders which cause weakness of the gracilis muscle. A recent study on the medium-term follow-up of these patients, erroneously labelled long-term in the article, has shown an improvement of 50% or more in episodes of incontinence at 24 months in 56% of patients without a pre-existing stoma and 43% in those with a stoma.[29]

Bilateral gracilis wraps have also been used particularly after the creation of a perineal colostomy following an abdominoperineal resection for cancer or after extensive perineal trauma. The muscles can be used separately, one to form a neosphincter and the other to form a sling to replace puborectalis. Alternatively, they can be used together to encircle the anus, coming from either side, around the back of the perineal colostomy and joined anteriorly. This latter method of reconstruction has been used with limited success even without stimulation.

ARTIFICIAL BOWEL SPHINCTER

The Acticon or artificial bowel sphincter (ABS) has been used now for more than 5 years. The artificial urinary sphincter (AUS) was introduced in 1972 and was reported to produce total or near-total urinary continence in over 75% of patients and improvement in a further 15% of patients.[30] Initially, it was this urinary sphincter (AMS Sphincter 800, American Medical Systems, Minneapolis, MN, USA), with or without some minor modifications, that was initially used for faecal incontinence, with good results reported by Christiansen and Sparso (12 patients),[31] Lehur et al. (13 patients),[32] and Wong et al. (12 patients).[33] The overall success rate was 73% with 54% of patients being totally continent of stool at all times and 19% having some loss of liquid stool only. The major complications were infection and mechanical failure, both occurring in 22% of the patients. Only one patient with previous irradiation and scarring had erosion of the device through the perineum. As with the graciloplasty, tightening of the anal canal sometimes results in difficulty with defecation after the procedure.

The operation to implant the Acticon is relatively simple. A hydraulic cuff encircles the anus, a balloon reservoir is placed in the pre-peritoneal plane in the lower abdomen and a valve pump in the labia or scrotum. These three components are connected by fully implanted silicone tubing and the device filled with a water-soluble contrast agent for ease of visibility on plain film. The pump is squeezed to achieve cuff deflation via a temporary transfer of fluid into the balloon. Continence is restored as the fluid passes passively back into the cuff with equilibration of pressures.

The results from a multicentre trial of 112 patients showed a success rate of 85% in patients with a functioning device, but there were 73 revisional operations and the success rate on an intention-to-treat basis was only 53%.[34] The incidence of infection and skin erosion has been higher than in the initial pilot studies, although mechanical failures are now rare. Late postoperative complications are frequent.[35]

Key point 6

- The more complex surgical options have a high complication and re-operation rate.

STOMAS AND IRRIGATIONS

The option of a colostomy for intractable incontinence should be reserved for those not suitable for conventional surgery, but should not be regarded as a treatment failure. For some patients, it is the optimal treatment, allowing return to as near normal a life-style as possible. Further improvement of quality-of-life can often be achieved by stoma irrigation. A note of caution when taking consent from patients is that they may still leak mucous from the anus if there is a residual rectum. An alternative strategy for faecal incontinence involves the creation of a proximal colonic stoma though which irrigation is performed to keep the distal bowel empty. The antegrade continence enema (ACE) has been used in children, especially in those with a congenital disorder, using antegrade irrigation through a reversed appendicostomy.[36] If the appendix is not available, then a tubularised caecal flap can be used. Long-term problems include stenosis at the muco-cutaneous junction, reflux of irrigation fluid into the ileum and loss of responsiveness to infused fluid. Retrograde per rectal irrigation, using a specially designed tube such as The Shandling Tube (CAMCARE Gels, UK), has been successful in some patients. The irrigation tube is fitted with a balloon with an easy

---

Key point 7

- A colostomy may provide a much improved quality-of-life, although per anal leakage of mucous can still be a problem.

---

inflation/deflation mechanism and this allows for sufficient retention of irrigation fluid in patients without an adequate sphincter complex.

CONCLUSIONS

Successful surgical treatment of faecal incontinence depends on the accurate characterisation of the motor, sensory and anatomical integrity of the anal sphincter mechanism. Prevention of sphincter damage should be a priority both in the obstetric setting and in anal surgery.

Key points for clinical practice

- There is a surprisingly high incidence of faecal incontinence, and it is not just a disability of the elderly.

- The biggest advance in incontinence has been endo-anal ultrasonography which allows for improved selection for surgery.

- Most cases of incontinence are due to defective or atrophic anal sphincter muscles.

- Conservative options should be used before consideration for surgery.

- Prevention is better than cure particularly in view of the disappointing long-term results of most therapies.

- The more complex surgical options have a high complication and re-operation rate.

- A colostomy may provide a much improved quality-of-life, although per anal leakage of mucous can still be a problem.

References

1. Nelson R, Norton N, Cautley E, Furner S. Community-based prevalence of anal incontinence. *JAMA* 1995; **274**: 559–561.
2. Engel AF, Kamm MA, Bartram CI, Nicholls RJ. Relationship of symptoms in faecal incontinence to specific sphincter abnormalities. *Int J Colorectal Dis* 1995; **10**: 152–155.
3. Parks AG, Swash M, Urich H. Sphincter denervation in anorectal incontinence and rectal prolapse. Gut 1977; **19**: 656–665.
4. Burnett SJ, Spence-Jones C, Speakman CT, Kamm MA, Hudson CN, Bartram CI. Unsuspected sphincter damage following childbirth revealed by anal endosonography. *Br J Radiol* 1991; **64**: 225–227.
5. Vaizey CJ, Bartram CI, Kamm MA. Primary degeneration of the internal anal sphincter as a cause of passive faecal incontinence. *Lancet* 1997; **349**: 612–615.
6. Briel JW, Zimmerman DD, Stoker J et al. Relationship between sphincter morphology on endoanal MRI and histopathological aspects of the external anal sphincter. *Int J Colorectal Dis* 2000; **15**: 87–90.

7. Briel JW, Stoker J, Rociu E, Lameris JS, Hop WC, Schouten WR. External anal sphincter atrophy on endoanal magnetic resonance imaging adversely affects continence after sphincteroplasty. *Br J Surg* 1999; **86**: 1322–1327.

8. deSousa N, Hall A, Puni R, Gilderdale DJ, Young JR, Kmiot WA. High resolution magnetic resonance imaging of the anal sphincter using a dedicated endoanal coil. Comparison of magnetic resonance imaging with surgical findings. *Dis Colon Rectum* 1996; **39**: 926–934.

9. Vaizey CJ, Carapeti E, Cahill J, Kamm MA. Prospective comparison of faecal incontinence grading systems. *Gut* 1999; **44**: 77–80.

10. Norton C, Kamm MA. Outcome of biofeedback for faecal incontinence. *Br J Surg* 1999; **86**: 1159–1163.

11. Malouf AJ, Norton CS, Engel AF, Nicholls RJ, Kamm MA. Long term results of overlapping anterior anal sphincter repair for obstetric trauma. *Lancet* 2000; **355**: 260–265.

12. Pinedo G, Vaizey CJ, Nicholls RJ, Roach R, Halligan S, Kamm MA. Results of repeat anal sphincter repair. *Br J Surg* 1999; **86**: 66–69.

13. Leroi AM, Kamm MA, Weber J, Denis P, Hawley PR. Internal anal sphincter repair. *Int J Colorectal Dis* 1997; **12**: 243–245.

14. Carapeti EA, Kamm MA, Evans BK, Phillips RKS. Topical phenylephrine increases anal sphincter resting pressure. *Br J Surg* 1999; **86**: 267–270.

15. Kumar D, Benson M, Bland J. Glutaraldehyde cross-linked collagen in the treatment of faecal incontinence. *Br J Surg* 1998; **85**: 978–979.

16. Kenefick NJ, Vaizey CJ, Malouf AJ, Norton CS, Marshall M, Kamm MA. Injectable silicone biomaterial for faecal incontinence due to internal anal sphincter dysfunction. *Gut* 2002; **51**: 225–228.

17. Matzel KE, Stadelmaier U, Hohenfeller M, Gall FP. Electrical stimulation of spinal nerves for treatment of faecal incontinence. *Lancet* 1995; **346**: 1124–1127.

18. Vaizey CJ, Kamm MA, Turner I, Nicholls RJ, Woloszko J. The results of short term sacral nerve stimulation in the treatment of faecal incontinence. *Gut* 1999; **44**: 407–412.

19. Vaizey CJ, Kamm MA, Roy AJ, Nicholls RJ. A double blind, cross over, study of sacral nerve stimulation for faecal incontinence. *Dis Colon Rectum* 2000; **43**: 298–302.

20. Ganio E, Ratto C, Masin A *et al*. Neuromodulation for fecal incontinence: outcome in 16 patients with definitive implant. The initial Italian Sacral Neurostimulation Group (GINS) experience. *Dis Colon Rectum* 2001; **44**: 965–970.

21. Leroi AM, Michot F, Grise P, Denis P. Effect of sacral nerve stimulation in patients with fecal and urinary incontinence. *Dis Colon Rectum* 2001; **44**: 779–789.

22. Salmons S, Henriksson J. The adaptive response of skeletal muscle to increased use. *Muscle Nerve* 1981; **4**: 94–105.

23. Kenefick NJ, Vaizey CJ, Cohen RC, Nicholls RJ, Kamm MA. Medium-term results of permanent sacral nerve stimulation faecal incontinence. *Br J Surg* 2002; **89**: 896–901.

24. Chapman AE, Geedes B, Hewett P *et al*. Systematic review of dynamic graciloplasty in the treatment of faecal incontinence. *Br J Surg* 2002; **89**: 138–153.

25. Baeten C, Geerdes BP, Adang EMM *et al*. Anal dynamic graciloplasty in the treatment of intractable fecal incontinence. *N Engl J Med* 1995; **332**: 1600–1605.

26. Williams NS, Patel J, George BD, Hallan RI, Watkins ES. Development of an electrically stimulated neoanal sphincter. *Lancet* 1991; **338**: 1166–1169.

27. Wexner S, Gonzalez-Padron A, Rius J *et al*. Stimulated gracilis neosphincter operation: initial experience, pitfalls and complications. *Dis Colon Rectum* 1996; **39**: 957–964.

28. Korgen S, Keighley M. Stimulated gracilis neosphincter – not as good as previously thought. Report of four cases. *Dis Colon Rectum* 1995; **38**: 1331–1333.

29. Wexner SD, Baeten C, Bailey R *et al*. Long-term efficacy of dynamic graciloplasty for fecal incontinence. *Dis Colon Rectum* 2002; **45**: 809–818.

30. Montague DK. The artificial urinary sphincter (AS 800): experience in 166 consecutive

patients. *J Urol* 1992; **142**: 380–382.

31. Christiansen J, Sparso B. Treatment of anal incontinence by an implantable prosthetic anal sphincter. *Ann Surg* 1992; **215**: 383–386.

32. Lehur P-A, Michot F, Denis P *et al*. Results of artificial sphincter in severe anal incontinence: report of 14 consecutive implantations. *Dis Colon Rectum* 1996; **39**: 1352–1355.

33. Wong WD, Jensen LL, Bartolo DCC, Rothenberger DA. Artificial anal sphincter. *Dis Colon Rectum* 1996; **39**: 1345–1351.

34. Wong WD, Congliosi SM, Spencer MP *et al*. The safety and efficacy of the artificial bowel sphincter for fecal incontinence. *Dis Colon Rectum* 2002; **45**: 1139–1153.

35. Ortiz H, Armendariz P, DeMiguel M, Ruiz MD, Alos R, Roig JV. Complications and functional outcome following artificial anal sphincter implantation. *Br J Surg* 2002; **89**: 877–881.

36. Malone PS, Ransley PG, Kiely EM. Preliminary report: the antegrade continence enema. *Lancet* 1990; **336**: 1217–1218.

Majid Hashemi

5

Postoperative complications following oesophagectomy

Ever since the first successful oesophagectomy by Torek in 1913, refinement of peri-operative care and surgical technique have helped to reduce the mortality of this procedure. Even though the frequency of many complications has not changed dramatically over time, patients are more likely to survive a complication when compared to previous decades,[1,2] and death in today's practice is most likely to be due to pulmonary complications.[2,3]

There are numerous variations in how oesophageal resections are performed in terms of approach (trans-thoracic, trans-hiatal or laparoscopic and thoracoscopic), conduit (gastric or colonic), site and type of anastomosis (cervical, intrathoracic, sutured or stapled), as well as extent of lymph-adenectomy (one, two or three field). All these variations are physiologically disruptive, particularly in a group of patients who often have life-long alcohol and tobacco exposure with associated cardiopulmonary co-morbidity and who are often debilitated at the time of presentation as a result of the primary malignancy. The complications that will be discussed are common to all oesophageal resections in their aetiology, presentation and principles of management although there are minor differences in their relative frequency.

IDENTIFYING RISK

Recognition of patients who may be at increased risk of complications is important for several reasons. First, the rationale for resection is put into perspective when palliation may offer a better alternative for an individual patient. Oesophageal resections are embarked on with curative intent, but most patients are at stage III at presentation and achieve a 5-year survival of 20%: non-resectional palliation may be a more appropriate option in the high-risk patient with confirmed T3 disease.

Majid Hashemi FRCS(Gen), Senior Lecturer/Consultant Surgeon, The Whittington Hospital, Whittington NHS Trust, Highgate Hill, London N19 5NF, UK

Second, the surgical approach itself may be modified: a trans-hiatal approach may be more suitable in a patient when a thoracotomy might not be tolerated.

Third, in obtaining informed consent, the likelihood of specific complications should be quantified, discussed and documented.

Finally, stratification of risk enables comparative audit between individual units and a proposed risk scoring model using Bayesian principles may have a role for the individual patient.[4]

Bartel and colleagues[5] identified four factors that predict a poor surgical outcome. A poor general status, poor cardiac, hepatic and respiratory function were independent predictors of a fatal postoperative course. By applying a composite score of these variables to help in the patient selection and in the tailoring of the surgical procedure, they were able to reduce the postoperative mortality from 9.4% to 1.6%. Others have identified a range of pre-operative variables that are associated with increased early morbidity or mortality including smoking,[2,6] age,[7] and diabetes.[8] Predicting risk by using POSSUM has been shown to over-estimate morbidity and mortality and to have little correlation with the observed outcome after oesophagectomy.[9]

NUTRITION

The prognostic nutritional index (PNI) was initially proposed by Ondera[10] and is based on the serum albumin and leukocyte count. It has been validated in a study of 258 patients undergoing oesophageal resection and shown to be predictive of postoperative complications.[11] Peri-operative supplementation by enteral nutrition influences cellular immunity. Nasojejunal or percutaneous jejunal feeding may be most effective in patients immunosuppressed from pre-operative chemotherapy;[12,13] postoperative enteral nutrition has greater immunomodulating effects than parenteral nutrition.[14]

BLOOD TRANSFUSION

As in surgery for other types of cancer, blood transfusions are associated with a reduced overall survival although not with early morbidity.[8] There seems to be a cut off of three units of blood below which there is no apparent effect.[15]

SPLENECTOMY

Splenectomy for iatrogenic damage is required in 0.7—9% of resections,[8,16,17] and leads to an increased likelihood of postoperative pneumonia, intra-abdominal sepsis, anastomotic leak and death.[18]

PERI-OPERATIVE CARE

Hypoxia within the first 24 h of surgery is associated with increased morbidity and mortality. Adequate tissue oxygenation relies on both adequate ventilation and cardiac output for the delivery of oxygen. Kusano *et al.* showed a significantly lower measured oxygen delivery and consumption at 6-h post-oesophagectomy in patients who went on to develop complications or die compared to uncomplicated survivors.[19]

PULMONARY COMPLICATIONS

Pulmonary complications occur in 20–30% of patients after oesophagectomy,[2,17,20–22] and pneumonia is associated with a greater than 4-fold risk of death.[23] The frequency of isolated atelectasis is hard to determine, with some reporting only cases where there is a delay in discharge (2%)[16] whilst others, with comparable overall outcome data, group atelectasis with pleural effusions and thus report a frequency of 87%.[24] Acute respiratory distress syndrome (ARDS) occurs in 15% of patients and has a mortality of 50%.[6]

AETIOLOGY

The aetiology of these frequent pulmonary complications is multifactorial.

Lung injury

Even without thoracotomy, major surgery is associated with an elevation of inflammatory mediators within the lungs with a concomitant increase in vascular permeability and fluid sequestration. Tsukada et al.[25] showed a significant elevation of granulocyte elastase and interleukin-8 levels in bronchial lavage fluid on days 1–3 in patients who develop pneumonia. Thoracotomy exacerbates these effects, and one lung ventilation adds further to the insult.

Oesophagectomy may also be followed by acute lung injury; the development of ARDS after elective oesophagectomy is influenced by factors that cause intra-operative cardiorespiratory instability including peri-operative hypoxaemia, prolonged one lung ventilation, peri-operative hypotension, increased fluid requirements and the need for inotropic support and surgical re-exploration.[6]

Reduced pulmonary injury is considered an important advantage of a trans-hiatal approach to the oesophagus. This is supported by a recent randomised prospective trial comparing trans-hiatal and trans-thoracic oesophagectomy[26] which revealed fewer pulmonary complications following trans-hiatal oesophagectomy. A trans-hiatal dissection, nevertheless, does carry a significant risk of pulmonary morbidity. There is often a breach of the pleura (77%)[16] and postoperative pleural fluid collections are common.[24]

Compromised ventilation

After a thoracotomy, the reduced lung volumes and spirometry may take more than 6 months to return to normal.[27] Painful abdominal and thoracic incisions further limit ventilatory effort and lead to atelectasis and predispose to pneumonia. By using a thoracic epidural, Watson et al.[28] were able to reduce pulmonary complications from 30% to 15% and fatal pulmonary complications from 5% to zero. Huge improvements in outcome have also been demonstrated following the introduction of an acute pain service after oesophagectomy with thoracotomy: in a retrospective outcome analysis, Tsui et al.[29] reported reduced pulmonary complications from 27% to 12% and reduced overall mortality from 14% to 8%.

Pulmonary oedema

Meticulous attention to fluid replacement and maintenance at the time of surgery, with cautious peri-operative fluid restriction results in a reduction of intensive care stay, fewer failed extubations, and a reduced need for both tracheostomies and regular postoperative bronchoscopies.[30]

A D2 abdominal nodal dissection is often combined with an extensive mediastinal and thoracic lymph node dissection. Sasako and colleagues[31] warn of the risk of fluid overload on the third postoperative day as the third space fluid loss resulting from extensive lymphatic dissection is re-absorbed. They recommend a reduction of fluid administered combined with diuretic use and particular close observation of urine output.

Early aspiration

This may occur in up to a third of patients after extubation, particularly with the reduction in the sensitivity and force of the cough reflex. Damage to the vagal nerve caused by dissection of the paratracheal lymph nodes, and injury to the diaphragm during operation for oesophageal cancer may be responsible for the inability to cough. Patients who have a good cough reflex in the immediate postoperative period have fewer pulmonary complications. The postoperative measurement of cough ability may be a useful indicator for safe extubation of the intratracheal tube.[32] Maintaining an endotracheal tube for the first 24 h may provide a degree of airway protection at this vulnerable stage.[33] Damage to the recurrent laryngeal nerve has a tremendous impact on the length of intubation and intensive care stay and leads to recurrent bouts of aspiration pneumonia.[34]

PREDICTORS OF PULMONARY RISK

Earlier studies of 170 oesophageal transthoracic resections by Nagawa[35] identified vital capacity, liver cirrhosis, and tumour stage as three significant factors that were predictive of the risk of postoperative pulmonary complications. Ferguson[7] identified age, forced expiratory volume (FEV1), and performance status as independent predictors of postoperative pulmonary and vascular complications.

Avendano found that an FEV1 of 65% or less predicted the need for ventilation for longer than 48 h and a higher frequency of lung complications, but not overall survival. Length of time on the ventilator, ARDS, older age (66.9 years fatal *versus* 60.9 years survivors) and a low albumin were all associated with a higher likelihood of death.[24]

Presently, there is no single validated scoring system that can be universally applied, although identifying individual factors facilitates patient selection.

PREVENTION AND TREATMENT

Some authors perform routine postoperative bronchoscopy and bronchial aspiration,[21,30,36] and the therapeutic role of bronchoscopy is supported by an observed significant reduction in mortality in patients receiving this treatment at regular intervals.[2]

Patients in acute respiratory distress benefit from brief periods of prone ventilation. Watanabe *et al.*[36] randomised eight patients each to ventilation in the supine and prone positions immediately following three field oesophagectomy. Five paramedical and nursing staff and one physician were needed to turn the patients to the prone position for 6 h every day for 4 days. Despite minor problems with facial oedema and lip bruising, there were marked improvements in oxygenation with an increase of the PaO_2/FiO_2 ratio and a significant reduction in the need for ventilatory support and intensive care stay.

Reactive pleural effusions are common and failure to drain a large collection can lead to acute respiratory distress and tamponade. Chest drainage is performed routinely after thoracotomy; the type of chest drain[37,38] or use of negative pressure suction drainage does not seem to influence outcome. Orringer[16] placed chest drains in 75% of patients after trans-hiatal oesophagectomy and an alternative is selective ultrasound-guided placement of fine pigtail catheters when an effusion develops. A chest drain should not be inserted blindly after an oesophagectomy.

Key point 1

- Pulmonary complications are the commonest cause of morbidity and death after oesophagectomy.

Key point 2

- Attention to fluid management, with cautious monitoring of intravenous maintenance fluids to avoid overload will reduce the risk of pneumonia.

Key point 3

- Recurrent laryngeal nerve damage is a major contributor to the risk of aspiration pneumonia and the need for re-intubation.

CARDIOVASCULAR COMPLICATIONS

Arrhythmias occur most commonly on postoperative days 2–4 and are often an early sign of an anastomotic leak, pulmonary complications or sepsis. Old age is a predictor of an increased risk of postoperative supraventricular tachydysrhythmias and these may be associated with an increased mortality.[39] Pre-operative digoxin does not seem to decrease the incidence of dysrhythmias.[40] Treatment of the underlying cause, correction of any associated electrolyte abnormality and pharmaceutical cardioversion with a cardiac glycoside if simple atrial fibrillation or with another anti-arrhythmic agent such as amiodorone is effective therapy in most cases.

Table 1 Grading of anastomotic leak[53]

Grade of leak	Clinical findings
Radiological	No clinical signs
Clinically minor	Neck wound inflammation, pyrexia, leukocytosis, contained leak on imaging
Clinically major	Sepsis, severe disruption on endoscopy, diffuse leak on contrast study
Conduit necrosis	Sepsis, endoscopic confirmation

ANASTOMOTIC LEAKS

Only 20% of leaks occur before the 7th postoperative day, with the median time to detection being about 12 days.[41–43] The true frequency of leaks is difficult to ascertain due to wide definitions of leakage and non-standardised reporting. Subclinical leaks are missed if contrast radiology is omitted and clinical leaks vary greatly in degree of severity and consequence (Table 1).

Efforts to understand the cause of anastomotic leaks continue. Technical failure results in early clinical leaks. Leak rates are increased if there are periods of intra-operative hypotension, and ischaemia of the conduit is likely to play a role: There is a definite drop in perfusion of the stomach with mobilisation and formation of a conduit and placement in the mediastinum causes a further reduction in blood flow.[44] Two observations suggest that there are other factors at play. First, patients with Doppler-detected reduced perfusion do not have increased leakage but may have some increased risk of anastomotic stricture formation.[45] Second, when Jacobi et al.[46] measured the tissue oxygen tension in the gastric mucosa near an anastomosis, they found an elevated oxygen tension in patients who went on to leak. They concluded that there are other causes for anastomotic leaks that are associated with a problem with oxygen utilisation.

For both hand-sutured and stapled anastomosis, surgical technique and experience seem to be the main determinants of a leak. Leaks occur in operations where there have been technical difficulties,[37,43] and collected results over several decades have shown a decrease in leak rates in the latter periods.[1,2,43,47]

Staplers do not result in a reduced leak rate but lead to a higher incidence of anastomotic stricture.[37] Leak rates do not relate to whether a trans-thoracic or trans-hiatal approach is used although the consequences of an intrathoracic anastomosis are more serious.[48] Routine placement of drains in cervical incisions does not reduce the incidence of infections, haematomas or collections and has no influence on the leak rate.[49]

DETECTION OF AN ANASTOMOTIC LEAK

A high index of clinical suspicion is essential. Water-soluble contrast radiology as a routine screening investigation is not accurate.[42] If there is still suspicion of a leak after a normal water-soluble contrast study, a repeat swallow with barium sulphate is safe and may reveal an undisclosed leak.[50] If a patient is unable to swallow, then CT scanning is an accurate alternative.[41] Early flexible endoscopy can be considered if radiology is inconclusive, and it can allow planning before surgical re-exploration. Endoscopy can also facilitate re-positioning of a nasogastric tube which may be required for treatment. Anastomotic leaks are proposed as a major aetiological factor in stricture formation and early endoscopic pneumatic dilatation may have the dual benefit of preventing the development of a stricture and of accelerating healing of the anastomosis.[16,51]

Elevation of salivary amylase in fluid drained from the neck wound may help confirm leakage from a cervical anastomosis.[52] The nature and colour of the fluid in the intercostal drains may suggest a leak, but is not necessarily always a representative or early sign, particularly if a trans-hiatal procedure has been carried out and the pleura are intact.

MANAGEMENT OF A LEAK

A radiological leak in an asymptomatic patient requires little specific treatment. Delaying oral intake for several days with frequent and regular observations and follow-up contrast radiology will suffice (Fig. 1).

The clinical presentation of a leak may be subtle and limited to erythema and cellulitis in the neck wound of a cervical anastomosis. If an infection is established in the neck, laying open of the wound will allow external drainage. A contained leak from a thoracic anastomosis may manifest with local thoracic symptoms or gastrointestinal bleeding, and with signs of a systemic inflammatory response combined with elevation of serum inflammatory markers. Many patients first develop symptoms when oral intake is resumed after surgery.

Once the diagnosis is established, feeding needs to be continued via an endoscopically sited nasojejunal tube or a percutaneous jejunostomy and the patient should be placed nil-by-mouth. Intravenous antibiotic and antifungal treatments are recommended even in the absence of positive cultures. Some supplement the above regimen with a somatostatin analogue and proton pump inhibitors, and avoid routine gastric tube decompression with a nasogastric tube,[53] although most recommend nasogastric decompression.[41,42] Inadequate drainage of any collection will result in deterioration and failure of medical therapy and inadequate radiological drainage is a frequent cause of death.[43] Drainage with underwater, sealed intercostal drains may be adequate, but early CT-guided placement of additional drains may be required.[41] Regular bed-side ultrasound of the chest will identify new pleural effusions and permit placement of percutaneous pigtail catheters, which are less restrictive for the patient.

These measures, combined with supportive nursing care and attention to hydration, chest physiotherapy, and careful monitoring will be sufficient treatment for the majority of patients with an anastomotic leak.[16,41,43,54]

Leaks seldom continue as the sole complication and inevitably further additional problems occur, in particular pneumonia often with the development of multi-resistant organisms. A persistently catabolic state ensues and nutritional support that is dependent on a tube is fraught with problems of blockage and dislodgement as well as local mechanical and infective irritations. A multidisciplinary approach is, therefore, indicated from the outset.

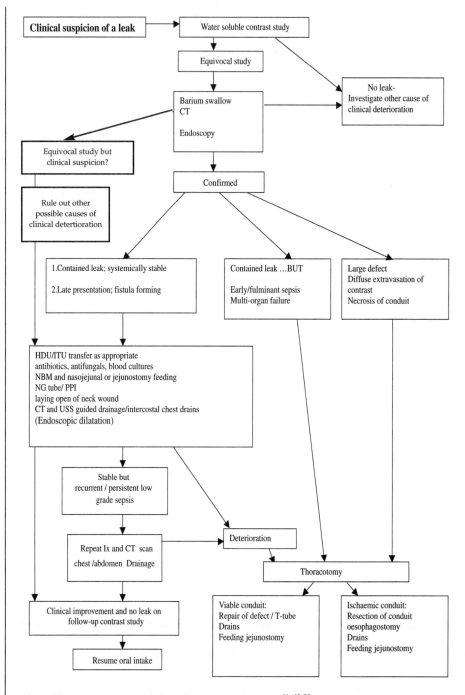

Fig. 1 The management of clinical anastomotic leaks.[41–43,53]

Once there is clinical evidence of resolution, contrast radiology can help confirm that the leak has sealed and oral intake can be resumed under a watchful eye. The feeding tubes allow valuable supplementation of oral intake and may still be required should any symptoms recur. This above conservative medical strategy may need to be continued for weeks or even months.[41–43,53]

Deterioration of the clinical condition whilst on medical treatment may be due to: (i) initial under-estimation of the size of defect; (ii) failure to identify an ischaemic focus in the conduit or anastomosis; (iii) extension of an area of ischaemia; or (iv) an inadequately drained collection. Uncorrected mediastinal contamination will result in sepsis and multi-organ failure.

A diffuse leak or rapidly developing sepsis in the presence of a confirmed leak is an indication for thoracotomy. The two broad options are: (i) if the defect is small and the conduit appears viable, it may be repaired directly and this may be done over a T-tube for added protection with placement of nearby intrathoracic drains; or (ii) if the conduit is ischaemic, then the anastomosis needs to be taken down, the ischaemic conduit excised, an oesophagostomy fashioned in the neck and a percutaneous jejunostomy placed, allowing a staged reconstruction at a later date with an alternative conduit.

Key point 4

- Most oesophageal anastomotic leaks can be managed non-operatively and are non-fatal.

Key point 5

- Precise definition of an anastomotic leak, using contrast radiology combined with early endoscopy allows timely re-operation for salvage before established multi-organ failure.

The death rate from a leak ranges from less than 10%[17] to 35%,[42,43] and the outcome from anastomotic leaks, as with other complications, is dependent on timely diagnosis and treatment and demands the expertise of a multidisciplinary team.

BLEEDING

Haemorrhage may present with variation in vital signs, as well as signs related to the volume effects of intrapleural blood displacing the lungs or causing a cardiac tamponade. Drainage from abdominal and chest drains in excess of 100 ml/h beyond the first 2–3 postoperative hours is a cardinal sign of haemorrhage and a drain fluid with a haemoglobin concentration that resembles that of the serum supports the diagnosis. Intrathoracic, intra-abdominal and intragastric haemorrhage carry a mortality of over 30%, death being associated with incomplete resuscitation and delay in intervention.[55] Urgent re-exploration is indicated. Haemorrhage after trans-thoracic resection may be from the wound itself, from intercostal or tracheobronchial vessels or from the anastomosis staple or suture lines.[22] Thoracic bleeding after a trans-hiatal resection is usually from an arterial source in the oesophageal bed. In Orringer's series of 1085 cases, urgent re-operation with thoracotomy was required in five patients (< 1%);[16] in this series, there were 3 deaths from bleeding during the primary operation.

CHYLOTHORAX

The cisternae chyli collect chyle from the liver and gastrointestinal tract and coalesce in the midline at the level of the 2nd lumbar vertebra to form the thoracic duct. The duct then runs alongside the aorta through the hiatus and crosses to the left of the oesophagus at the level of the 5th thoracic vertebra. It enters the root of the neck on the left and drains as much as four litres of immunoglobulin and fat-rich chyle into the left subclavian vein. Damage to the main duct can occur at any point along its route and can result in leakage into any body cavity, most commonly the chest.

Strategies employed to reduce the risk of thoracic duct injury include routine *en bloc* ligation at the time of surgery and the administration of cream meals before surgery to make the ducts more prominent and easier to protect. Nevertheless, injuries occur in 1–8% of resections.[22,56,57]

DETECTION AND TREATMENT

Chyle is easily recognised as turbid, creamy fluid in the chest drain. Any straw-coloured pleural effusion greater than 500 ml should arouse suspicion and prompt biochemical analysis. Examination of chyle will reveal chylomicrons and elevated levels of triglycerides (> 100 mg/dl), a lymphocyte count more than 90% of the total white blood cell count, and a total protein concentration approaching that of the serum. There is often a refractory period of 1–2 days post-resection before the drainage of chyle becomes noticeable. In situations where there is no intercostal drainage, the mass effect of a gradually accumulating large volume effusion of several litres leads to acute respiratory distress, cardiac tamponade and a drop in cardiac output. More rarely, there may be a predominantly intra-abdominal collection initially and, in very rare instances, a chylous ascites may occur without any significant thoracic collection (Fig. 2).

Percutaneous, image-guided localisation and embolisation of the thoracic duct using platinum coils appears safe and a success rate of over 70% has been achieved by one unit with a large experience.[58] If there is local expertise, then this should be a first-line measure, performed soon after diagnosis and combined with appropriate medical treatment.

Orringer has made a strong case for early thoracotomy and duct ligation, achieving successful resolution of the leak with no mortality in all 11 patients in his series. However, none of these patients had undergone a prior thoracotomy for their oesophagectomies.[56] In studies where a period of conservative treatment is tried initially, the mortality is 8–23%%,[57,59] but was as high as 46% when the mean duration of conservative treatment was 35 days.[60] Death is often due to a combination of septic and surgical complications that develop on a background of progressively worsening debility, often associated with a surgical re-intervention several weeks after the onset of the leak. It is

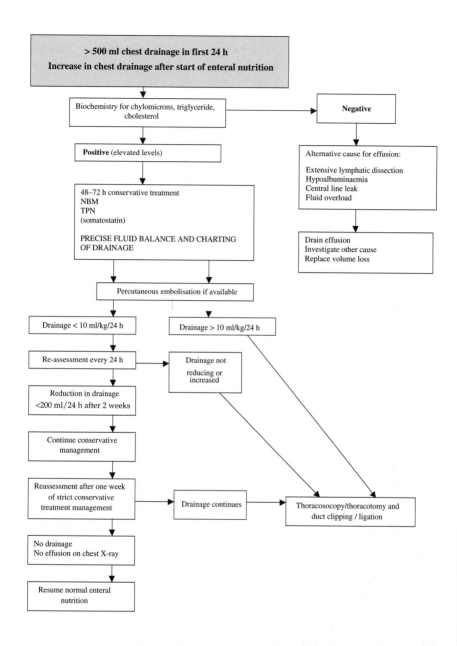

Fig. 2 The management of chylothorax.

imperative that patients who have a persistently high output and who are unlikely to resolve with medical treatment are identified early and selected for surgical duct ligation. This is particularly so today with the availability of thoracoscopic techniques which make re-operation less daunting. However, it is also clear that 41–80% of patients will settle with medical treatment and a period of conservative treatment has now become accepted as a safe adjunct to surgical re-exploration and ligation.[57,59,61]

The mainstays of modern medical management are reduction of chyle production, maintenance of nutrition, the prevention of septic complications, drainage of pleural collections and precise documentation of on-going drainage. The criteria for surgical re-exploration need to be defined at the outset of treatment and daily re-appraisal of the success of medical treatment is required.

A fat-free enteral diet with medium-chain triglyceride supplementation will lead to reduction of chyle output, but most advise total intestinal rest and total parenteral nutrition from the outset. Octreotide and more latterly etilefrine, an α-adrenergic, have been reported as effective in reducing chyle leakage.[62] Just as there is variation in the degree of damage to the duct or its branches, there is difficulty in predicting when a leak may or may not resolve. A drainage of less than 10 ml/kg/day by the fifth day is an indication that there will be spontaneous closure,[57] drainage stopping altogether by 14 days in most cases.[57-59] Once drainage has stopped, enteral nutrition, which may be enriched with medium-chain triglycerides, can be cautiously introduced, observing for signs of re-accumulation of chyle.

Undue delay in surgical ligation can be avoided by adopting a low threshold for persistent drainage of greater than 200 ml/day after two weeks of medical treatment. Surgical options are either to attempt a repair of the duct or to ligate the duct caudal to the site of leakage. Imaging may be useful to plan intervention, but is of limited practical application. Lymphangiography may help to localise the site of duct damage. Technetium-labelled lymphoscintigraphy may confirm the diagnosis, but poses practical difficulties.

A right thoracotomy provides access for an *en bloc* ligation of the duct and its surrounding tissue although thoracoscopic ligation or clipping is now an established alternative.[61] Precise localisation of the damaged segment of duct can present a challenge, particularly with postoperative adhesion formation and pleural thickening. Methylene blue or cream administered through a nasogastric or jejunostomy tube an hour before surgery may occasionally help to identify a leak. A persistent leak occurs after 10% of surgical ligations and a range of additional manoeuvres such as spraying the damaged duct with fibrin glue and a pleurodesis have been tried. Interruption of the thoracic duct does not lead to chylous ascites as the numerous lymphaticovenous communications with the lumbar, intercostal and azygos veins allow continued circulation.

RECURRENT LARYNGEAL NERVE INJURIES

Injuries are most common and severe in patients who have had three field lymph node dissections.[63] Injuries can also occur during the mediastinal dissection in the aortopulmonary window on the right, but are commoner after trans-hiatal oesophagectomy possibly due to traction during the course of the mediastinal dissection and from compression in the tracheo-oesophageal groove from retractor placement during the cervical anastomosis.[16] Awareness of the anatomy of the supralaryngeal and the recurrent laryngeal nerve (RLN) is essential, and identification of the nerve during surgery by using nerve stimulation may aid this.

Key point 6

• Untreated chylothorax carries a high mortality and early detection is essential.

Key point 7

• Large volume pleural effusions, particularly if opaque, require biochemical analysis for triglycerides and cholesterol.

Key point 8

• There is a place for conservative management of a chylothorax.

DETECTION AND SIGNIFICANCE

Even partial and subtle degrees of RLN injury can impair the patient's swallowing and ability to cough efficiently, leading to loss of airway protection and early pulmonary morbidity.[34] Hoarseness is not always obvious, and may be multifactorial in the early postoperative period. Repeated ineffective coughing, particularly once established on oral intake, should arouse suspicion and an initial bed-side assessment is a useful screen. A contrast video pharyngo-oesophagram may identify aspiration,[64] and flexible laryngoscopy provides information on the degree of vocal cord paralysis and abduction.

Initial re-training of speech and swallowing by a speech therapist may be beneficial, and the chin tuck manoeuvre[64] will reduce the incidence of aspiration. Bilateral palsy results in life-threatening stridor and a tracheostomy is required to maintain an airway and improve pulmonary toilet. The majority of nerve injuries are unilateral and transient, with 80% of patients having resolution of their hoarseness within one year, but prolonged or permanent impairment has a significant impact on the quality-of-life.[63] Vocal cord medialisation or teflon injections into the vocal cord are reserved for symptomatic patients where there is no improvement with conservative measures and such remedial treatment is required in less than 10% of patients with nerve injuries.[16,34]

TRACHEAL INJURIES AND TRACHEO-OESOPHAGEAL FISTULA

Injuries to the major airways occur as a result of direct trauma, devascularisation during surgery, or due to pressure necrosis associated with the cuff of an endotracheal tube or tracheostomy. In a recent report, the incidence of isolated major airway injury was 1.8% and 0.8% following trans-hiatal and trans-thoracic resection, respectively. Most of these injuries were discovered at the time of surgery and all defects were closed primarily. Despite further pulmonary complications in most, there was no associated mortality.[65]

Table 2 Complications following oesophageal resection, selected series

	n	Approach (gastric conduit unless specified) (%)	Pulmonary atelectasis# pneumonia air leak ARDS (%)	Cardiac arrhythmia (%)	Cardiac MI (%)	Anastomotic leak (%)	Conduit necrosis (%)	Haemorrhage requiring re-operation (%)	Chylothorax (%)	RLN palsy (%)	Mortality (%)
Orringer (2001)[16]	1085	TH	217 (2)*	N/S	4 (<1)	146 (13)	9 (0.8)	5 (<1)	18 (<1)	74 (7)	44 (4)
Obertop (2002)[17]	115	TH	27 (23)	15 (13)	N/S	10 (9)**	2 (2)	2 (2)	2 (2)	28 (24)	4 (3.5)
DeMeester (2001)[19]	100	TT (72% colon) 2 field	20 (20)	6 (6)	1 (1)	10 (10)**	6 (6)	7 (7)	6 (6)	4 (4)	6 (6)
Wong (2001)[3]	710	TT (TH)	227 (32)	164 (23)	8 (1)	25 (3.5)	6 (0.8)	16 (2.2)	12 (1.7)	N/S	79 (11)
Heitmiller (2002)[12]	120	TH (TH)	6 (5)	9 (7.5)	1 (0.8)	1 (0.8)	0	0	2 (1.7)	4 (3.3)	1 (0.8)
Altorki (2001)[21]	111	TT 2 field	30 (27)	10 (9)	1 (1)	10 (9)	5 (4.5)	0	2 (2)	4 (3.6)	6 (5.4)
Karl (2000)[8]	143	TT	20 (13)	19 (13)	0	5 (3.5)**	0	N/S	0	N/S	3 (2.1)
Luketich (2000)[71]	77	Min inv	16 (21)	8 (10)	2 (2.5)	7 (10)	0	0	3 (4)	2 (2.5)	0

TT, transthoracic, usually with en bloc 2 field lymphadenectomy; TH, transhiatal; Min inv, minimally invasive; N/S, not specified; ARDS, acute respiratory distress syndrome; MI, myocardial infarct; RLN, recurrent laryngeal nerve palsy.

#Clinically significant, excluding radiological atelectasis.

*Only those clinically significant leading to delay in discharge beyond 10 days reported.

**Radiological and clinical leak.

Tracheo-oesophageal fistulae may also develop as a result of an inadequately drained cervical anastomotic leak.[47,66] The presentation may be with acute respiratory failure requiring re-intubation or more insidious with repeated coughs and bouts of aspiration pneumonia. Early recognition and careful assessment of the airway and the anastomosis with conduit by bronchoscopy and endoscopy can be followed by a brief period of conservative management accompanied by a tailored ventilator regimen, which includes reduced ventilatory pressures. If there is an associated cervical or mediastinal collection, this needs drainage and an attempt can be made to cover the defect in the airway by application of endoscopic clips and fibrin glue or an endotracheal stent can be inserted.[66]

Most cases will require re-operation to close the defect in the airway and to excise any devitalised part of the conduit, exteriorising proximally with an oesophagostomy in the first instance, and re-fashioning a new conduit (colon) through an alternative route (retrosternally or subcutaneously) as a staged second procedure.[67]

GASTRIC OUTLET OBSTRUCTION

Recurrent vomiting and aspiration after oesophagectomy requires investigation with contrast radiology. Delayed gastric emptying may be functional, but mechanical hold up, particularly in the absence of a pyloroplasty, requires early identification and treatment. The importance of a gastric drainage procedure is illustrated by Whooley et al.[2] who, in reporting a series of 710 oesophagectomies, encountered symptomatic gastric outlet obstruction in 17 of the 21 patients that had not had a pyloroplasty. Endoscopic transluminal balloon dilatation can be tried in the first instance, but a re-operation may be required. There is no apparent difference in results when comparing a pyloroplasty and a pyloromyotomy.[68]

Diaphragmatic herniation is rare, but, if symptomatic, early re-operation and reduction of the herniated intrathoracic viscera and repair of the diaphragmatic defect is indicated.[69] There has been a report of intrapleural herniation of the gastric conduit after trans-hiatal oesophagectomy which required urgent correction by incising the full length of the mediastinal pleura and plicating a redundant portion of the conduit.[70]

BENIGN ANASTOMOTIC STRICTURE

There is a wide variation in the reporting and definition of benign anastomotic strictures. Most report patients with symptomatic dysphagia requiring dilatation.[17,47] Others routinely perform early dilatation in over 75% of their patients.[16] Strictures may present as early as one month after surgery,[17,37] and can be safely treated by endoscopic pneumatic dilatations with the majority requiring 3–7 sessions (Table 2).[17,37,47]

SUMMARY

The peri-operative management of oesophagectomy patients is challenging and complex. RLN injury, thoracic duct damage and some anastomotic leaks can be ascribed to technical failure which may be avoidable, and, although

Key point 9

• Treatment of complications requires a multidisciplinary team.

pulmonary complications and many other serious medical problems seem inevitable, recent evidence suggests these too can be predicted and their frequency reduced.[12,28–30]

The management of the majority of postoperative problems is primarily non-operative, at least initially. It is the oesophageal surgeon's role to co-ordinate the team of specialists and varied health professionals in providing supportive treatment to these patients and forward planning is essential: Explanation at the outset of the proposed duration of treatment, which can take months, is essential to reduce disappointment and frustration for the patient, their relatives and health workers. Second, the patient and the remainder of the team need to understand the criteria for abandoning a medical approach and opting for a surgical exploration. Most complex postoperative problems are rare and integrated networks linking geographically separate units may allow pooling of experience and sharing of expertise, thus allowing optimum care for the more challenging patients.

Key points for clinical practice

• Pulmonary complications are the commonest cause of morbidity and death after oesophagectomy.

• Attention to fluid management, with cautious monitoring of intravenous maintenance fluids to avoid overload will reduce the risk of pneumonia.

• Recurrent laryngeal nerve damage is a major contributor to the risk of aspiration pneumonia and the need for re-intubation.

• Most oesophageal anastomotic leaks can be managed non-operatively and are non-fatal.

• Precise definition of an anastomotic leak, using contrast radiology combined with early endoscopy allows timely re-operation for salvage before established multi-organ failure.

• Untreated chylothorax carries a high mortality and early detection is essential.

• Large volume pleural effusions, particularly if opaque, require biochemical analysis for triglycerides and cholesterol.

• There is a place for conservative management of a chylothorax.

• Treatment of complications requires a multidisciplinary team.

References

1. Hofstetter W, Swisher SG, Correa AM *et al*. Treatment outcomes of resected esophageal cancer. *Ann Surg* 2002; **236**: 376–384.
2. Whooley BP, Law S, Murthy SC, Alexandrou A, Wong J. Analysis of reduced death and complication rates after esophageal resection. *Ann Surg* 2001; **233**: 338–344.
3. Gray AJG, Hoile RW, Ingram GS, Sherry K. (eds) *Management of Patients Undergoing Oesophagectomy. The Report of the National Confidential Enquiry Into Peri-Operative Deaths 1996/1997 (National CEPOD)*. London: Department of Health, 2002; 57–61.
4. Griffin SM, McCulloch P, Davies S, Kinsman R. *Augis Database Report 2002*. London: AUGIS. 2002.
5. Bartels H, Stein HJ, Siewert JR. Preoperative risk analysis and postoperative mortality of oesophagectomy for resectable oesophageal cancer. *Br J Surg* 1998; **85**: 840–844.
6. Tandon S, Batchelor A, Bullock R *et al*. Peri-operative risk factors for acute lung injury after elective oesophagectomy. *Br J Anaesth* 2001; **86**: 633–638.
7. Ferguson MK, Durkin AE. Preoperative prediction of the risk of pulmonary complications after esophagectomy for cancer. *J Thorac Cardiovasc Surg* 2002; **123**: 661–669.
8. Karl RC, Schreiber R, Boulware D, Baker S, Coppola D. Factors affecting morbidity, mortality, and survival in patients undergoing Ivor Lewis esophagogastrectomy. *Ann Surg* 2000; **231**: 635–643.
9. Zafirellis KD, Fountoulakis A, Dolan K, Dexter SP, Martin IG, Sue-Ling HM. Evaluation of POSSUM in patients with oesophageal cancer undergoing resection. *Br J Surg* 2002; **89**: 1150–1155.
10. Onodera T, Goseki N, Kosaki G. Prognostic nutritional index in gastrointestinal surgery of malnourished cancer patients. *Nippon Geka Gakkai Zasshi* 1984; **85**: 1001–1005.
11. Nozoe T, Kimura Y, Ishida M, Saeki H, Korenaga D, Sugimachi K. Correlation of pre-operative nutritional condition with post-operative complications in surgical treatment for oesophageal carcinoma. *Eur J Surg Oncol* 2002; **28**: 396–400.
12. Doty JR, Salazar JD, Forastiere AA, Heath EI, Kleinberg L, Heitmiller RF. Postesophagectomy morbidity, mortality, and length of hospital stay after preoperative chemoradiation therapy. *Ann Thorac Surg* 2002; **74**: 227–231.
13. Takagi K, Yamamori H, Morishima Y, Toyoda Y, Nakajima N, Tashiro T. Preoperative immunosuppression: its relationship with high morbidity and mortality in patients receiving thoracic esophagectomy. *Nutrition* 2001; **17**: 13–17.
14. Aiko S, Yoshizumi Y, Sugiura Y *et al*. Beneficial effects of immediate enteral nutrition after esophageal cancer surgery. *Surg Today* 2001; **31**: 971–978.
15. Langley SM, Alexiou C, Bailey DH, Weeden DF. The influence of perioperative blood transfusion on survival after esophageal resection for carcinoma. *Ann Thorac Surg* 2002; **73**: 1704–1709.
16. Orringer MB, Marshall B, Iannettoni MD. Transhiatal esophagectomy for treatment of benign and malignant esophageal disease. *World J Surg* 2001; **25**: 196–203.
17. Van Sandick JW, Van Lanschot JJ, ten Kate FJ, Tijssen JG, Obertop H. Indicators of prognosis after transhiatal esophageal resection without thoracotomy for cancer. *J Am Coll Surg* 2002; **194**: 28–36.
18. Kyriazanos ID, Tachibana M, Yoshimura H, Kinugasa S, Dhar DK, Nagasue N. Impact of splenectomy on the early outcome after oesophagectomy for squamous cell carcinoma of the oesophagus. *Eur J Surg Oncol* 2002; **28**: 113–119.
19. Kusano C, Baba M, Takao S *et al*. Oxygen delivery as a factor in the development of fatal postoperative complications after oesophagectomy. *Br J Surg* 1997; **84**: 252–257.
20. Hagen JA, DeMeester SR, Peters JH, Chandrasoma P, DeMeester TR. Curative resection for esophageal adenocarcinoma: analysis of 100 *en bloc* esophagectomies. *Ann Surg* 2001; **234**: 520–530.
21. Altorki N, Skinner D. Should *en bloc* esophagectomy be the standard of care for esophageal carcinoma? *Ann Surg* 2001; **234**: 581–587.
22. Griffin SM, Shaw IH, Dresner SM. Early complications after Ivor Lewis subtotal esophagectomy with two-field lymphadenectomy: risk factors and management. *J Am Coll Surg* 2002; **194**: 285–297.

23. Ferguson MK, Martin TR, Reeder LB, Olak J. Mortality after esophagectomy: risk factor analysis. *World J Surg* 1997; **21**: 599–603.

24. Avendano CE, Flume PA, Silvestri GA, King LB, Reed CE. Pulmonary complications after esophagectomy. *Ann Thorac Surg* 2002; **73**: 922–926.

25. Tsukada K, Hasegawa T, Miyazaki T *et al.* Predictive value of interleukin-8 and granulocyte elastase in pulmonary complication after esophagectomy. *Am J Surg* 2001; **181**: 167–171.

26. Hulscher JB, Van Sandick JW, de Boer AG *et al.* Extended transthoracic resection compared with limited transhiatal resection for adenocarcinoma of the esophagus. *N Engl J Med* 2002; **347**: 1662–1669.

27. Maruyama K, Kitamura M, Izumi K *et al.* Postoperative lung volume calculated by chest computed tomography in patients with esophageal cancer. *Jpn J Thorac Cardiovasc Surg* 1999; 47: 193–198.

28. Watson A, Allen PR. Influence of thoracic epidural analgesia on outcome after resection for esophageal cancer. *Surgery* 1994; **115**: 429–432.

29. Tsui SL, Law S, Fok M *et al.* Postoperative analgesia reduces mortality and morbidity after esophagectomy. *Am J Surg* 1997; **173**: 472–478.

30. Kita T, Mammoto T, Kishi Y. Fluid management and postoperative respiratory disturbances in patients with transthoracic esophagectomy for carcinoma. *J Clin Anesth* 2002; **14**: 252–256.

31. Sasako M, Katai H, Sano T, Maruyama K. Management of complications after gastrectomy with extended lymphadenectomy. *Surg Oncol* 2000; **9**: 31–34.

32. Sugimachi K, Ueo H, Natsuda Y, Kai H, Inokuchi K, Zaitsu A. Cough dynamics in oesophageal cancer: prevention of postoperative pulmonary complications. *Br J Surg* 1982; **69**: 734–736.

33. Gillinov AM, Heitmiller RF. Strategies to reduce pulmonary complications after transhiatal esophagectomy. *Dis Esophagus* 1998; **11**: 43–47.

34. Hulscher JB, Van Sandick JW, Devriese PP, Van Lanschot JJ, Obertop H. Vocal cord paralysis after subtotal oesophagectomy. *Br J Surg* 1999; **86**: 1583–1587.

35. Nagawa H, Kobori O, Muto T. Prediction of pulmonary complications after transthoracic oesophagectomy. *Br J Surg* 1994; **81**: 860–862.

36. Watanabe I, Fujihara H, Sato K *et al.* Beneficial effect of a prone position for patients with hypoxemia after transthoracic esophagectomy. *Crit Care Med* 2002; **30**: 1799–1802.

37. Law S, Fok M, Chu KM, Wong J. Comparison of hand-sewn and stapled esophagogastric anastomosis after esophageal resection for cancer: a prospective randomized controlled trial. *Ann Surg* 1997; **226**: 169–173.

38. Lau H, Law S, Wong J. Prospective evaluation of vacuum pleural drainage after thoracotomy in patients with esophageal carcinoma. *Arch Surg* 1997; **132**: 749–752.

39. Amar D, Burt ME, Bains MS, Leung DH. Symptomatic tachydysrhythmias after esophagectomy: incidence and outcome measures. *Ann Thorac Surg* 1996; **61**: 1506–1509.

40. Ritchie AJ, Whiteside M, Tolan M, McGuigan JA. Cardiac dysrhythmia in total thoracic oesophagectomy. A prospective study. *Eur J Cardiothorac Surg* 1993; **7**: 420–422.

41. Sauvanet A, Baltar J, Le Mee J, Belghiti J. Diagnosis and conservative management of intrathoracic leakage after oesophagectomy. *Br J Surg* 1998; **85**: 1446–1449.

42. Griffin SM, Lamb PJ, Dresner SM, Richardson DL, Hayes N. Diagnosis and management of a mediastinal leak following radical oesophagectomy. *Br J Surg.* 2001; **88**: 1346–1351.

43. Whooley BP, Law S, Alexandrou A, Murthy SC, Wong J. Critical appraisal of the significance of intrathoracic anastomotic leakage after esophagectomy for cancer. *Am J Surg* 2001; **181**: 198–203.

44. Boyle NH, Pearce A, Hunter D, Owen WJ, Mason RC. Intraoperative scanning laser Doppler flowmetry in the assessment of gastric tube perfusion during esophageal resection. *J Am Coll Surg* 1999; **188**: 498–502.

45. Pierie JP, de Graaf PW, Poen H, Van Der Tweel I, Obertop H. Impaired healing of cervical oesophagogastrostomies can be predicted by estimation of gastric serosal blood perfusion by laser Doppler flowmetry. *Eur J Surg* 1994; **160**: 599–603.

46. Jacobi CA, Zieren HU, Zieren J, Muller JM. Is tissue oxygen tension during esophagectomy a predictor of esophagogastric anastomotic healing? *J Surg Res* 1998; **74**: 161–164.

47. Heitmiller RF, Fischer A, Liddicoat JR. Cervical esophagogastric anastomosis: results following esophagectomy for carcinoma. *Dis Esophagus* 1999; **12**: 264–269.

48. Blewett CJ, Miller JD, Young JE, Bennett WF, Urschel JD. Anastomotic leaks after esophagectomy for esophageal cancer: a comparison of thoracic and cervical anastomoses. *Ann Thorac Cardiovasc Surg* 2001; **7**: 75–78.

49. Choi HK, Law S, Chu KM, Wong J. The value of neck drain in esophageal surgery: a randomized trial. *Dis Esophagus* 1998; **11**: 40–42.

50. Tanomkiat W, Galassi W. Barium sulfate as contrast medium for evaluation of postoperative anastomotic leaks. *Acta Radiol* 2000; **41**: 482–485.

51. Trentino P, Pompeo E, Nofroni I *et al*. Predictive value of early postoperative esophagoscopy for occurrence of benign stenosis after cervical esophagogastrostomy. *Endoscopy* 1997; **29**: 840–844.

52. Machens A, Busch C, Bause H, Izbicki JR. Gastric tonometry and drain amylase analysis in the detection of cervical oesophagogastric leakage. *Br J Surg* 1996; **83**: 1614–1615.

53. Lerut T, Coosemans W, Decker G, De Leyn P, Nafteux P, Van Raemdonck D. Anastomotic complications after esophagectomy. *Dig Surg* 2002; **19**: 92–98.

54. Griffin SM, Lamb PJ, Dresner SM, Richardson DL, Hayes N. Diagnosis and management of a mediastinal leak following radical oesophagectomy. *Br J Surg*. 2001; **88**: 1346–1351.

55. Kun L, Yun-Jie W, Qing-Shu C, Dao-Xi W, Zhen-Yuan Z. Emergency re-operation for postoperative hemorrhage following partial esophagectomy for carcinoma of the esophagus and cardia of the stomach. *Dis Esophagus* 2001; **14**: 251–253.

56. Orringer MB, Bluett M, Deeb GM. Aggressive treatment of chylothorax complicating transhiatal esophagectomy without thoracotomy. *Surgery* 1988; **104**: 720–726.

57. Dugue L, Sauvanet A, Farges O, Goharin A, Le Mee J, Belghiti J. Output of chyle as an indicator of treatment for chylothorax complicating oesophagectomy. *Br J Surg* 1998; **85**: 1147–1149.

58. Cope C, Kaiser LR. Management of unremitting chylothorax by percutaneous embolization and blockage of retroperitoneal lymphatic vessels in 42 patients. *J Vasc Interv Radiol* 2002; **13**: 1139–1148.

59. Alexiou C, Watson M, Beggs D, Salama FD, Morgan WE. Chylothorax following oesophagogastrectomy for malignant disease. *Eur J Cardiothorac Surg* 1998; **14**: 460–466.

60. Bolger C, Walsh TN, Tanner WA, Keeling P, Hennessy TP. Chylothorax after oesophagectomy. *Br J Surg* 1991; **78**: 587–588.

61. Fahimi H, Casselman FP, Mariani MA, van Boven WJ, Knaepen PJ, van Swieten HA. Current management of postoperative chylothorax. *Ann Thorac Surg* 2001; **71**: 448–450.

62. Guillem P, Billeret V, Houcke ML, Triboulet JP. Successful management of post-esophagectomy chylothorax/chyloperitoneum by etilefrine. *Dis Esophagus* 1999; **12**: 155–156.

63. Baba M, Aikou T, Natsugoe S *et al*. Quality of life following esophagectomy with three-field lymphadenectomy for carcinoma, focusing on its relationship to vocal cord palsy. *Dis Esophagus* 1998; **11**: 28–34.

64. Lewin JS, Hebert TM, Putnam Jr JB, DuBrow RA. Experience with the chin tuck maneuver in postesophagectomy aspirators. *Dysphagia* 2001; **16**: 216–219.

65. Hulscher JB, ter Hofstede E, Kloek J, Obertop H, De Haan P, Van Lanschot JJ. Injury to the major airways during subtotal esophagectomy: incidence, management, and sequelae. *J Thorac Cardiovasc Surg* 2000; **120**: 1093–1096.

66. Bartels HE, Stein HJ, Siewert JR. Tracheobronchial lesions following oesophagectomy: prevalence, predisposing factors and outcome. *Br J Surg* 1998; **85**: 403–406.

67. Buskens CJ, Hulscher JB, Fockens P, Obertop H, Van Lanschot JJ. Benign tracheo-neo-esophageal fistulas after subtotal esophagectomy. *Ann Thorac Surg* 2001; **72**: 221–224.

68. Law S, Cheung MC, Fok M, Chu KM, Wong J. Pyloroplasty and pyloromyotomy in gastric replacement of the esophagus after esophagectomy: a randomized controlled trial. *J Am Coll Surg* 1997; **184**: 630–636.

69. Van Sandick JW, Knegjens JL, Van Lanschot JJ, Obertop H. Diaphragmatic herniation following oesophagectomy. *Br J Surg* 1999; **86**: 109–112.

70. Frank A, Montgomery RC, LeVoyer TE, Goldberg M. Pleural incarceration of the gastric graft after trans-hiatal esophagectomy. *Ann Thorac Surg* 1999; **68**: 250–252.

71. Pierre AF, Luketich JD. Technique and role of minimally invasive esophagectomy for premalignant and malignant diseases of the esophagus. *Surg Oncol Clin North Am* 2002; **11**: 337–350.

Timothy A. Rockall

6

Endoscopic treatment of bleeding duodenal ulcers and assessment of risk

ENDOSCOPIC TREATMENT

The application of endoscopic therapy to bleeding duodenal ulcers is now an accepted and widely practised form of therapy. The aim of such therapy is to arrest haemorrhage and prevent re-bleeding with the ultimate purpose of reducing transfusion requirements, operative intervention rate, morbidity, and mortality.

Endoscopic therapy is effective in a number of situations. For oesophageal varices, banding has superseded injection sclerotherapy as the treatment of choice. Peptic ulcers with major stigmata of recent haemorrhage should all be treated and, where adherent clot is present, this should be removed by washing and the underlying lesion treated as appropriate. The importance of washing the ulcer base has been a source of controversy in the past, but a recent study randomising patients with adherent clot to injection therapy, removal of clot and coagulation plus standard medical therapy or standard medical therapy alone revealed a significant reduction in re-bleeding from 34% to 4.8% with endoscopic treatment.[1] Other more rare lesions are also amenable to endoscopic haemostatic therapy including vascular lesions, Dieulafoy lesions and Mallory-Weiss tears. Thermal methods are often recommended in these cases.

Key point 1

- Many endoscopic haemostatic therapies are effective in reducing re-bleeding.

Mr Timothy A. Rockall MD FRCS, Senior Lecturer/Honorary Consultant, Department of Surgical Oncology and Technology, Division of Surgery Anaesthetics and Intensive Care, Faculty of Medicine, Imperial College of Science, Technology and Medicine, 10th floor QEQM, St Mary's Hospital, Praed Street, London W2 1NY, UK

Endoscopic therapy has been in clinical practice for many years and a large number of different modalities, both alone and in combination, have been studied. These broadly take the form of injecting substances, applying thermal energy and mechanical haemostatic devices.

INJECTION

A number of substances have been studied including adrenaline and a variety of sclerosing agents such as Polidocanol, ethanolamine and absolute alcohol. The British Society of Gastroenterology guidelines[2] recommend dilute adrenaline as the substance of choice because of the lack of added benefit from using a sclerosant and the small, but potentially serious, complication of sclerosant-associated necrosis and perforation of the bowel wall. Adrenaline injection in sufficient volume provides an initial tamponade which, together with the arterial constriction, leads to a physiological thrombosis of the vessel. It has been suggested that the main effect is one of tamponade and that normal saline injection is equally effective, although a recent study showed normal saline injection to be less effective than bipolar electrocoagulation.[3] The volume of adrenaline used has been the subject of another recent study which concluded a larger volume (average 16.5 ml *versus* 8.0 ml) significantly reduced the re-bleeding rate from 30.8% to 15.4%.[4]

Fibrin glue and thrombin are both more expensive and more difficult to use, but are effective in inducing thrombosis in the vessel and preventing re-bleeding. A large randomised trial of 854 cases has compared the safety and efficacy of repeated fibrin glue injection with that of a single injection of fibrin glue or a single injection of Polidocanol.[5] All patients were pretreated with an injection of 1:10,000 adrenaline. Repeated injection with fibrin glue had a significantly reduced overall failure rate (7.7%) compared to a single injection of Polidocanol (13%) or single injection of fibrin glue (12.4%). In patients with Forrest type Ia lesions (spurting haemorrhage), repeated fibrin glue injection reduced the re-bleeding rate from 42% in the other two groups to 15%. Additionally, the study confirmed the safety of fibrin glue with no episodes of necrosis or perforation compared to three such cases in the Polidocanol group. Other smaller studies, however, have not demonstrated that a single injection of fibrin glue is any more effective than adrenaline alone,[6] whilst others have shown a significant reduction in re-bleeding with fibrin glue compared to adrenaline but no improvement in other outcomes including mortality.[7] The key to reducing re-bleeding may be repeated endoscopic treatments which has also been demonstrated in studies of other modalities.[8]

THERMAL TECHNIQUES

Thermal energy is applied to a bleeding vessel with the purpose of coagulating the vessel. A heater probe consists of a Teflon-coated catheter that is heated with a pre-set amount of energy. The ulcer base is cleaned with a water jet and the probe is placed in contact with the bleeding point providing both immediate tamponade and thermal coagulation.

By contrast, bipolar diathermy utilises electrocoagulation to apply thermal energy. Nd:YAG laser and argon plasma coagulators are both non-contact methods of delivering thermal energy. All these methods seem to be equally efficacious in reducing re-bleeding. There is some evidence that combining heater probe treatment with injection therapy is more efficacious than injection alone for the actively bleeding vessel.[9]

MECHANICAL METHODS

Some recent advances have been made in the development of physical haemostatic methods that might be more effective especially for the larger bleeding vessels that would traditionally require surgery or angiographic embolisation. Vessel size in patients studied at post mortem following upper gastrointestinal haemorrhage range up to 3.2 mm in diameter, beyond the ability of injection and thermal methods to achieve haemostasis. Hemoclips are not new,[10] but have recently received further attention. Hemoclips (Olympus) are endoscopically placed titanium clips that are located directly on the bleeding vessel. They are shed into the lumen of the bowel a few days later. There is no doubt that they can be effective, but there are problems associated with their application that limits their use and it can be technically challenging to place the clips appropriately. A randomised, control trial involving 124 patients with visible vessels allocated patients to injection with hypertonic saline and adrenaline, or to Hemoclip, or to a combination arm. Re-bleeding was lowest (2.3%) in the Hemoclip group with combined therapy offering no advantage.[11]

Key point 2

- Hemoclips may play an important role in the management of larger vessels and those with active arterial bleeding. Their use is currently limited by technical difficulties and by availability.

Key point 3

- Repeated therapy with fibrin glue or with the heater probe may also reduce re-bleeding in high-risk lesions.

A trial of 113 cases randomised to heater probe or Hemoclip application revealed a significant reduction in re-bleeding from 21% to 1.8%.[12] By contrast, another recent study randomising 101 patients to injection therapy or Hemoclip revealed significantly higher initial and overall failure rate with both Hemoclip alone and Hemoclip combined with injection than with injection alone.[13]

ASSESSMENT OF RISK

Analysis of risk factors following acute upper gastrointestinal haemorrhage has been approached in a number of different ways. Most studies have concentrated on mortality as an outcome measure but, with the advent of endoscopic therapies, re-bleeding scores have been developed with a view to assessing the impact of treatment. More recently, a scoring system has been developed that assesses the risk of need for treatment rather than predicting outcome, on the basis that treatment conferred is likely to alter outcome.

RISK OF FURTHER HAEMORRHAGE

Further haemorrhage, comprising both continued bleeding and re-bleeding, has an established association with poor outcome and is predominantly predicted on the basis of endoscopic findings including the diagnosis and the presence of stigmata of recent haemorrhage. Forrest *et al.*[14] described endoscopic criteria in the 1970s and they are still widely quoted today. In peptic ulcer disease, the characteristics of the ulcer base are clearly related to risk of further haemorrhage which, in the absence of treatment, may be up to 90% with active spurting arterial haemorrhage (Forrest Ia). The identification of Forrest criteria is important as it selects out suitable lesions for endoscopic therapy (Forrest Ia, Ib, IIa, IIb). These stigmata of recent haemorrhage are not the only predictive factors, however, and less lesion-specific criteria also independently predict the likelihood of further haemorrhage. Several attempts have been made to combine the endoscopic characteristics with other clinical factors to determine risk of re-bleeding. An example of this is the Baylor score.[15] It combines the endoscopic criteria with age and co-morbidity to give a simple integer score that predicts the likelihood of further haemorrhage.

Factors associated with failure of endoscopic therapy have been identified in a recent prospective study of 427 cases receiving adrenaline injection therapy. The re-bleeding rate was 20.1% and significant factors associated with this were presence of shock at presentation, ulcer size, posterior duodenal position, type Ia stigmata of recent haemorrhage, chronic ulcers and stomal ulcers.[16]

RISK OF REQUIRING INTERVENTION

A risk score has been developed to predict the need for treatment based on the premise that clinical treatment aims to prevent the adverse outcomes of further haemorrhage and death and so it logical to develop a score that can predict the need for such treatment rather than the likelihood of a poor outcome. A large Scottish study analysed 1748 cases and subsequently validated their score in a further 197 cases. The risk was calculated on the basis of admission haemoglobin, blood urea, pulse, systolic blood pressure, as well as presentation with syncope or melaena and evidence of hepatic disease or cardiac failure (Table 1). The authors also developed a fast-track screening tool

---

Key point 4
- Validated risk scoring systems for the prediction of need for treatment and for adverse outcomes exist and are suitable for use in the clinical setting.

Table 1 Admission risk markers and associated score component values for prediction of need for treatment

	Admission risk marker	Score component value
Blood urea (mmol/l)		
	≥ 6.5 <8.0	2
	≥ 8.0 <10.0	3
	≥ 10.0 <25.0	4
	≥ 25.0	6
Haemoglobin (g/l) for men		
	≥ 120 <130	1
	≥ 100 <120	3
	< 100	6
Haemoglobin (g/l) for women		
	≥ 100 <120	1
	< 100	6
Systolic blood pressure (mmHg)		
	100–109	1
	90–99	2
	< 90	3
Other markers		
	Pulse ≥ 100 beats/min	1
	Presentation with melaena	1
	Presentation with syncope	2
	Hepatic disease	2
	Cardiac failure	2

and concluded that if, at presentation, the blood urea was less than 6.5 mmol/l, the haemoglobin was greater than 13 g/dl (men) or 12 g/dl (women), the systolic blood pressure was greater than 110 mmHg and the pulse less than 100 beats/min, the patients were at low risk of requiring surgical intervention. This abbreviated score (without endoscopic information) identified 99% of serious bleeds that required treatment and 32% of the minor bleeds that did not require treatment. Therefore, it has poor specificity for the identification of patients not requiring intervention. Although internally validated, this system has yet to be externally validated.

RISK OF DEATH

Further haemorrhage has an established association with increased mortality, but the relationship between these factors is not direct. Death following an upper gastrointestinal haemorrhage, more so than re-bleeding, is multifactorial and is certainly not restricted to factors that reflect the magnitude of the initial bleed or further haemorrhage. A relatively small acute bleed in an elderly patient with severe co-morbidity may be a more serious event in terms of eventual outcome than a much larger bleed in a fit, young patient. This is supported by data that reveal that mortality from upper gastrointestinal haemorrhage, regardless of severity, under the age of 60 years and in the absence of major co-morbidity is of the order of 0.1%.[17]

Table 2 Risk score for mortality

Variable	Score			
	0	1	2	3
Age	< 60 years	60–79 years	≥ 80 years	
Shock	'No shock' Systolic BP ≥ 100 Pulse < 100	'Tachycardia' Systolic BP ≥ 100 Pulse ≥ 100	'Hypotension' Systolic BP < 100	
Co-morbidity	No major co-morbidity		Cardiac failure Ischaemic heart disease Any major co-morbidity	Renal failure Liver failure Disseminated malignancy
Diagnosis	Mallory-Weiss tear	All other diagnoses	Malignancy of upper GI tract	No lesion identified & no SRH
Major stigmata of recent haemorrhage	None or dark spot only	Blood in upper GI tract	Adherent clot Visible or spurting vessel	

Many attempts have been made to categorise these variables to give some sense of the relative contribution and to confirm the independent predictive nature of each factor. Some of these analyses have resulted in the development of scoring systems, but many have been derived from small datasets and have not been validated. The score based on the largest population-based datasets and the one that has been most extensively validated was derived from data collected during

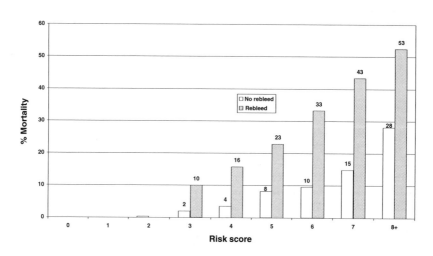

Fig. 1 Mortality by risk score.

the UK National Audit of Acute Upper Gastrointestinal Haemorrhage.[18] An initial analysis of 4185 cases using logistical regression analysis determined independently significant risk factors. A simple integer score was then devised with reference to the co-efficients in the analysis (Table 2). A pre-endoscopy score based purely upon clinical factors of age, co-morbidity and shock gives a score of 0–7 with a step-wise increase in mortality. A post-endoscopy score includes the further endoscopic criteria of diagnosis and stigmata of recent haemorrhage and gives a total score of 0–11 (Fig. 1). Once again, this reveals a step-wise increase in mortality with zero mortality when the score is two or less. Re-bleeding results in a 2–5-fold increase in mortality depending on the initial risk category. This scoring system has been validated in a number of ways including in a second population of 1621 cases. Subsequently, others have further validated the model in independent populations and in a variety of sub-groups.[19–22] Scoring systems of this nature have a number of potential uses including prognostication, comparative audit, and case selection for studies and treatment. One area that has received some attention recently is the use of such systems to identify patients of very low risk in whom out-patient treatment or limited admission can be safely carried out with the potential for resource savings.[23]

Key points for clinical practice

- Many endoscopic haemostatic therapies are effective in reducing re-bleeding.

- Hemoclips may play an important role in the management of larger vessels and those with active arterial bleeding. Their use is currently limited by technical difficulties and by availability.

- Repeated therapy with fibrin glue or with the heater probe may also reduce re-bleeding in high-risk lesions.

- Validated risk scoring systems for the prediction of need for treatment and for adverse outcomes exist and are suitable for use in the clinical setting.

References

1. Bleau BL, Gostout CJ, Sherman KE *et al.* Recurrent bleeding from peptic ulcer associated with adherent clot: a randomized study comparing endoscopic treatment with medical therapy. *Gastrointest Endosc* 2002; **56**: 1–6.
2. British Society of Gastroenterology. Non-variceal upper gastrointestinal haemorrhage: guidelines. *Gut* 2002; **51 (Suppl IV)**: iv1–iv6.
3. Laine L, Estrada R. Randomized trial of normal saline solution injection versus bipolar electrocoagulation for treatment of patients with high-risk bleeding ulcers: is local tamponade enough? *Gastrointest Endosc* 2002; **55**: 6–10.
4. Lin HJ, Hsieh YH, Tseng GY, Perng CL, Chang FY, Lee SD. A prospective, randomized trial of large- *versus* small-volume endoscopic injection of epinephrine for peptic ulcer bleeding. *Gastrointest Endosc* 2002; **55**: 615–619.

5. Rutgeerts P, Rauws E, Wara P et al. Randomised trial of single and repeated fibrin glue compared with injection of Polidocanol in treatment of bleeding peptic ulcer. *Lancet* 1997; **350**: 692–696.

6. Pescatore P, Jornod P, Borovicka J et al. Epinephrine *versus* epinephrine plus fibrin glue injection in peptic ulcer bleeding: a prospective randomized trial. *Gastrointest Endosc* 2002; **55**: 348–353.

7. Lin HJ, Hsieh YH, Tseng GY, Perng CL, Chang FY, Lee SD. Endoscopic injection with fibrin sealant *versus* epinephrine for arrest of peptic ulcer bleeding: a randomized, comparative trial. *J Clin Gastroenterol* 2002; **35**: 218–221.

8. Saeed ZA, Cole RA, Ramirez FC, Schneider FE, Hepps KS, Graham DY. Endoscopic re-treatment after successful initial hemostasis prevents ulcer rebleeding: a prospective randomized trial. *Endoscopy* 1996; **28**: 288–294.

9. Chung SCS, Lau JY, Sung JL. Randomised comparison between adrenaline injection alone and adrenaline injection plus heat probe treatment for actively bleeding peptic ulcers. *BMJ* 1997; **314**: 1307–1311.

10. Binmoeller KF, Thonke T, Soehendra N. Endoscopic Hemoclip treatment for gastrointestinal haemorrhage. *Endoscopy* 1993; **25**: 167–170.

11. Chung IK, Ham JS, Kim HS, Park SH, Lee MH, Kim SJ. Comparison of the haemostatic efficacy of the endoscopic Hemoclip method with hypertonic saline-epinephrine injection and a combination of the two for the management of bleeding peptic ulcer. *Gastrointest Endosc* 1999; **49**: 13–18.

12. Cipolletta L, Bianco MA, Marmo R. Endoclips versus heater probe in preventing early recurrent bleeding from peptic ulcer: a prospective and randomised trial. *Gastrointest Endosc* 2001; **53**: 147–151.

13. Gevers AM, De Goede E, Simoens M, Hiele M, Rutgeerts P. A randomized trial comparing injection therapy with Hemoclip and with injection combined with Hemoclip for bleeding ulcers. *Gastrointest Endosc* 2002; **55**: 466–469.

14. Forrest JAH, Finlayson NDC, Shearman DJC. Endoscopy in gastrointestinal bleeding. *Lancet* 1974; **2**: 394–397.

15. Saeed ZA, Ramirez FC, Hepps KS, Cole RA, Graham DY. Prospective validation of the Baylor bleeding score for predicting the likelihood of rebleeding after endoscopic hemostasis of peptic ulcers. *Gastrointest Endosc* 1995; **41**: 561–565.

16. Thomopoulos KC, Mitropoulos JA, Katsakoulis EC et al. Factors associated with failure of endoscopic injection haemostasis in bleeding peptic ulcers. *Scand J Gastroenterol* 2001; **36**: 664–668.

17. Rockall TA, Logan RF, Devlin HB, Northfield TC. Incidence of and mortality from acute upper gastrointestinal haemorrhage in the United Kingdom. Steering Committee and Members of the National Audit of Acute Upper Gastrointestinal Haemorrhage [see comments]. *BMJ* 1995; **311**: 222–226.

18. Rockall TA, Logan RF, Devlin HB, Northfield TC. Risk assessment after acute upper gastrointestinal haemorrhage [see comments]. *Gut* 1996; **38**: 316–321.

19. Vreeburg EM, Terwee CB, Snel P et al. Validation of the Rockall risk scoring system in upper gastrointestinal bleeding. *Gut* 1999; **44**: 331–335.

20. Sanders DS, Carter MJ, Goodchap RJ, Cross SS, Gleeson DC, Lobo AJ. Prospective validation of the Rockall risk scoring system for upper GI hemorrhage in subgroups of patients with varices and peptic ulcers. *Am J Gastroenterol* 2002; **97**: 630–635.

21. Ch'ng CL, Kingham JG. Scoring systems and risk assessment for upper gastrointestinal bleeding. *Eur J Gastroenterol Hepatol* 2001; **13**: 1137–1139.

22. Church NI, Palmer KR. Relevance of the Rockall score in patients undergoing endoscopic therapy for peptic ulcer haemorrhage. *Eur J Gastroenterol Hepatol* 2001; **13**: 1149–1152.

23. Rockall TA, Logan RF, Devlin HB, Northfield TC. Selection of patients for early discharge or outpatient care after acute upper gastrointestinal haemorrhage. National Audit of Acute Upper Gastrointestinal Haemorrhage [see comments]. *Lancet* 1996; **347**: 1138–1140.

Brendan J. Moran

7

Management of pseudomyxoma peritonei

Pseudomyxoma peritonei is a disease characterized by copious production of mucinous ascites that, over time, fills the peritoneal cavity. Pseudomyxoma peritonei (PMP) is a rare condition, with a reported incidence of approximately one per million per year, and classically presents at laparotomy with 'jelly belly'.[1] Increasingly, the diagnosis is made prior to laparotomy, by awareness of the condition, advances in cross-sectional imaging and percutaneous biopsy techniques.

In 1884, Werth[2] coined the term 'pseudomyxoma peritonei' when he described the condition in association with a mucinous carcinoma of the ovary. In 1901, Frankel[3] described a case of pseudomyxoma peritonei in association with a cyst of the appendix. Ever since, controversy has continued as to the aetiology of PMP, particularly in women.

Synchronous disease is found in the ovary and appendix in most females with PMP and the disease is reported to be more prevalent in females.[4]

The available scientific and clinical evidence suggests that the appendix is the most likely primary. Ronnett *et al.*[5] used immunohistochemistry to identify the origin of PMP in females. In a total of 13 cases of PMP, appendiceal mucinous adenomas and ovarian tumours from the same patients were stained. They concluded that most ovarian tumours in PMP are immunophenotypically identical to the associated appendiceal tumours and distinct from mucinous ovarian tumours. Young *et al.*[6] and Prayson *et al.*[7] came to similar conclusions in 22 and 17 cases, respectively. However, Chuaqui *et al.*[8] concluded that the ovarian disease represented second primaries.

From a clinical viewpoint, if the appendix theory of origin were correct, sex distribution should be similar as it would be reasonable to speculate that there is unlikely to be huge differences in the pathological behaviour of the appendix in females as compared to males. An analysis of the male/female distribution of 4

Mr Brendan J. Moran MCh FRCSI(Gen) FRCS, Consultant Surgeon, Director NSCAG Pseudomyxoma Peritonei Centre, The North Hampshire Hospital, Aldermaston Road, Basingstoke RG24 9NA, Hampshire, UK

Key point 1

- Pseudomyxoma peritonei (PMP) is a rare disease usually arising from a tumour of the appendix and presents as 'jelly belly'. Mucinous adenocarcinoma from any condition can simulate PMP clinically, radiologically, and at operation.

---

reported case series[9–12] suggests a similar incidence in men. In 393 cases treated, 182/393 (46%) were males.

In addition to the association of PMP with appendiceal and ovarian tumours, there are case reports suggesting occasional origin from other intra-abdominal organs such as the colon and rectum,[13] stomach,[14] gallbladder and bile ducts,[15] small intestine and urinary bladder,[13] lung,[16] breast,[17] fallopian tube,[18] and pancreas.[19] With the exception of colorectal mucinous adeno-carcinoma, which often simulates PMP, these are rare and only account for less than 5% of the total cases.

A similar clinical, radiological and surgical presentation to PMP can be seen in mucinous adenocarcinoma of any origin, particularly from the colon and from the ovaries in females. This may account for the perception that PMP is commoner in females.

Whilst PMP is most commonly applied to a slowly progressive disease process, most clinicians, including oncologists and pathologists, apply the term to any condition that leads to extensive mucus accumulation within the abdomen and pelvis, thus incorporating a spectrum of disease varying from a mucinous cystadenoma of the appendix to a mucinous adenocarcinoma, arising anywhere within the abdominal cavity. The difficulty in accurately defining PMP, together with the historical lumping together of tumours of various sites with significant biological behaviours, has resulted in on-going confusion in many aspects of optimal management of PMP.

Sugarbaker and colleagues[20] have tried to clarify the uncertainty by defining that *'the term pseudomyxoma peritonei syndrome be strictly applied to a pathologically and prognostically homogenous group of cases characterised by histologically benign peritoneal tumours that are frequently associated with an appendiceal mucinous adenoma'*. Cases of peritoneal carcinomatosis, regardless of the presence of abundant extracellular mucus production, are excluded from this precise definition of PMP.

Although PMP is not considered biologically aggressive, as it does not invade or metastasise, the disease is nevertheless invariably fatal as the space required within the abdomen for nutritional function is eventually replaced by

---

Key point 2

- There is a spectrum of disease varying from 'borderline malignant' adenomucinosis to mucinous adenocarcinoma. The behaviour and prognosis vary depending on the nature of the cells producing mucin.

---

mucinous tumour, resulting in death unless the disease is definitively treated. The median survival with PMP is approximately 6 years, with 5-year survival ranging from 53–75%.[4]

Unfortunately, there is currently no experimental animal model to help to elucidate the origin, natural history and management aspects of PMP. Furthermore, the current trend towards evidence-based medicine with a particular emphasis on randomised trials is devoid of hard evidence in PMP. This is not surprising given the rarity and heterogeneity of the condition.[21]

CLINICAL PRESENTATION

The clinical presentation of PMP is variable due to few reports of any quantity. A recent publication by Esquivel and Sugarbaker[11] is the most enlightening. In a series of 410 patients with appendiceal tumours, 217 had the diagnosis of PMP with histological confirmation. Overall, 27% presented with suspected acute appendicitis, 23% presented with increasing abdominal distension, and 14% a new onset hernia, the majority being inguinal.

In women, a diagnosis of PMP was most commonly made while being evaluated, or treated, for an ovarian mass (39% of women).

Whilst these are the common presentations, the majority of patients are diagnosed at, or after, a laparotomy performed for either suspected appendicitis or peritonitis, or at surgery for suspected gynaecological cancer in women.

The increasing availability of reliable cross-sectional imaging has resulted in an increasing number in which the diagnosis is suspected at imaging alone, particularly based on the classical features on CT.[22] Image-guided percutaneous biopsies may be useful, though the relatively acellular material is often difficult to diagnose with certainty. Commonly, tumour markers are measured and, based on the CA-125 in women and the CEA levels in either sex, many patients are erroneously diagnosed as advanced ovarian cancer or advanced metastatic intestinal adenocarcinoma.

Upper and lower gastrointestinal tract investigations, when performed, are normal and the diagnosis of PMP comes to light, in time, due to the longer than expected survival and the findings, often at repeat laparotomy of mucinous ascites. Due to the rarity of the condition, few clinicians, even gynaecologists and abdominal surgeons, will encounter more than a handful of cases during a clinical career. A delay in diagnosis is common and many patients are labelled as irritable bowel syndrome for a number of years prior to definitive diagnosis.

PATHOLOGICAL FEATURES AND TUMOUR BEHAVIOUR

In PMP, the mucus is the predominant factor and contains sparse cells, which are generally histologically categorized as having the features of low grade adenocarcinoma. Invasion and lymph node metastases are invariably absent. This has led to the misconception that the condition is 'benign' and can be safely, and adequately, treated by evacuation of the mucus in the form of debulking, on a repeated basis as necessary. Repeated debulking is increasingly dangerous due to the difficulty in avoiding bowel injury in a debilitated patient with numerous adhesions.

A continuing problem is how to categorize patients at clinical presentation and how to plan appropriate management. As for many abdominal tumours, a surgical approach with complete tumour removal is likely to be optimal and much recent work has emanated from Sugarbaker's group on the details of a radical surgical approach to PMP.

By analysing the detailed pathology and outcomes in a series of patients with abdominal mucinous tumours presenting as pseudomyxoma peritonei, who had undergone complete tumour removal, Ronnett and colleagues[23] have retrospectively categorized the tumours into three broad categories: (i) adenomucinosis; (ii) a hybrid group; and (iii) mucinous adenocarcinoma.

The prognosis, with regard to recurrence and survival, was heavily dependent on the histological type, with the favourable patients with adenomucinosis having an approximately 80%, 10-year survival.

In the author's opinion, there is a spectrum of disease ranging from adenomucinosis to adenocarcinoma, and it is often impossible to categorize the majority of patients with 'PMP-like conditions' into distinct categories prior to laparotomy. It is also conceivable that there may be an 'adenoma-carcinoma sequence' such that the tumour may at some stage undergo a malignant transformation to a more aggressive variant. This opinion is supported by a personal experience of over 100 operative cases, together with on-going follow-up.

From a clinical/pathological point of view, PMP should always be regarded as 'borderline malignant' in that tumour recurrence and progression is almost inevitable in the absence of definitive surgical treatment. Interestingly, lymphatic and haematogenous spread may not occur, even in the terminal stages of the disease. Lymph node or other metastases indicate mucinous adenocarcinoma rather than PMP *per se*, but most cases do not fit neatly into either of these two categories at the ends of the spectrum.

There are some features which may point towards disease type and aggressiveness: (i) time interval from first to subsequent presentation(s); (ii) general condition of the patient as more aggressive disease tends to result in more systemic symptoms, with muscle wasting, cachexia, *etc.*; (iii) clinical findings at examination with multiple solid lumps indicating aggressive disease; and (iv) markedly elevated tumour markers (CEA, CA-125 and CA-19-9).

PATHOPHYSIOLOGY OF DISEASE SPREAD BY THE 'REDISTRIBUTION PHENOMENON'

Current opinion regarding the pathophysiology of PMP suggests that PMP usually originates as an adenoma in the submucosa of the appendix. With progressive growth, the lumen of the appendix becomes occluded resulting in distension of the appendix by both mucus and mucinous tumour cells. The appendix eventually ruptures, often initially by a 'blow out' and then a slow leak of mucus-containing epithelial cells from the adenoma. In many cases, appendicular adenoma perforation is an occult event and not diagnosed clinically; the perforation may reseal, only to extrude more epithelial cells at a later date. Over the course of years, the primary lesion grows little in size, whereas the epithelial cells within the peritoneal cavity continue to proliferate and produce large quantities of mucus.

Most of the tumour cells in the peritoneal cavity are surrounded by mucus and move with the normal flow of peritoneal fluid. The tumour cell surfaces do not have the adhesion molecules and the distinctive feature of PMP is its tendency to 'redistribute' around the peritoneal cavity.[24] Adenomatous epithelial cells surrounded by mucus accumulate at specific abdominal and pelvic sites. Two factors determine peritoneal distribution of PMP.

DISTRIBUTION RELATED TO PERITONEAL FLUID ABSORPTION

Adenomatous cells concentrate at the normal sites of peritoneal fluid absorption, namely the under surface of the right hemi-diaphragm and the greater and lesser omentum. Bulky accumulations occur as fluid is absorbed and cells are 'filtered'. From a clinical perspective, the 'omental cake' may be visualized at imaging and is the characteristic finding at laparotomy. Thick accumulations of tumour are present under the right hemi-diaphragm and, as the disease becomes generalized, the redistribution process extends to the left hemi-diaphragm, engulfs the spleen and spreads throughout the abdomen.

DISTRIBUTION BY GRAVITY

The other main mechanism of tumour redistribution is gravity, such that tumour cells concentrate in line with gravitational forces. Dependent portions of the abdomen and pelvis such as the recto-vesical pouch, the right retro-hepatic space and the paracolic gutters, accumulate tumour cells.[24]

VISCERAL SPARING OF PMP

One of the features of favourable PMP is the complete, or nearly complete, absence of mucinous tumours on the intestinal surfaces. The exceptions to this are the antrum of the stomach and pylorus, the ileo-caecal valve region, and the recto-sigmoid colon. These sites are fixed to the retro-peritoneum, and not actively and freely moving by normal peristaltic mechanisms. The almost continuous small bowel peristalsis prevents mucinous implantations on the mesentery or serosa. To a lesser extent, peristalsis prevents disease on the stomach and colon.

This characteristic distribution of PMP, and the 'redistribution' away from bowel surfaces is a crucial feature of PMP that permits complete tumour removal and, thereby, a possibility of cure.

TUMOUR CELL ENTRAPMENT

Tumour cell entrapment, as a result of prior surgery, is an important aspect of the natural history of PMP. Tumour cells adhere to abraded surfaces on the

---

Key point 3

- CT is the best method for predicting operability. Extensive small bowel involvement precludes complete cytoreduction. Small bowel obstruction or separation of loops of bowel by tumour masses indicate poor outcome.

bowel that result from laparotomies, particularly where debulking procedures have been performed. The small bowel serosa and mesenteric surfaces become coated with tumour and complete cytoreduction becomes dangerous, or impossible, because of the risk of fistulation. Extensive involvement of the small bowel and its mesentery are critical in the planning of a surgical strategy for the disease and such involvement will make complete tumour removal impossible.

Key point 4

- PMP spreads within the abdomen by 'redistribution' whereby absorption of peritoneal fluid and thus cell filtering, by the omentum and by peritoneum on the undersurface of the diaphragm, together with gravitational forces, results in characteristic distribution of tumour. Peristalsis protects the small bowel and to a lesser extent the colon and stomach.

TREATMENT OF PMP AND PMP-LIKE CONDITIONS

The treatment of PMP and PMP-like conditions is controversial and lacking in hard scientific evidence; nor is such evidence likely to ever be available,[21] due to the rarity and heterogeneity of the problem.

As for all tumours, there are four main strategies – radiotherapy, chemotherapy, expectant treatment with symptom control, and surgery.

Radiotherapy has little place due to unacceptable side-effects from such a wide-field tumour. Systemic chemotherapy is not reliably effective, due to the 'borderline malignancy' of the cells, and the relatively poor blood supply such that side-effects almost always outweigh benefits. There are some anecdotal reports, including personal experience, of benefits from COX II inhibitors, with some on-going small trials in PMP. For all patients, symptom management is an essential part of treatment and may be the optimal treatment for many. Symptom control may require appropriate palliative surgery.

SURGICAL APPROACHES TO THE MANAGEMENT OF PMP

There are two broad approaches in surgical management. The traditional and still universally practised approach is 'debulking' whereby, at laparotomy, as much as possible of the mucus and tumour is removed by blunt dissection and by limited procedures such as a right hemi-colectomy and partial omentectomy, or these combined with bilateral oophorectomy and hysterectomy in females. The disease eventually recurs, although in many cases the patient can remain asymptomatic for many years. Symptomatic recurrence, resulting in small bowel obstruction or gross distension, is treated by further laparotomy and debulking. Each repeated procedure becomes more ineffective and dangerous due to the risk of bowel injury resulting in fistula formation, or death from peritonitis. Anecdotally, the author has seen a few such cases referred with a long interval from the primary surgery (10 years and above), only to then undergo repeated and more ineffective laparotomies. Complete tumour removal becomes impossible due to small bowel involvement, either due to cell entrapment in small bowel adhesions, or perhaps due to malignant transformation analogous to an 'adenoma-carcinoma sequence'.

The alternative surgical approach is complete tumour removal, based on an understanding of the behaviour of the disease and the position of the intra-abdominal tumour. Because the mucinous tumours associated with PMP are minimally invasive and yet extensively coat parietal peritoneal surfaces, Sugarbaker[20] has developed a series of peritonectomy procedures, with the addition of adjunctive, intra-peritoneal, chemotherapy.

The surgery involves stripping of parietal peritoneum and resecting intra-abdominal structures at fixed sites that contain tumour-laden visceral peritoneum to accomplish a complete cytoreduction. Sugarbaker has advocated dissection and tumour evaporation by laser mode electrosurgery using a ball tipped (2.5 mm) hand piece. The electrosurgical generator is placed on pure cut at high voltage. A smoke evaporator is used to protect the operating theatre environment and to facilitate vision for dissection.

SURGICAL PROCEDURES IN COMPLETE CYTOREDUCTION

The abdomen is opened by a long mid-line incision extending from the xiphisternum to the symphysis pubis. A careful assessment of the abdominal cavity is performed. The small bowel and stomach are inspected. A crucial factor is the amount of disease-free small bowel, especially if a gastrectomy is required for complete cytoreduction. A decision has to be made as to whether complete cytoreduction is likely to be achievable prior to embarking on irreversible, high-risk procedures.

Key point 5

- Optimal outcomes result from peritonectomy, which takes on average 10 h, combined with intraperitoneal, intra-operative heated chemotherapy. Intraperitoneal chemotherapy has a direct effect and is only effective when residual disease nodules are less than 3 mm in size.

PERITONECTOMY PROCEDURES

The principles of complete cytoreduction in PMP revolve around six peritonectomy procedures as described by Sugarbaker[20], usually performed in the following order.

1. Greater omentectomy with splenectomy.

2. Stripping of the left hemi-diaphragm.

3. Stripping of the right hemi-diaphragm.

4. Cholecystectomy and lesser omentectomy.

5. Distal gastrectomy(antrectomy).

6. Pelvic peritonectomy with resection of the recto-sigmoid by anterior resection.

In addition, diseased parietal peritoneum on the anterior abdominal wall requires excision and a right hemi-colectomy is usually required due to the concentration of disease around the ileo-caecal region. At the end of the procedure, the ileum can be anastomosed to the remaining colon or brought out as an end ileostomy.

Not all patients require all six peritonectomies as described and it is often possible to avoid having to remove the gastric antrum. The detail of the greater omentectomy involves ligation of the gastric branches inside the gastro-epiploic arcade such that when all disease is removed from the antrum (with or without distal gastrectomy), the sole remaining blood supply is via the left gastric artery. Occasionally, the left gastric artery is completely surrounded by tumour and has to be ligated to achieve complete cytoreduction. In this situation, a total gastrectomy is required and the stomach replaced by a Roux-en-Y jejunal interposition. The oesophago-jejunal anastomosis is at high risk of leakage due to the long operative time, oedematous small bowel, intra-operative and postoperative chemotherapy and, often, a long postoperative ileus with reflux of pancreatic and biliary juice. Sugarbaker[25] has advocated that such patients should have diversion of the pancreatic and biliary juice away from the gastrointestinal tract into a high jejunostomy for 6 months during which time the patient is maintained on home TPN. More evidence is needed prior to the definitive management of patients who require a total gastrectomy.

With regards to other aspects of the surgery, we have been able to perform a complete pelvic peritonectomy, excising the recto-vesical pouch but, nevertheless, preserving the rectum in a number of cases. The rectum has to be mobilized completely and the peritoneal reflexion carefully removed. The preservation of the rectum is important, as both our experience and that of Sugarbaker[20] is that an anterior resection in these situations should be defunctioned due to the unacceptably high risks of anastomotic leakage. Thus, if the rectum is preserved, a stoma can be avoided. In Sugarbaker's[20] and the author's experience, complete cytoreduction takes, on average, over 10 h.

INTRAPERITONEAL CHEMOTHERAPY

Systemic chemotherapy, by oral or intravenous routes, is of limited effectiveness in the treatment of intra-abdominal mucinous tumours. This is a consequence of the peritoneal/plasma barrier,[20] the relatively poor blood

---

Key point 6

• Morbidity and mortality from complete cytoreduction is high and is best concentrated in specialized centres. A surgeon encountering a case of PMP at laparotomy should take biopsies, remove the appendix if accessible, and refer patients to a specialized centre.

supply to the tumour, and the tendency for such tumours to be 'slow-growing'. Sugarbaker has proposed strong arguments in favour of intraperitoneal chemotherapy instillation, especially if the treatment is given intra-operatively when all macroscopic tumour has been removed, all intra-abdominal adhesions have been broken down, and the surgeon can ensure access to the entire abdomen. Whilst randomised controlled trial (RCT) evidence to support chemotherapeutic treatment in PMP is non-existent, recent evidence in gastric cancer is very exciting.[26] In an RCT, 248 patients with gastric cancer were randomised to receive surgery alone *versus* surgery and intra-peritoneal mitomycin C and 5-fluorouracil (5-FU), along similar protocols as for PMP. The 5-year survival was 23% in surgery alone compared to 54% in the combined group.[26]

Similarly, a prospective study in patients with gastric cancer treated with early postoperative intraperitoneal chemotherapy demonstrated a reduction in local recurrence and an improved 5-year survival compared to patients treated with surgery alone.[27]

The rationale behind intraperitoneal chemotherapy is that direct delivery can eradicate cells and small volume intraperitoneal disease by a local effect without relying on systemic delivery. In this context, chemotherapy enters tumour cells by simple diffusion and can probably only penetrate residual nodules up to 2–3 mm in size. Attempts to instil intraperitoneal chemotherapy when there is gross residual macroscopic disease, or there are multiple adhesions, is likely to do more harm that good and any possible benefit is likely to be a systemic effect following absorption.

Traditionally in PMP, mitomycin C has been given at operation, followed by 4–5 days of postoperative intraperitoneal 5-FU. Newer agents, particularly platinum-based therapies, are currently being evaluated.

Current practise is to heat the chemotherapeutic agent to 41°C within the patient's abdomen with perfusion of 'hyperthermic' intraperitoneal chemo-therapy (HIPC).[20] Heat alone has anticancer effects, it may synergize cytotoxicity of chemotherapy and augment the penetration of drug into tissues.[20,28]

There is little hard evidence to support the benefits of the heating with regard to cytotoxic benefits; however, there are likely to be substantial physiological benefits to the patient whose abdomen has often been exposed and open for up to 10 h, with a resultant drop in body temperature. Experience has shown a significant rise in the patient's core body temperature during the 60–90 min perfusion. There are undoubtedly complications associated with HIPC; Sugarbaker[20] has documented an increase in postoperative fistula complications and possibly in anastomotic leakage, especially in colorectal anastomosis.

Serious postoperative neutropenia occurs in approximately 5% of patients,[10,12,20] and usually does not manifest until the second postoperative week and beyond. It may be associated with infection. The treatment involves early detection, appropriate antibacterial and antifungal treatment as needed, and early use of granulocyte colonizing stimulating factor (GCSF).

SELECTION OF CASES FOR SURGICAL INTERVENTION

Surgical intervention for PMP should only be considered for two indications: (i) where complete tumour removal is likely to be achievable and can be combined with intraperitoneal chemotherapy; and (ii) for the relief of symptoms (*i.e.* palliative surgery).

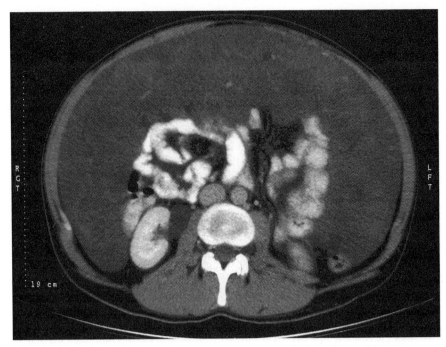

Fig. 1 CT scan of male aged 35 years. The contrast enhanced small bowel is compartmentalized by an omental cake. The patient had a complete cytoreduction in a 12 h laparotomy.

The morbidity and mortality of the surgery, together with the spectrum of disease, makes careful selection of patients for complete cytoreduction critical. Many such patients will be asymptomatic, with uncertainty about their prognosis even if no treatment is performed. However, most patients will undergo disease progression, often over a number of years, and will eventually succumb. The current best method to assess operability is contrast enhanced CT. A number of favourable, and unfavourable, features have been described by Jacquet and colleagues[22] and have been validated by the author's group.[29] The main aims are to differentiate PMP (adenomucinosis) from mucinous adenocarcinoma, and to predict likely benefit from surgery.

The CT findings in PMP are 'pathognomic' with appropriate radiological techniques and a combination of oral, rectal and intravenous contrast.[22,29] In most cases, the striking feature is the relative sparing of the small bowel and mesentery with the small bowel 'compartmentalized' in the centre of the abdominal cavity by a large omental cake (Fig. 1). The small bowel lumen is of normal calibre, and its configuration does not show obstructed segments.

Key point 7

- Techniques used in PMP, particularly intra-operative intraperitoneal chemotherapy and extensive local surgery, may be applicable in many intra-abdominal tumours where local failure is still a common cause of recurrence and death.

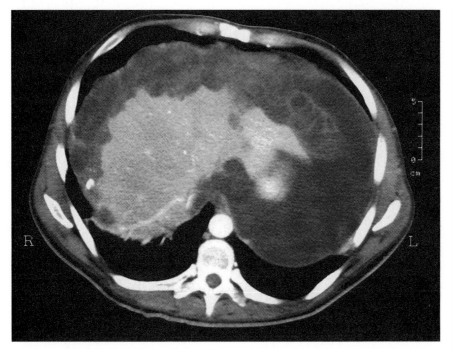

Fig. 2 Upper abdominal CT scan in a male aged 42 years showing pathognomic 'scalloping' of the liver with engulfment of the spleen and stomach. The patient had a palliative 5-h laparotomy involving removal of a subtotal colectomy and omentectomy. The small bowel was also extensively involved.

There is a characteristic layer of tumour surrounding and 'scalloping' the diaphragmatic surface of the liver (Fig. 2).

Progression of the disease at both ends of the abdomen eventually results in encasement of the stomach (Fig. 2) and recto-sigmoid. Gradually, redistribution ceases, and the small bowel and its mesentery become progressively involved by mucinous tumour masses.

Jacquet and colleagues[22] retrospectively analysed a group of patients who underwent complete cytoreduction and compared them with a matched group who had incomplete cytoreduction. The two radiological findings that predicted that complete cytoreduction would be unlikely were: (i) segmental obstruction of the small bowel; and (ii) tumour masses greater than 5 cm on small bowel and small bowel mesentery in the jejunum and proximal ileum.

These features are the best predictors of suitability for surgical intervention (Fig. 3). Focal narrowing of the small bowel indicates an invasive component (*i.e.* a mucinous adenocarcinoma). Whilst these radiological features are very helpful at the extremes, like the disease itself there is a spectrum of radiological appearances. Prior surgery can also alter the appearances and make interpretation difficult.

TUMOUR MARKERS IN PMP

There is little published information concerning the significance of tumour markers in PMP. We routinely measure CEA, CA-19-9 and CA-125. A few

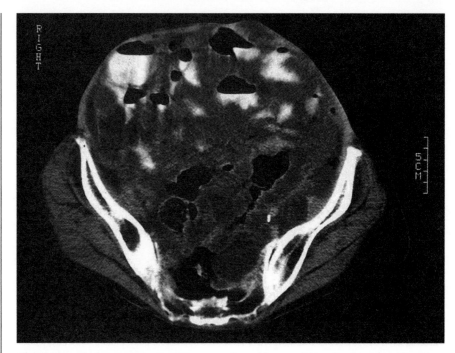

Fig. 3 CT scan of a women aged 58 years referred for consideration for cytoreduction. The contrast enhanced small bowel has air fluid levels with large masses of tumour between the loops. The patient was deemed inoperable and died 3 weeks later from bronchopneumonia.

points of interest emerge. CA-125, normally regarded as a marker of ovarian cancer, is commonly elevated in PMP, including in males where the primary tumour is appendiceal. Thus, elevations in CA-125 should not be used to target ovarian-type chemotherapy in patients with PMP, or PMP-type syndromes. Intestinal type chemotherapy, that is 5-FU and derivatives thereof, are likely to be more appropriate.

Our own unpublished results suggest that marked elevations of tumour markers are indicators of advanced and invasive disease, and signify that complete cytoreduction is less likely to be achievable compared to low or normal levels. In those patients who are secretors, monitoring of the levels is a sensitive predictor of recurrence and disease progression.

COMPLICATIONS OF PMP SURGERY

In patients who have complete cytoreduction, the complex surgery lasting approximately 10 h,[12,20] together with the associated risks of HIPC, combine to result in significant serious morbidity and mortality. The mortality rate in experienced centres is in the region of 3–5%[10,12,20] mainly from sepsis, often associated with intestinal fistula, and cardiovascular and respiratory complications.

The risk of serious morbidity is in the region of 30–40% with sepsis (chest, intra-abdominal, wound and urinary infections) fistula and anastomotic leakage, re-operative surgery for bleeding, and thrombo-embolic complications being the commonest.[10,12,20]

Thrombo-embolism is a particular risk. A high index of suspicion, aggressive investigation, and judicious use of anticoagulation is essential.

CONCLUSIONS

Pseudomyxoma peritonei is a rare condition which, though of 'borderline malignancy', is invariably fatal. Difficulties exist with the definition of PMP. It has been broadly applied to include a heterogeneous group of pathological lesions that present clinically with 'jelly belly' due to mucinous ascites. The relatively few reports in the literature commonly use different pathological definitions and there is no consensus on the point of separation between PMP and carcinomatosis secondary to a mucinous adenocarcinoma. Sugarbaker has suggested 'the term pseudomyxoma peritonei syndrome be strictly applied to a pathologically and prognostically homogenous group of cases characterised by histologically benign peritoneal tumours that are frequently associated with an appendiceal mucinous adenoma'. This definition excludes all cases with mucinous adenocarcinoma.

The optimal treatment is undoubtedly complete tumour excision, by complex surgical peritonectomy procedures, taking on average 10 h. Surgery is usually combined with intraperitoneal, and now intra-operative, chemotherapy. These techniques have a high morbidity and mortality. The rarity of the condition together with the risks associated with definitive treatment suggest that such treatment ought to be centralized into a few centres, covering a large population. The search continues for safer, less aggressive treatments, but is hampered by a lack of hard evidence and the absence of an experimental model to evaluate emerging strategies.

Key points for clinical practice

- Pseudomyxoma peritonei (PMP) is a rare disease usually arising from a tumour of the appendix and presents as 'jelly belly'. Mucinous adenocarcinoma from any condition can simulate PMP clinically, radiologically, and at operation.

- There is a spectrum of disease varying from 'borderline malignant' adenomucinosis to mucinous adenocarcinoma. The behaviour and prognosis vary depending on the nature of the cells producing mucin.

- CT is the best method for predicting operability. Extensive small bowel involvement precludes complete cytoreduction. Small bowel obstruction or separation of loops of bowel by tumour masses indicate poor outcome.

- PMP spreads within the abdomen by 'redistribution' whereby absorption of peritoneal fluid and thus cell filtering, by the omentum and by peritoneum on the undersurface of the diaphragm, together with gravitational forces, results in characteristic distribution of tumour. Peristalsis protects the small bowel and to a lesser extent the colon and stomach.

Key points for clinical practice (continued)

- Optimal outcomes result from peritonectomy, which takes on average 10 h, combined with intraperitoneal, intra-operative heated chemotherapy. Intraperitoneal chemotherapy has a direct effect and is only effective when residual disease nodules are less than 3 mm in size.

- Morbidity and mortality from complete cytoreduction is high and is best concentrated in specialized centres. A surgeon encountering a case of PMP at laparotomy should take biopsies, remove the appendix if accessible, and refer patients to a specialized centre.

- Techniques used in PMP, particularly intra-operative intraperitoneal chemotherapy and extensive local surgery, may be applicable in many intra-abdominal tumours where local failure is still a common cause of recurrence and death.

References

1. Fann JI, Vierra M, Fisher D *et al*. Pseudomyxoma peritonei. *Surg Gynecol Obstet* 1993; **177**: 441–447.
2. Werth R. Klinische and Anatomische Untersuchungen zur Lehre von der Bauchgeschwullsten and der Laparotomie. *Arch Gynecol Obstet* 1884; **84**: 100–118.
3. Frankel E. Uber das sogenanute Pseudomyxoma Peritonei. *Med Wochenschr* 1901; **48**: 965–970.
4. Hinson FL, Ambrose NS. Pseudomyxoma peritonei. *Br J Surg* 1998; **85**: 332–339.
5. Ronnett BM, Shmookler BM, Diener-West M *et al*. Immunohistochemical evidence supporting the appendiceal origin of pseudomyxoma peritonei in women. *Int J Gynecol Pathol* 1997; **16**: 1–9.
6. Young RH, Gilks CB, Scully RE. Pseudomyxoma peritonei. *Am J Surg Pathol* 1993; **17**: 1068–1071.
7. Prayson RA, Hart WR, Petras RE. Pseudomyxoma peritonei: a clinicopathologic study of 19 cases with emphasis on site of origin and nature of associated ovarian tumours. *Am J Surg Pathol* 1994; **18**: 591–603.
8. Chaqui RF, Zhuang Z, Emmert-Buck MR *et al*. Genetic analysis of synchronous mucinous tumours of ovary and appendix. *Hum Pathol* 1996; **27**: 165–171.
9. Gough DB, Donohue JH, Schutt AJ, Gonchoroff N, Goellner JR, Wilson TO. Pseudomyxoma peritonei. Long-term patient survival with an aggressive regional approach. *Ann Surg* 1994; **219**: 112–119.
10. Witkamp AJ, de Bree E, Kagg MM, Van Slooten GW, Van Coevorden F, Zoetmulder FAN. Extensive surgical cytoreduction and intraoperative hyperthermic intraperitoneal chemotherapy in patients with pseudomyxoma peritonei. *Br J Surg* 2001; **88**: 458–463.
11. Esqviel J, Sugarbaker PH. Clinical presentation of pseudomyxoma peritonei syndrome. *Br J Surg* 2000; **87**: 1414–1418.
12. Parvaiz A, Amin AI, Howell R, Sexton R, Moran BJ. First one hundred referrals, predominantly of pseudomyxoma peritonei, to a peritoneal surface malignancy unit: operability and early outcome. *Br J Surg (Suppl)* 2002; **89**: 3.
13. Costa MJ. Pseudomyxoma peritonei. Histologic predictors of patient survival. *Arch Pathol Lab Med* 1994; **118**: 1215–1219.
14. Ikejiri K, Anai H, Kitmura K, Yakabe S, Saku M, Yoshida K. Pseudomyxoma peritonei concomitant with early gastric cancer: report of a case. *Surg Today* 1996; **26**: 923–925.
15. Young RH, Scully RE. Ovarian metastasis from the carcinoma of gall bladder and extra hepatic bile ducts simulating primary tumour of ovary. A report of six cases. *Int J Gynecol Pathol* 1990; **9**: 60–72.

16. Kurita M, Komatsu H, Hata Y *et al*. Pseudomyxoma peritonei due to adenocarcinoma of lung: case report. *J Gastroenterol* 1994; **29**: 344–348.

17. Hawes D, Robinson R, Wira R. Pseudomyxoma peritonei from metastatic colloid carcinoma of the breast. *Gastrointest Radiol* 1991; **16**: 80–82.

18. McCarthy JH, Aga R. A fallopian tube lesion of borderline malignancy associated with pseudomyxoma peritonei. *Histopathology* 1988; **13**: 223–225.

19. Chejfec G, Rieker WJ, Jablokow VR, Gould VE. Pseudomyxoma peritonei associated with colloid carcinoma of pancreas. *Gastroenterology* 1986; **90**: 202–205.

20. Sugarbaker PH, Ronnett BM, Archer A *et al*. Pseudomyxoma peritonei syndrome. *Adv Surg* 1997; **30**: 233–280.

21. McCulloch P, Taylor I, Sasako M, Lovett B, Griffin D. Randomised trials in surgery: problems and possible solutions. *BMJ* 2002; **324**: 1448–1451.

22. Jacquet P, Jelinek J, Sugarbaker PH. Use of abdominal computerized tomogram to select peritoneal carcinomatosis patients for the cytoreductive approach. *J Am Coll Surg* 1995; **181**: 530–538.

23. Ronnett BM, Zahn CM, Kurman RJ *et al*. Disseminated peritoneal adenomucinosis and peritoneal mucinous carcinomatosis: a clinicopathological analysis of 109 cases with emphasis on distinguishing pathologic features, site of origin, prognosis, and relationship to 'pseudomyxoma peritonei'. *Am J Surg Pathol* 1995; **19**: 1390–1408.

24. Sugarbaker PH. Pseudomyxoma peritonei: a cancer whose biology is characterized by a redistribution phenomenon. *Ann Surg* 1994; **219**: 109–111.

25. Sugarbaker PH. Cytoreduction, including gastrectomy for pseudomyxoma peritonei. *Br J Surg* 2002; **89**: 208–212.

26. Yu W, Ilwoo W, Young Chung H *et al*. Indications for early postoperative chemotherapy of advanced gastric cancer: results of a prospective randomized trial. *World J Surg* 2001; **25**: 985–990.

27. Lamb PJ, Dresner SM, Immanuel A *et al*. Early postoperative chemotherapy (EPIC) for gastric carcinoma – a prospective study. *Br J Surg* 2002; **89**: 87.

28. Los G, Smals OA, Van Vight MJ. A rationale for carboplatin treatment and abdominal hyperthermia in cancers restricted to the peritoneal cavity. *Cancer Res* 1992; **52**: 1252–1258.

29. Sulkin TVC, Oneill H, Amin AI, Moran B. CT in pseudomyxoma peritonei: a review of 17 cases. *Clin Radiol* 2002; **57**: 608–613.

Charles H. Knowles Peter J. Lunniss

Risk assessment and classification in septic diverticular disease

While government initiatives continue to focus on improving the lot of the patient with suspected colorectal cancer, diverticular disease, along with many other areas of benign coloproctological pathology remains rather neglected. This is not to say that diverticular disease may not be associated with just as great an impact to the individual. In nearly all hospitals providing an acute general surgical service around the country at any time, there is likely to be one patient on the intensive care unit struggling to recover from recent major surgery for complicated acute diverticulitis, another on the general surgical ward slowly returning to physiological normality, and yet another patient on the rehabilitation ward facing up to returning to the community with an end colostomy of perhaps suboptimal quality.

Department of Health Episode statistics re-inforce the suggestion that diverticulitis is becoming more common, with a parallel increase in the numbers of patients undergoing surgery, but with no improvements in overall mortality rates (Table 1).[1] Similar increases in prevalence have also been identified in Scandinavia.[2] Diverticulosis is predominantly a disease of the elderly. In Western societies, where diverticulosis and its complications are most commonly seen, populations are becoming increasingly elderly, carrying with them the non-specific and specific co-morbidities associated with ageing. Complicated diverticulitis, however, is also seen in the younger individual, in whom the diagnosis may not be so high in the differential. Although diverticulitis is more prevalent in females, these data suggest that there is a greater rise in prevalence in the male population.[1]

Dr C.H. Knowles PhD FRCS, Specialist Registrar and Clinical Lecturer in Surgery, Academic Department of Surgery, The Royal London Hospital, London, UK

Mr P.J. Lunniss MS FRCS, Senior Lecturer and Honorary Consultant Surgeon, Academic Department of Surgery, 4th Floor Alexandra Wing, The Royal London Hospital, Whitechapel, London E1 1BB, UK (for correspondence), and Homerton Hospital, London, UK

Key point 1

• The prevalence of complicated diverticulitis is increasing.

Table 1 Demography of diverticulitis based on Department of Health Episode statistics[1]

	1989/1990		1999/2000		Change (%)	
Colonic diverticulitis	M	F	M	F	M	F
Admission rate/100,000 population	20.1	28.6	23.2	31.9	16	12
Admissions with an operation (%)	22.9	20	27	22	16	14
Case fatality rate	3.1	3.2	3.4	3.4	11	5

There is no doubt that morbidity and mortality rates for patients undergoing surgery for diverticular disease as a whole are influenced by the presence and degree of complication, in particular sepsis. Closely audited data relating to sigmoid diverticulitis in a population of 150,000 served by 6 general surgeons in a district general hospital about 30 km from Amsterdam over a 10-year period are shown in Table 2 (Oomen & Engel, Zaans Medical Centre, Amsterdam, The Netherlands, personal communication). As in England, surgery for diverticulitis is more common in females than males. Postoperative mortality for elective resection reaches nearly 5% with a 50% complication rate (6.7% anastomotic breakdown) with over 1 in 10 patients requiring a second operation during the same admission. For those in whom surgery is performed in the acute setting, mortality rises to 17% (10% for low risk, 29% for high risk patients), with a 70% complication rate (33% respiratory, 37% urinary, 12% wound infections, 5% intra-abdominal abscess), and 16% re-operation rate.

Table 2 Audit of outcomes of surgery for sigmoid diverticular disease in a Dutch district general hospital serving a population of 150,000 over a 10-year period to 2001

	Elective (*n* = 149)	Acute (*n* = 114)
Average age (years)	64 (M 61; F 66)	67 (M 62; F 70)
Female/male	98/51	67/47
Possum score completeness	> 95%	> 95%
Predicted possum mortality	4.9%	23.4%
Mortality	4.7%	17%
	(M 7.8%; F 3.1%)	(M 15%; F 18%)
Complication	53.7%	71.1%
Re-operation at first admission	12.1%	15.8%
Operations after discharge	15.4%	61.4%
Surgery		
Resection and anastomosis	88%	8%
Hartmann's procedure	5%	71%
Other	8%	21%

Data kindly provided by JLT Oomen and AF Engel, Zaans Medical Centre, Amsterdam, The Netherlands (2002).

> **Key point 2**
> - Complicated diverticulitis is associated with significant morbidity and mortality.

Similar statistics are observed in other continental European,[3] UK,[4-6] and American[7] series.

SCOPE OF THE REVIEW

A number of classification systems or scores that aim to predict outcome in specific conditions are familiar to all surgeons (*e.g* Glasgow coma score in head injury, Ranson's score in acute pancreatitis, and Child's classification in liver failure). In addition to these 'disease-specific' scores are those that are applicable generally to all pre-operative surgical patients to predict morbidity and mortality. These vary from the relatively simple grading of the patient's overall health (*e.g.* American Society of Anesthesiologists [ASA] grading) or cardiac/respiratory status (*e.g.* Goldman Cardiac Risk Index), to complex so-called 'physiological scores of severity of illness' (*e.g.* Acute Physiology and Chronic Health Evaluation II [APACHE II], Physiological and Operative Severity Score for enUmeration of Mortality and morbidity [POSSUM]). It must, however, be noted that some disease-specific scores also incorporate general indices of co-morbidity (*e.g.* Mannheim Peritonitis Index [age, sex, organ failure]) and that implicit within physiological scores is the effect of the severity of disease itself on the physiological parameters measured.

This chapter reviews the application of disease-specific classification systems and physiological scores of severity of illness in the risk assessment of patients with septic complications of diverticular disease. Whilst such topics may be less glamorous than the surgical aspects of the condition, the influence of appropriate initial management in determining outcome cannot be overestimated.

DISEASE-SPECIFIC CLASSIFICATIONS

In essence, all diverticulitis is perforated diverticulitis with a presumed microperforation even when a macroperforation is not evident.[8] However, the

Table 3 Hinchey[9] and modified Hinchey[10] classifications of diverticulitis

Hinchey classification	
Stage I	Pericolic abscess or phlegmon
Stage II	Pelvic, intra-abdominal or retroperitoneal abscess*
Stage III	Generalised purulent peritonitis
Stage IV	Faecal peritonitis
*Modified Hinchey classification	
Stage IIa	Distant abscess amenable to surgical drainage
Stage IIb	Complex abscess associated with/without fistula

Table 4 Mannheim Peritonitis Index[12]

Risk factor		Weighting if present
Age > 50 years		5
Female sex		5
Organ failure		7
Malignancy		4
Pre-operative duration of peritonitis > 24 h		4
Origin of sepsis not colonic		4
Diffuse generalized peritonitis		6
Exudate	Clear	0
	Cloudy, purulent	6
	Faecal	12

clinicopathological spectrum of the patient with acute diverticulitis clearly varies and forms the basis of several classification systems. The most commonly applied classification system in current practice is still that of Hinchey (Table 3).[9] This is similar to that described by Hughes in 1963,[11] but importantly subdivides peritonitis into purulent and faecal types. With the greater use of contrast CT, further modification has been made to the Hinchey classification to distinguish complexity of abscess.[10] Another system is the Mannheim Peritonitis Index (Table 4),[12] which incorporates the type, duration and degree of peritonitis as well as some non-disease specific findings such as age, sex, and associated other organ failure to determine prognosis.

For the patient admitted with acute left lower abdominal discomfort, low fever, with normal pulse and blood pressure, and with left iliac fossa tenderness only on examination (Hinchey I), management centres on bowel rest, intravenous antibiotics and fluids and DVT prophylaxis in the expectation that the acute inflammation will settle, and the diagnosis be confirmed after complete resolution, normally by barium enema, but also by endoscopy if diagnostic confidence is less high. Both inflammatory bowel disease and malignancy may each co-exist with diverticular disease and acute vascular insufficiency may initially be difficult to distinguish from complicated diverticulitis. Gynaecological causes (pelvic inflammatory disease, endometriosis) usually are associated with specific histories and findings on pelvic examination.

The patient with an associated abscess (Hinchey II) will usually have more severe pain, fever, anorexia and a tender fullness or mass palpable with localized guarding and rebound tenderness. Pelvic examination may be positive. Investigations will reveal a leukocytosis and raised acute inflammatory markers (*e.g.* C-reactive protein), no free gas on a plain radiograph, but perhaps features of an ileus. Initial management involves more aggressive fluid resuscitation and monitoring together with more detailed imaging.

The widespread availability of computed tomography (CT) has revolutionised assessment of patients with complicated diverticular disease and supplanted contrast studies. In addition to confirming the diagnosis with high sensitivity and specificity (especially when rectal and oral contrast are used),[13] CT allows accurate assessment of disease severity and the potential for radiological interventions.[14] In most centres, this method of imaging is

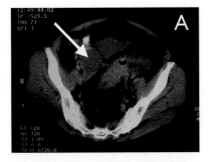
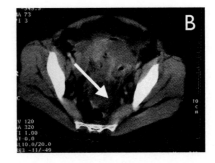
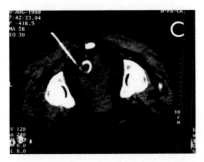

Fig. 1 CT images of a paracolic (A) and pelvic abscess (B) (arrowed) in association with sigmoid diverticulitis drained successfully by CT-guided percutaneous drainage (C). The patient subsequently underwent uneventful elective sigmoid colectomy.

preferred to ultrasonography, despite the ionising radiation (resources allowing). The request for further imaging should come from a senior member of the surgical team and be put to a senior radiologist. A CT scan performed early clarifies any diagnostic difficulty and gives the team confidence that they are managing the patient appropriately. Furthermore, if an abscess is seen which is amenable to percutaneous drainage then this may occur without undue delay (Fig. 1). Success rates for CT-guided percutaneous drainage vary from 70–90% and are higher for modified Hinchey stage IIa disease.[8,15,16]

Numerous reports suggest that the sensitivity and specificity of gradient pressure ultrasound scanning are similar to those of CT in experienced hands.[17] From continental Europe, evidence has been published suggesting that surgical trainees, trained in ultrasound scanning of the abdomen, can diagnose acute diverticulitis accurately.[18] This is a potentially dangerous strategy; just as surgery, if indicated, should at least be supervised by a senior surgeon, so diagnostic radiology, in this scenario, should be undertaken or supervised by a senior radiologist. Furthermore, CT is superior in the visualization of other organs and for guiding drainage procedures.[19]

Key point 3

- Early imaging by contrast-enhanced CT should be considered, both for diagnosis and therapy.

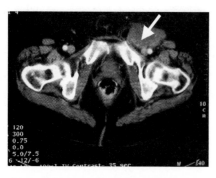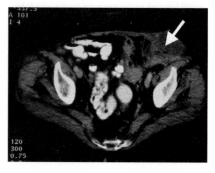

Fig. 2 CT images of an elderly lady who presented with severe left iliac fossa pain, sepsis, and an abscess pointing in the left groin (arrowed). The abscess originated from the sigmoid colon, affected by diverticulosis. After drainage of the abscess via the groin, further investigations (contrast studies, endoscopy) yielded no more information. Histology of the resected colon, excised electively during the same admission unfortunately revealed malignancy within the diverticular sigmoid. One year later, the patient developed an enterovesical fistula residing in recurrent malignancy.

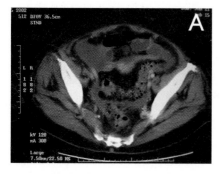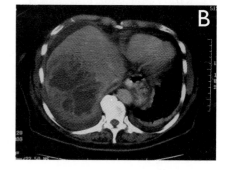

Fig. 3 Axial CT images demonstrating purulent peritonitis with free gas, multiple collections and sick looking fat in a young female immunocompromised patient in whom the clinical findings, vital signs chart and results of serological investigations (CRP, white cell count) did not reflect the gravity of the intra-abdominal pathology.

It should be noted that neither CT nor ultrasonography can confidently distinguish between inflammatory and neoplastic masses (Fig. 2).[18] The indication for early imaging is even greater in patients who are immunocompromised for whatever reason, as their clinical state and indeed results of serological investigations may appear much better than the true intra-abdominal situation (Fig. 3).[20]

The patient admitted with purulent (Hinchey stage III) or faecal peritonitis (stage IV) will be obviously severely unwell with signs of both peritonitis and sepsis or septic shock (Table 4). Priorities in management include:

Key point 4

• Diverticulitis and malignancy may co-exist.

Table 5 Microbiology of acute diverticulitis. Antibiotic policy must cover anaerobic and aerobic Gram-negative bacteria

Enterobacteriaceae	*E. coli*, *Serratia* spp., *Klebsiella* spp., *Proteus* spp.
Bacteroides spp.	
Enterococci	

1. Restoration of tissue perfusion by supplementary oxygen and intravenous fluids (colloids are preferred currently to crystalloids).

2. If restoration of circulating volume is insufficient to restore tissue perfusion, and once circulating volume has been restored, the use of inotropes and vasoconstrictors to optimize cardiac output and the cardiac index.

3. Appropriate analgesia (neither insufficient nor excessive).

4. Intravenous antibiotics. Hospitals have differing antibiotic policies, but in the context of complicated diverticulitis, those prescribed must cover both aerobic and anaerobic Gram-negative bacilli (Table 5).

5. Ventilation; correction of anaemia and coagulopathy, renal support.

Such interventions cannot be performed on a general ward, but rather in the high dependency/intensive care setting, where the level of intervention, both therapeutic and for monitoring, can be instituted and adjusted appropriately according to the patient's condition and progress.

Key point 5

- The level of pre-operative intervention, both for therapy and monitoring, should be appropriate to the patient's clinical condition and response to treatment.

For those patients with peritonitis, laparotomy remains the mainstay of definitive therapy although decisions have to be made with respect to the timing of surgical intervention. The decision, in the minority, that attempts at resuscitation would be futile and that management should be purely palliative, can only be made by combined assessment at a senior level, and with the patient (if possible) and their loved ones involved in the decision making process, which should be collective. For the majority, surgery will be offered on the basis that recovery may ensue once the source of continued infection and systemic sequelae are removed. The decision that a patient has undergone optimal resuscitation and that they can no further be improved without surgery is again a joint decision between senior intensivist, anaesthetist and surgeon. As in all aspects of our professional lives, frequent, honest and realistic communication is paramount, the patient being managed in a

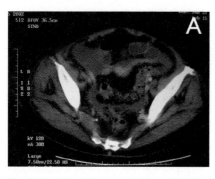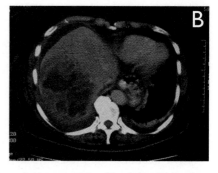

Fig. 4 A patient, known to have diverticulosis and who presents with abdominal pain and sepsis, does not necessarily have diverticulitis. (A) Shows typical CT appearances of marked diverticulosis, but no pericolic inflammation or abscess. The symptoms of pain, fever, anorexia and diarrhoea originated in a massive hepatic abscess (B).

multidisciplinary approach involving, of course, nurse specialists (including those trained in counselling in stoma care), as the likelihood will be that the patient returns from the operating theatre with an end colostomy which will be permanent in 60–70% of such patients.[7,21] A discussion of the preferred surgical procedure, especially the debate regarding primary anastomosis in patients with Hinchey III stage disease, is beyond the scope of this article and in any case is not supported by any consensus in the current literature.

RISK AND DISEASE-SPECIFIC CLASSIFICATIONS

Several studies have addressed the outcome of emergency surgery for septic complications of diverticular disease in terms of disease-based classification systems. It is well documented in several audit-based reviews that perforated diverticular disease with peritonitis (Hinchey III/IV) is associated with higher mortality rates (20–50%) than with abscess formation (5–10%).[4-6] For example, the national audit of diverticular disease[5] demonstrates that operative mortality rises from 4% to 48% for Hinchey II-IV respectively. Data utilizing the Hughes' classification show a similar ascendancy of morbidity (28–57%) and mortality (2–12%) for grades I–III.[22] The Mannheim Peritonitis Index has been employed to produce a polynomial curve of increasing mortality with increasing score.[23] In terms of utilising classification systems of disease severity, it should be stressed that like physiological scores (below), these may assist in predicting outcome to compare institutions, but do not often aid decision-making for the individual. For instance, according to the Mannheim Peritonitis index, a lady of 50 years of age, previously well, with 24 h generalised purulent peritonitis (Hinchey III) would score a value

---

Key point 6

- Disease-specific and more general scoring systems exist which may predict morbidity and mortality, but which should not necessarily be used to influence clinical management in an individual.

indicative of a 95% mortality,[3] not in reality consistent with the aggressive management that all would deem appropriate, and in whom ultimate demise would not be expected. Emergency surgery for right-sided diverticulitis is associated with less morbidity and mortality than left-sided,[24] reflecting the younger age of these patients and the predominantly lower Hinchey stage (usually only stages I and II) of disease.

GENERAL AND PHYSIOLOGICAL SCORING

The institution and development of intensive care units (ICUs) has undoubtedly saved lives and allowed critically ill patients resumption of a normal life-style. Synchronously, however, debate has grown over issues such as mortality rates within and between ICUs, survival of those patients discharged from them, costs, patient selection for admission, setting limits of treatment, etc.[25]

The outcome of critical illness is determined by:

1. Severity of the acute illness.

2. The patient's previous state of health.

3. Nature of the underlying disease.

4. The treatment given.

5. The patient's response to treatment.

These factors, to varying degrees, form the basis of several scoring systems (Table 6) the details of which are reviewed elsewhere.[26] The broad division of such scores into the simple, easily applicable, and complex physiological has been alluded to in the introduction. Regardless of which is used, their role is

Table 6 Non disease-specific scoring systems

Pre-operative scores
    American Society of Anesthesiologists grading (ASA)
    Goldman Cardiac Risk Index (CRI)
    Hospital Prognosis Index (HPI)
    Prognostic Nutritional Index (PNI)

Physiological scores of severity of illness
    Acute Physiology, Age, Chronic Health Evaluation (APACHE I, II, III)
    Mortality Prediction Model (MPM)
    Physiologic & Operative Severity Score for the nUmeration of
        Morbidity & Mortality (POSSUM, p-POSSUM)
    Simplified Acute Physiology Score (SAPS)
    Therapeutic Intervention Scoring System (TISS)
    Trauma Score & Revised Trauma Score (TS, RTS)

principally to allow some comparison between individual units and, as is increasingly the vogue, individual surgeon performances rather than in the prediction of outcome in an individual. Thus, they should not be used primarily to direct individual patient management. In addition, physiological scores are perhaps too unwieldy for use in routine surgical practice and remain very much, at least at present, the remit of the intensivist with a research interest.

RISK AND NON-DISEASE-SPECIFIC CLASSIFICATIONS

In some large series of patients undergoing surgery for complicated diverticulitis, it is evident that nearly all deaths occurred in patients with co-existing disease.[3] Similarly, Elliot *et al.*[6] showed that the mortality from Hartmann's procedure for diverticular peritonitis was related to the patient's age, presence of co-existent medical disease, ASA score, and presence of shock on admission.

Some of the specific physiological scoring systems outlined above have been applied to the field of gastrointestinal/colonic surgery and can predict mortality with reasonable accuracy. In colorectal surgery, the use of POSSUM scoring has been demonstrated in predicting outcome, especially mortality.[27] However, the tendency of this score to overpredict mortality has lead to the development of the Portsmouth predictor equation[28] which, when applied to the original POSSUM score (p-POSSUM), provides more accurate mortality prediction – as recently demonstrated pre-operatively in gastrointestinal surgery.[29] Few studies specifically address the use of physiological scoring systems with respect to septic complicated diverticular disease alone. In the Dutch study, as with those above, mortality rates in both elective and emergency settings are slightly lower than predicted from POSSUM scoring (Oomen & Engel, personal communication). An Italian group[30] showed that APACHE II scores were the best predictor of mortality (compared with other prognostic factors including Hinchey grade) in patients undergoing surgery for complications of diverticulitis and this score has been similarly applied by other groups.[31]

CONCLUSIONS

The clinical and physiological status of the patient admitted with presumed diverticulitis is extremely variable. Initial resuscitation should be combined with a low threshold for CT imaging, both for diagnostic and possibly therapeutic reasons. The level of intervention, both therapeutic and for monitoring the efficacy of therapy, depends upon the clinical state. In cases of peritonitis, surgery will usually be offered once the patient has been deemed resuscitated optimally, the decision concerning surgery and its timing being combined and at a senior level. Malignancy may co-exist within a diverticular segment, and its identification, both by imaging and endoscopy, but also at laparotomy, may be extremely difficult.

Disease-specific and general-grading systems have been developed which may be used to predict outcome in populations of patients with complicated diverticulitis, and which may also be used to compare outcomes between institutions (especially intensive care units), but which should not be used in the direct management of an individual.

Key points for clinical practice

- The prevalence of complicated diverticulitis is increasing.
- Complicated diverticulitis is associated with significant morbidity and mortality.
- Early imaging by contrast-enhanced CT should be considered, both for diagnosis and therapy.
- Diverticulitis and malignancy may co-exist.
- The level of pre-operative intervention, both for therapy and monitoring, should be appropriate to the patient's clinical condition and response to treatment.
- Disease-specific and more general scoring systems exist which may predict morbidity and mortality, but which should not necessarily be used to influence clinical management in an individual.
- Clinical decisions should be combined and at a senior level, with close involvement of the patient and relatives.

ACKNOWLEDGEMENT

The authors are extremely grateful to Drs Oomen and Engel for allowing their data to be included in this review.

References

1. Subramanian S, Tinto A, Majeed A *et al*. Colonic diverticulitis: a disease on the rise. *Gut* 2002; **50**(Suppl 2): A59.
2. Mäkelä J, Kiviniemi H, Laitinen S. Prevalence of perforated sigmoid diverticulitis is increasing. *Dis Colon Rectum* 2002; **45**: 955–961.
3. Wedell J, Banzhaf G, Chaoui R, Fischer R, Reichmann J. Surgical management of complicated colonic diverticulitis. *Br J Surg* 1997; **84**: 380–383.
4. Berry AR, Turner WH, Mortensen NJMcC *et al*. Emergency surgery for complicated diverticular disease. A five-year experience. *Dis Colon Rectum* 1989; **32**: 849–854.
5. Tudor RG, Farmakis N, Keighley MRB. National audit of complicated diverticular disease: analysis of index cases. *Br J Surg* 1994; **81**: 730–732.
6. Elliot TB, Yego S, Irvin TT. Five-year audit of the acute complications of diverticular disease. *Br J Surg* 1997; **84**: 535–539.
7. Belmonte C, Klas JV, Perez JJ *et al*. The Hartmann procedure. First choice or last resort in diverticular disease? *Arch Surg* 1996; **131**: 616–617.
8. Novak L, Hyman N. Surgery for complicated diverticulitis. *Semin Colon Rectal Surg* 2000; **11**: 214–217.
9. Hinchey EJ, Schaal PG, Richards GK. Treatment of perforated diverticular disease of the colon. *Adv Surg* 1978; **12**: 85–109.
10. Sher M, Agachan F, Bortal M *et al*. Laparoscopic surgery for diverticulitis. *Surg Endosc* 1997; **1**: 264–267.
11. Hughes ESR, Cuthbertson AM, Garden ABG. The surgical management of acute diverticulitis. *Med J Aust* 1963; **1**: 780–782.
12. Linder M, Wach H. Der Peritonitis-Index – Grundlage zur Bewertung der Periitoitiskrankung? *Fortchr Antimickrob Chemother* 1983; **2–3**: 511–516.

13. Rao PM, Rhea JT, Novelline RA. Helical CT with only colonic contrast material for diagnosing diverticulitis. *AJR Am J Roentgenol* 1998; **170**: 1445–1449.
14. Stabile BE, Puccio E, van Sonnenberg E *et al*. Preoperative percutaneous drainage of diverticular abscess. *Am J Surg* 1990; **159**: 99–104.
15. Thompson DA, Bailey HR. Management of acute diverticulitis with abscess. *Semin Colon Rectal Surg* 1990; **1**: 74–80.
16. Ambrossetti P, Robert J, Witzig JA *et al*. Incidence, outcome, and proposed management of isolated abscess complicating acute left-sided diverticulitis. *Dis Colon Rectum* 1992; **35**: 1072–1076.
17. Schwerk WB, Schwarz S, Rothmund M. Sonography in acute colonic diverticulitis. A prospective study. *Dis Colon Rectum* 1992; **35**: 1077–1084.
18. Zielke A, Hasse C, Nies C *et al*. Prospective evaluation of ultrasonography in acute colonic diverticulitis. *Br J Surg* 1997; **84**: 385–388.
19. Eggesbø HB, Jacobsen T, Kolmannskog F *et al*. Diagnosis of acute left-sided colonic diverticulitis by three radiological modalities. *Acta Radiol* 1998; **39**: 315–321.
20. Roberts P, Abel M, Rosen L *et al*. Practice parameters for sigmoid diverticulitis. The Standards Task Force American Society of Colon and Rectal Surgeons. *Dis Colon Rectum* 1995; **38**: 126–132.
21. Navara G, Occhionorelli S, Marcello D *et al*. Gasless video-assisted reversal of Hartmann's procedure. *Surg Endosc* 1995; **9**: 687–689.
22. Illert B, Engemann R, Thiede A. Success in treatment of complicated diverticular disease is stage related. *Int J Colorectal Dis* 2001; **16**: 276–279.
23. Billing A, Fröhlich D, Schildberg FW and the Peritonitis Study Group. Prediction of outcome using the Mannheim peritonitis index in 2003 patients. *Br J Surg* 1994: **81**: 209–213.
24. Law WL, Lo CY, Chu KW. Emergency surgery for colonic diverticulitis: differences between right-sided and left-sided lesions. *Int J Colorectal Dis* 2001; **16**: 280–284.
25. Hinds C, Watson D. Planning, organisation and management. In: Hinds C, Watson D. (eds) *Intensive Care. A Concise Textbook*. London: WB Saunders, 1996; 1–18.
26. Jones HJS, de Cossart L. Risk scoring in surgical patients. *Br J Surg* 1999; **86**: 149–157.
27. Whiteley MS, Prytherch DR, Higgins B, Weaver PC, Prout WG. An evaluation of the POSSUM surgical scoring system. *Br J Surg* 1996; **83**: 1483–1484.
28. Prytherch DR, Whiteley MS, Higgins B *et al*. POSSUM and Portsmouth POSSUM for predicting mortality. Physiological and Operative Severity Score for the enUmeration of Mortality and morbidity. *Br J Surg* 1998; **85**: 1217–1220.
29. Tekkis PP, Kocher HM, Bentley AJE *et al*. Operative mortality rates among surgeons. Comparison of POSSUM and p-POSSUM scoring systems in gastrointestinal surgery. *Dis Colon Rectum* 2000; **43**: 1528–1534.
30. Setti Carraro PG, Magenta A, Segala M *et al*. Predictive value of pathophysiological score in the surgical management of perforated diverticular disease. *Chir Ital* 1999; **51**: 31–36.
31. Khan AL, Ah-See AK, Crofts TJ, Heys SD, Eremin O. Surgical management of the septic complications of diverticular disease. *Ann R Coll Surg Engl* 1995; **77**: 233–234.

Wendy Atkin John Northover

9

Screening for colorectal cancer

THE DISEASE AS A WORLD HEALTH ISSUE

World-wide, the large bowel is the fourth commonest site for cancer after lung, stomach and breast and the fourth cause of cancer death after lung, stomach and liver cancer. There were 943,000 new cases diagnosed and 510,000 large bowel cancer deaths in 2000. Highest incidence rates occur in North America, Northern Europe and Australasia; lowest rates are found in sub-Saharan Africa and India. There have been marked increases in incidence rates in Asian populations adopting a Western life-style; however, in higher risk areas, such as the UK, rates are increasing more slowly or have stabilised. According to latest estimates, there are around 34,000 new diagnoses and 19,000 deaths from colorectal cancer in the UK each year. In the US, a pronounced decrease in incidence and mortality rates in white men and women began in the 1980s, but only very small reductions have been recorded in black men and women. Some researchers have speculated that the increased use of sigmoidoscopy and polypectomy have played an important role, although there is some evidence that the increased consumption of fruit and vegetables, non-steroidal anti-inflammatory drugs and hormone replacement therapy may also be playing a part.

In the US and the UK the estimated probability at birth of eventually developing colorectal cancer is 6% and the probability of dying from the disease is around 3%. Cancer of the colon is equally frequent in men and women while cancer of the rectum occurs 20–50% more frequently in men.

Dr Wendy Atkin MPH PhD, Deputy Director, Colorectal Cancer Unit, Cancer Research UK, and Honorary Reader in Epidemiology, Imperial College of Science, Technology and Medicine, St Mark's Hospital, Watford Road, Harrow, Middlesex HA1 3UJ, UK (for correspondence)

Prof. John Northover MS FRCS, Professor of Intestinal Surgery, Imperial College of Science, Technology and Medicine, London, Director, Colorectal Cancer Unit, Cancer Research, and Chair, Department of Surgery, St Mark's Hospital, Watford Road, Harrow, Middlesex HA1 3UJ, UK

NATURAL HISTORY IN RELATION TO POTENTIAL FOR EARLY DETECTION

Survival rates in the US improved substantially during the 1980s and now exceed 60% of all cases diagnosed (SEER cancer statistics 1973–1999). In the late 1980s, 5-year survival rates in the UK were 5% lower for colon and 3% lower for rectal cancer than the average for Europe (47% and 45%, respectively).[1] The wide differences in colorectal cancer survival across Europe in the 1980s[1] were found to depend largely on the stage at diagnosis in different countries. Five-year survival rates for localised disease are 85–90%, compared with 55–60% for regional disease and only 5–8% for cases with distant disease at primary diagnosis.

Epidemiological, pathological and molecular genetic studies[2,3] have provided convincing evidence that most colorectal cancers arise in adenomatous polyps and that their ablation arrests the development of cancer at that site.[4] People with familial adenomatous polyposis (FAP) typically develop hundreds or thousands of adenomas in their teens and have an almost 100% risk of developing cancer by age 40 years. In sporadic bowel cancer, the risk of developing metachronous adenomatous polyps or colorectal cancer increases with the number of adenomas detected initially. It is common to see a focus of malignancy within a large adenoma or to see remnant adenomatous tissue adjacent to a carcinoma in early stage cancers; this finding is rarely seen in advanced cancers, suggesting that the invasive tissue overgrows the adenomatous element. The chance of finding a focus of malignancy within an adenoma grows with increasing size, and with more advanced histology (tubular to tubulovillous to villous) and dysplasia.[2] Molecular genetic studies[3] have provided further evidence for the concept of the adenoma–carcinoma sequence by demonstrating that the adenoma accumulates genetic mutations as it grows and becomes more severely dysplastic.

The average duration of the adenoma–carcinoma sequence in both FAP and sporadic disease is around 10 years.[2] In a retrospective study[5] in which patients with unresected ≥ 1 cm colon polyps were followed radiologically, the cumulative risk of developing cancer was 2.5% at 5 years, 8% at 10 years and 24% at 25 years. The progression of the disease may be faster for flat or depressed adenomas; these have been reported frequently in Japanese colons but less frequently in Western patients.[6] The proportion of cancers that develop from flat or depressed adenomas is unknown.

APPROPRIATE GROUPS FOR PROPHYLACTIC TREATMENT OR FOR ASYMPTOMATIC SCREENING

A number of groups have an increased risk of developing colorectal cancer. At highest risk are those with either of the dominantly inherited conditions, FAP and hereditary non-polyposis colorectal cancer (HNPCC). Prophylactic colectomy is performed in teenagers and young adults affected by FAP since the cumulative risk of developing cancer by age 40 years approaches 100%. In HNPCC, the lifetime risk of colorectal cancer in mutation carriers is 80%,[7] so close surveillance is advised; prophylactic colectomy may be offered to those developing their first cancer, or who have wide-spread synchronous or recurrent adenomas. Other groups at moderately increased risk include those with long-standing ulcerative colitis or Crohn's disease,[8] individuals with a personal history of colorectal cancer or large, villous or multiple adenomas,[4] and those with a 'non-dominant' family history of colorectal cancer. It has been estimated using life-table methods[9] that risk is increased 2–3-fold in those with a single affected first degree relative (FDR) and 5–6-fold in those with two FDRs.

At least 75% of colorectal cancers develop in people with no known risk factors apart from older age. Colorectal cancer is infrequent below age 40 years, but incidence increases rapidly from age 50 years, with an approximate doubling with each decade of life. It is probably not worth screening asymptomatic average risk people below age 50 years. The age at which to stop screening is more contentious. Of all cases, 50% are diagnosed at age ≥ 70 years, and 25% at ≥ 80 years. Of course, with increasing age, life expectancy decreases, as does the number of life-years saved as a result of screening-initiated treatment of the disease. Therefore, most colorectal cancer screening initiatives have focused on the age-group 50–74 years.

TREATMENT OPTIONS FOLLOWING DIAGNOSIS BY SCREENING

Around 20% of cancers detected during endoscopic screening[10] will be malignant polyps that have only invaded locally and can be removed during endoscopy or by local surgical excision (LE). The others will require open abdominal surgery. At least 50% of colorectal cancers detected at screening will be localized, and then treated by endoscopic polypectomy, LE or open radical resection.[10,11] This compares with around 10% Dukes' stage A cases amongst patients presenting after symptom onset.[11]

The vast majority of adenomatous polyps are small enough to be removed safely at endoscopy. Only those which are sufficiently large and sessile to make endoscopic removal impossible or ill-advised require surgical excision. There are a variety of methods available for endoscopic polypectomy (for a detailed review of methods, see Cotton and Williams, chapter 10[12]). The main aims are to remove the lesion completely without perforating the bowel wall or causing bleeding. The method used in individual cases will depend largely on the size and shape of the polyp. It is desirable to retain all or part of the polyp for histological examination.

The US National Polyp Study has shown that within 3 years of removal of adenomas, around 30–50% of people will have a further neoplasm identified at repeat examination.[13] Some lesions are truly metachronous, while others found at repeat endoscopy are adenomas missed at the initial examination.[14] On this basis, it is customary to offer colonoscopic surveillance at 3-yearly intervals to all patients following adenoma detection. Because adenomas are very common and colonoscopy is costly and not without risk, it is gradually becoming accepted that people with adenomas should be stratified according to their risk of being found to have an advanced adenoma or cancer at follow-up.[4] This risk is increased if adenomas are multiple, large or have villous histology, in contrast to single, small, tubular adenomas.[4] Data from the US National Polyp Study suggest that subsequent surveillance intervals can be extended to 6 years in the low-risk group; in the context of a mass screening programme, it may be appropriate to offer no follow-up surveillance to this group.

EFFECTIVENESS OF SCREENING OPTIONS IN TERMS OF INCIDENCE/MORTALITY REDUCTION

FAECAL OCCULT BLOOD TEST (FOBT)

Haemoccult is the most extensively examined method for colorectal cancer screening. It is a guaiac-based test designed to detect an elevated level of blood in stool, assumed to be shed from a bleeding neoplasm. The test sensitivity is around 30–50% for colorectal cancers but < 20% for adenomas.[15] It has high specificity of around 98%.[11,16] In practice, this translates into about one case of cancer and three or four with adenomas for every 10 positive tests.

The test requires collection of two samples from each of three consecutive stools, which are smeared onto cards and mailed to a laboratory for processing. Colonoscopy is recommended if any of the six card 'windows' is positive as up to 50% will be found to have a cancer or large adenoma (≥ 1 cm). False positive results may be caused by components of the diet, including vegetables and some fruits, red meat, aspirin or horseradish; dietary restriction is sometimes advised before and during testing, but, when requested, tends to reduce compliance rates. Occasionally, a positive result is due to a bleeding lesion proximal to the colon.

FOBT has been shown in three large randomised trials (in the US,[17,18] Denmark[16,19] and the UK[11]) to reduce colorectal cancer mortality by up to 20% if offered biennially, and possibly up to 33% if offered every year (Table 1). In the US study,[20] colorectal cancer incidence rates were reduced, respectively, by 20% and 17% in the annually and biennially screened groups. In the US trial,[17] most of the test samples were rehydrated to increase sensitivity by adding a drop of water to each sample during processing; this led to an increase in the positivity rates from 2% to 10% and a cumulative colonoscopy rate at 13 years of 38% in the annual and 29% in the biennially screened groups (compared with only 4% in the Danish study[19]). It has been suggested that the reduction in cancer incidence rate observed in the US study was in part due to the chance detection of adenomas in the excess colonoscopies.[21]

Haemoccult is a relatively insensitive test; in a case-control study,[22] only 36% of FOBTs performed within the year prior to diagnosis of fatal colorectal cancer yielded positive results. This represents the maximum efficacy of the test even if 100% compliance rates are achieved. Immunochemical tests for haemoglobin or other blood components show greater sensitivity for both colorectal cancer and adenomas but at the expense of lower specificity, limiting its usefulness. Immunochemical tests are used routinely in Japan,[23] but there is only limited experience elsewhere.

The feasibility and acceptability of FOBT screening are now being examined in a UK pilot project in England and Scotland, each with around 200,000 people in the age-range 50–69 years.[24] A guaiac test similar to Haemoccult is

---

Key point 3

- Evidence from randomised, controlled trials has shown that detection of asymptomatic, early-stage, colorectal cancers by annual or biennial faecal occult blood testing is an effective means of reducing mortality rates.

---

being offered on a single occasion. The results of this 2-year study are due in 2003 after which a decision will be made on whether to offer this form of screening in a programme within the National Health Service.

FLEXIBLE SIGMOIDOSCOPY (FS)

The 60 cm flexible sigmoidoscope routinely examines the sigmoid colon and rectum, where two-thirds of colorectal cancers and adenomas are located; the examination is usually without sedation or analgesia performed in an endoscopy unit. A single phosphate enema, self-administered around 1 h before leaving home for the test, is required to clear the distal bowel.[10] The technique is sensitive for the detection of both adenomas and colorectal cancers within its reach. Those with 'high-risk' adenomas (see below) may be referred for subsequent examination of the rest of the colon by colonoscopy.

Prevalence rates of distal adenomas increase with age during the 50s but level off after age 60 years.[25] Distal adenoma prevalence rates in men are approximately double those in women.[10]

Evidence from case-control and cohort studies indicates that screening by FS reduces incidence and mortality rates of distal colorectal cancer[26-28] by around 60%. Without randomised trial evidence, most countries have been unwilling to introduce endoscopic screening. Three RCTs are in progress (in the UK,[29] Italy[30] and the US[31]) to address this issue (Table 1).

A 5-year interval is recommended by several professional organisations in the US,[32] although the protection afforded by a single FS may last for up to 10 years[26] or even longer depending on the age at which it is undertaken.[25] The UK and Italian trials are examining the efficacy of a single FS screen at around age 60 years while the US trial is examining the efficacy of 5-yearly screening.

In the UK and Italian trials, small polyps are removed during FS, a practice that has been shown to be safe.[10] Colonoscopy is offered only to those found to have adenomas with features associated with increased risks of synchronous

Key point 4

- Evidence from epidemiological studies has shown that sigmoidoscopy screening, with removal of adenomas detected, reduces both incidence and mortality rates of colorectal cancer. Several randomised trials are in progress.

or metachronous cancer (≥ 3 adenomas, size ≥ 1 cm, villous histology, severe dysplasia or malignancy). On these criteria, only 5% of people screened are offered colonoscopy compared with 24% if all people found to have any type of polyp are referred.

The three randomised trials have all reached their recruitment targets, but several more years of follow-up will be required to determine fully the effects on incidence and mortality. Meanwhile, a population experiment has been in progress in Northern California where for the past decade the Health Maintenance Organization, Kaiser Permanente, has been offering FS screening at 10-yearly intervals to its members aged over 50 years.[33] The uptake rate has been 70%. Colorectal cancer incidence rates have fallen steadily in California and the decrease in left-sided tumours is about twice that of right-sided tumours (24.3% *versus* 11.6%).[34]

Table 1 Randomised trials of efficacy of faecal occult blood testing and flexible sigmoidoscopy screening in reducing colorectal cancer incidence and mortality

Place	No. in trial	Start date	Years of follow-up	Regimen	Mortality reduction (%)	Incidence reduction (%)
Faecal occult blood testing						
Minnesota, USA[*17,18,20]	46,551	1975	18	Annual	33	20
				Biennial	6	17
Nottingham, UK[11]	152,850	1985	10	Biennial	15	No reduction
Odense, Denmark[16]	137,485	1985	13	Biennial	18	No reduction
Flexible sigmoidoscopy screening						
Telemark, Norway[44] NORCCAP	799	1983	13	Single exam	50	80
Multicentre, UK[10]	170,432	1996		Single exam	Not reported	Not reported
Multicentre, Italy, SCORE[30]	34,292	1995		Single exam	Not reported	Not reported
Multicentre, USA, PLCO[31]	148,000	1994	Not reported	5 yearly	Not reported	Not reported

COLONOSCOPY SCREENING

A limitation of FS screening is that it does not examine the proximal colon, where 40% of adenomas and cancers occur. The finding of a distal adenoma at sigmoidoscopy is associated with an increased likelihood of having adenomas in the proximal colon, so colonoscopy in people with distal neoplasia should enable detection of some proximal disease. A recent study[35] suggested that around 70% of all advanced colorectal neoplasia will be detected with this strategy.

A proportion of advanced proximal neoplasia occurs without a distal marker lesion, so some experts in the US[32] have advocated colonoscopy screening to avoid missing these lesions. There is little data to support the efficacy of colonoscopy in preventing proximal colon cancer, but for the motivated individual, whole colon screening by colonoscopy may give the greatest re-assurance. It is not, however, suitable for mass population screening because of the personal commitment required of the screenee, the considerable provider resources required, and the morbidity likely to result from wide-spread delivery of colonoscopy. Bowel preparation for colonoscopy requires participants to take a laxative and consume a liquid-only diet on the day before screening. The procedure can be painful, so sedation and analgesia are usually necessary. As a result, colonoscopy screening requires of the screenee at least 36 h of commitment and time off work, compared with only a couple of hours for flexible sigmoidoscopy. Complication rates are also higher (see below). Flexible sigmoidoscopy can be performed competently by nurses,[36] while colonoscopy requires the skills of an experienced endoscopist.

IMAGING TECHNIQUES

In the precolonoscopy era, barium enema (BE) was the only method available to examine areas of the bowel proximal to the distal sigmoid colon, apart from surgery. The advent of double-contrast barium enema improved the ability to detect polyps. Barium enema has been shown to be relatively insensitive compared with colonoscopy,[37] detecting only 21%, 42% and 46% respectively of polyps ≤ 5 mm, 6–10 mm or > 10 mm in size.

Computed tomography (CT) and magnetic resonance (MR) colography are new techniques for imaging the bowel that may find application in screening. Virtual colonoscopy (CT colography)[38] applies complex image rendering techniques to create 3D-graphical images of the colon that simulate colonoscopy (Fig. 1). These techniques require satisfactory bowel cleansing and temporary paralysis of the colon using a muscle relaxant. The technology is advancing rapidly and the performance characteristics are improving. Differentiation of faeces from mural lesions can be difficult, but that oral contrast, taken the day before screening, may obviate the need for bowel preparation by differentiating faeces from polyps. The techniques appear to have high sensitivity for colorectal cancer and large polyps, but are less sensitive for flat lesions and for smaller polyps.[39] A major limitation at present is the time required to interpret the output (~15–20 min) although computer algorithms under development may allow automatic detection and label suspicious regions, alerting the radiologist to the presence of a lesion. If

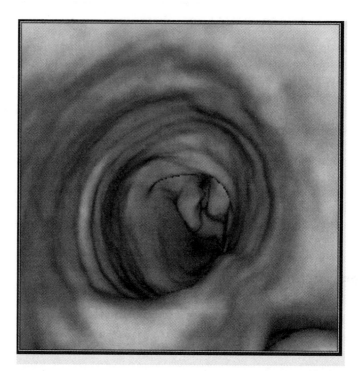

Fig. 1 Virtual colonoscopy. 3D rendering of spiral CT data, giving an intraluminal view of a colon cancer.

accuracy improves, if costs can be reduced, and if bowel preparation becomes unnecessary, there may be a role for these methods in screening average-risk people.

DNA-BASED STOOL TESTS

Stool tests have the advantage that they are non-invasive and, despite the universal distaste for handling faecal material, are potentially more convenient for the participant. The past decade has seen enormous advances in the ability to detect the tiny amounts of DNA present in stool, derived from cells shed from neoplastic lesions. DNA extraction from stool presents special problems as human DNA is often degraded and food digestion products and bacterial contaminants inhibit the polymerase chain reaction. The quantity and quality of the DNA extracted from stool are generally increased in the presence of colorectal neoplasia, probably because there is less efficient degradation by apoptosis of neoplastic cells compared with that of fully differentiated cells. However, several recent studies have reported that it is now possible, although still technically difficult, to extract epithelial DNA from 100% of stool samples, including those with no neoplasia. Mutations in several genes have been examined including k-ras, APC, p53 and BAT26.[40–42]

Using a panel of DNA markers, three research groups[40–42] have reported high sensitivity for cancers and large adenomas. Data so far suggest that, with the exception of k-ras, these markers are highly specific and, therefore, represent a significant improvement over FOBT. Whether stool-based DNA tests will replace or supplement existing screening methods has yet to be determined.

ACCEPTABILITY OF SCREENING METHODS

In the European trials of FOBT,[11] around 60% of participants completed at least one screening test, and around 40% completed all biennial tests offered.

Reported compliance rates with FS screening are highly variable. In a US Army screening initiative,[43] attendance was 95%, perhaps related to FS screening being a requirement for overseas posting! An attendance rate of 81% was achieved in Norway,[44] 49% in the UK,[45] 38% in Ireland,[46] and 29% in Italy.[30] The lowest of these rates are still higher than the 6% compliance in a study inviting physicians, dentists and their spouses to undergo colonoscopic screening.[47]

In a survey undertaken in 1999 among Americans aged over 50 years,[48] 21% had had an FOBT within the previous year and 34% had a sigmoidoscopy within previous 5 years as recommended; 44% had had either sigmoidoscopy or FOBT during the recommended period.

MORBIDITY ASSOCIATED WITH SCREENING AND THE SUBSEQUENT MANAGEMENT PROCESS

The main complications of screening are associated with colonoscopy, flexible sigmoidoscopy and surgery. Generally, flexible sigmoidoscopy is a much lower risk procedure than colonoscopy, particularly the perforation rate, which is around 1 in 50,000 examinations.[10,49] In contrast, there is a higher risk of perforation at colonoscopy of around 1 in 500 examinations.[10,49]. However, in one screening colonoscopy study in average-risk men, there were no perforations reported in over 3000 examinations.[35]

Haemorrhage, the next most important complication, is most likely to follow polypectomy. Waye,[50] using data from several prospective studies, estimated the rate to be 1% if polypectomy had been performed. Risk of bleeding following polypectomy is minimised by discontinuing any anticoagulant therapy several days beforehand.

Endoscopic procedures can induce transient bacteraemia, but prophylactic antibiotics are only needed for patients who are immunosuppressed or who have an implanted mechanical heart valve. Inadequately disinfected endoscopic equipment poses a potential risk of infectious transmission; cases of hepatitis acquired through endoscopy have been reported.[51]

Cardiac morbidity secondary to laxative or sedative use has been reported in up to 15% of people undergoing colonoscopy.[52]

Another source of morbidity and mortality is the surgical treatment of early cancers and adenomas too large to be removed endoscopically. Data are scarce, but the mortality from elective colorectal surgery varies between 1% and 7%.

Key point 5

- Colorectal cancer screening has been recommended in the US for the past decade and incidence rates are falling. Incidence rates have not fallen in the UK, where screening is not recommended.

Key point 6

- The UK Government has announced plans to introduce colorectal cancer screening. In preparation, an urgent training programme is required to increase the number of doctors and nurses capable of delivering high quality flexible sigmoidoscopy and colonoscopy.

CONCLUSIONS

Randomised trials have demonstrated that early detection of colorectal cancer by screening can reduce disease-specific mortality. Evidence from case-control studies is highly suggestive that removal of adenomas reduces colorectal cancer incidence rates. The US is the only country that has advocated endoscopic screening for the purpose of detecting the neoplasia in the premalignant phase, and is the only country in which incidence rates are falling.

There are many methods now available for colorectal cancer screening, with adequate evidence of benefit. The precise choice of screening regimen within a particular healthcare setting will depend on issues of acceptability, safety, feasibility and cost-effectiveness. Whatever method is chosen, it will be necessary to perform colonoscopy to a high standard. It is, therefore, essential that training and quality assurance programmes are in place before screening is implemented.

Key points for clinical practice

- Colorectal cancer is an important cause of death in Western and industrialised countries.

- Survival rates in the UK are improving but are still amongst the lowest in Europe, probably due to the late stage at diagnosis.

- Evidence from randomised, controlled trials has shown that detection of asymptomatic, early-stage, colorectal cancers by annual or biennial faecal occult blood testing is an effective means of reducing mortality rates.

- Evidence from epidemiological studies has shown that sigmoidoscopy screening, with removal of adenomas detected, reduces both incidence and mortality rates of colorectal cancer. Several randomised trials are in progress.

- Colorectal cancer screening has been recommended in the US for the past decade and incidence rates are falling. Incidence rates have not fallen in the UK, where screening is not recommended.

- The UK Government has announced plans to introduce colorectal cancer screening. In preparation, an urgent training programme is required to increase the number of doctors and nurses capable of delivering high quality flexible sigmoidoscopy and colonoscopy.

References

1. Gatta G, Capocaccia R, Sant M *et al*. Understanding variations in survival for colorectal cancer in Europe: a EUROCARE high resolution study. *Gut* 2000; **47**: 533–538.

2. Muto T, Bussey H, Morson B. The evolution of cancer of the colon and rectum. *Cancer* 1975; **36**: 2251–2270.

3. Vogelstein B, Fearon E, Hamilton S *et al*. Genetic alterations during colorectal-tumor development. *N Engl J Med* 1988; **319**: 525–532.

4. Atkin W, Morson B, Cuzick J. Long-term risk of colorectal cancer after excision of rectosigmoid adenomas. *N Engl J Med* 1992; **326**: 658–662.

5. Stryker S, Wolff B, Culp C, Libbe S, Ilstrup D, MacCarty R. Natural history of untreated colonic polyps. *Gastroenterology* 1987; **93**: 1009–1013.

6. Rembacken B, Fujii T, Cairns A *et al*. Flat and depressed colonic neoplasms: a prospective study of 1000 colonoscopies in the UK. *Lancet* 2000; **355**: 1211–1214.

7. Dunlop M, Farrington S, Carothers A *et al*. Cancer risk associated with germline DNA mismatch repair gene-mutations. *Hum Mol Genet* 1997; **6**: 105–110.

8. Itzkowitz S. Inflammatory bowel-disease and cancer. *Gastroenterol Clin North Am* 1997; **26**: 129–139.

9. John DS, McDermott F, Hopper J, Debney E, Johnson W, Hughes E. Cancer risk in relatives of patients with common colorectal cancer. *Ann Intern Med* 1993; **118**: 785–790.

10. Atkin W and UK Flexible Sigmoidoscopy Screening Trial Investigators. Single flexible sigmoidoscopy screening to prevent colorectal cancer; baseline findings of a UK multicentre randomised trial. *Lancet* 2002; **359**: 1291–1300.

11. Hardcastle J, Chamberlain J, Robinson M *et al*. Randomised controlled trial of faecal-occult-blood screening for colorectal cancer. *Lancet* 1996; **348**: 1472–1477.

12. Cotton P, Williams C. *Practical Gastrointestinal Endoscopy*, 4th edn. London: Blackwell Science; 1999.

13. Winawer S, Zauber A, O'Brien M, Ho M, Gottlieb L, Sternberg S. Randomized comparison of surveillance intervals after colonoscopic removal of newly diagnosed adenomatous polyps. *N Engl J Med* 1993; **328**: 901–906.

14. Rex D, Cutler C, Lemmel G *et al*. Colonoscopic miss rates and adenomas determined by back-to-back colonoscopies. *Gastroenterology* 1997; **112**: 24–28.

15. Ahlquist D, Wieand H, Moertal C *et al*. Accuracy of fecal occult blood screening for colorectal neoplasia: a prospective study using Hemoccult and Hemoquant. *J Am Med Assoc* 1993; **269**: 1262–1267.

16. Kronborg O, Fenger C, Olsen J, Jorgensen O, Sondergaard O. Randomised study of screening for colorectal cancer with faecal-occult-blood test. *Lancet* 1996; **348**: 1467–1471.

17. Mandel J, Bond J, Church T, Snover D, Bradley M, Schuman L. Reducing mortality from colorectal cancer by screening for fecal occult blood. *N Engl J Med* 1993; **328**: 1365–1371.

18. Mandel J, Church T, Ederer F, Bond J. Colorectal cancer mortality: effectiveness of biennial screening for fecal occult blood. *J Natl Cancer Inst* 1999; **91**: 434–437.

19. Jorgensen O, Kronborg O, Fenger C. A randomised study of screening for colorectal cancer using faecal occult blood testing: results after 13 years and seven biennial screening rounds. *Gut* 2002; **50**: 29–32.

20. Mandel J, Church T, Bond J *et al*. The effect of fecal occult blood screening on the incidence of colorectal cancer. *N Engl J Med* 2000; **343**: 1603–1607.

21. Lang C, Ransohoff D. Fecal occult blood screening for colorectal cancer: is mortality reduced by chance selection for screening colonoscopy? *JAMA* 1994; **271**: 1011–1013.

22. Selby J, Friedman G, Quesenberry C, Weiss N. Effect of fecal occult blood testing on mortality from colorectal cancer. A case-control study. *Ann Intern Med* 1993; **118**: 1–6.

23. Saito H. Screening for colorectal-cancer by immunochemical fecal occult blood testing. *Jpn J Cancer Res* 1996; **87**: 1011–1024.

24. Steele R, Parker R, Patnick J *et al*. A demonstration pilot trial for colorectal cancer screening in the United Kingdom: a new concept in the introduction of healthcare strategies. *J Med Screen* 2001; **8**: 197–203.

25. Atkin W, Cuzick J, Northover J, Whynes D. Prevention of colorectal cancer by once-only sigmoidoscopy. *Lancet* 1993; **341**: 736–740.

26. Selby J, Friedman Jr G, Weiss N. A case-control study of screening sigmoidoscopy and mortality from colorectal cancer. *N Engl J Med* 1992; **326**: 653–657.

27. Newcomb P, Norfleet R, Storer B, Surawicz S, Marcus P. Screening sigmoidoscopy and colorectal cancer mortality. *J Natl Cancer Inst* 1992; **84**: 1572–1575.

28. Muller A, Sonnenberg A. Prevention of colorectal cancer by flexible endoscopy and polypectomy. A case-controlled study of 32,702 veterans. *Ann Intern Med* 1995; **123**: 904–910.

29. Atkin W, Edwards R, Wardle J *et al*. Design of a multicentre randomised trial to evaluate flexible sigmoidoscopy in colorectal cancer screening. *J Med Screen* 2001; **8**: 137–144.

30. Segnan N, Senore C, Andreoni B *et al*. Baseline findings of the Italian Multicenter Randomized Controlled Trial of Once-Only Sigmoidoscopy – SCORE. *J Natl Cancer Inst* 2002; **94**: 1763–1772.

31. Prorok P, Andriole G, Bresalier R *et al*. Design of the Prostate, Lung, Colorectal and Ovarian (PLCO) Cancer Screening Trial. *Controlled Clin Trials* 2000; **21 (6 Suppl)**: 273S–309S.

32. US Preventive Services Task Force. Screening for colorectal cancer: recommendation and rationale. *Ann Intern Med* 2002; **137**: 129–131.

33. Levin T, Palitz A. Flexible sigmoidoscopy; an important screening option for average-risk individuals. *Gastrointest Endosc Clin North Am* 2002; **12**: 23–40.

34. Inciardi J, Lee J, Stijnen T. Incidence trends for colorectal cancer in California: implications for current screening practices. *Am J Med* 2000; **109**: 277–281.

35. Lieberman D, Weiss D, Bond J, Ahnen D, Garewal H, Chejfec G. Use of colonoscopy to screen asymptomatic adults for colorectal cancer. *N Engl J Med* 2000; **343**: 162–168.

36. Schoenfeld P, Piorkowski M, Allaire J, Ernst R, Holmes L. Flexible sigmoidoscopy by nurses: state of the art 1999. *Gastroenterol Nurs* 1999; **22**: 254–261.

37. Winawer S, Stewart E, Zauber A *et al*. A comparison of colonoscopy and double-contrast barium enema for surveillance after polypectomy. *N Engl J Med* 2000; **342**: 1766–1772.

38. Vining D, Gelfand D, Bechtold R, Scharing E, Grishaw E, Shifrin R. Technical feasibility of colon imaging with helical CT and virtual reality. *AJR Am J Roentgenol* 1994; **162 (Suppl)**: 104.

39. Fenlon H. Virtual colonoscopy. *Br J Surg* 2002; **89**: 1–3.

40. Ahlquist D, Skoletsky J, Boynton K *et al*. Colorectal cancer screening by detection of altered human DNA in stool: feasibility of a multitarget assay panel. *Gastroenterology* 2000; **119**: 1219–1227.

41. Rengucci C, Maiolo P, Saragoni L, Zoli W, Amadori D, Calistri D. Multiple detection of genetic alterations in tumors and stool. *Clin Cancer Res* 2001; **7**: 590–593.

42. Dong S, Traverso G, Johnson C *et al*. Detecting colorectal cancer in stool with the use of multiple genetic targets. *J Natl Cancer Inst* 2001; **93**: 858–865.

43. Wherry D, Thomas W. The yield of flexible fiberoptic sigmoidoscopy in the detection of asymptomatic colorectal neoplasia. *Surg Endosc* 1994; **8**: 393–395.

44. Thiis-Evensen E, Hoff G, Sauar J, Langmark F, Majak B, Vatn M. Population-based surveillance by colonoscopy: effect on the incidence of colorectal cancer. Telemark Polyp Study I. *Scand J Gastroenterol* 1999; **34**: 414–420.

45. Verne J, Aubrey R, Love S, Talbot I, Northover J. Population based randomised study of uptake and yield of screening by flexible sigmoidoscopy compared with screening by faecal occult blood testing. *BMJ* 1998; **317**: 182–185.

46. Foley D, Dunne P, Dervan P, Callaghan T, Crowe J, Lennon J. Left-sided colonoscopy and Haemoccult screening for colorectal neoplasia. *Eur J Gastroenterol Hepatol* 1992; **4**: 925–936.

47. Rex D, Lehman G, Hawes R, Ulbright T, Smith J. Screening colonoscopy in asymptomatic average-risk persons with negative fecal occult blood tests. *Gastroenterology* 1991; **100**: 64–67.

48. CDC. Trends in screening for colorectal cancer – United States, 1997 and 1999. *MMWR* 2001; **50**: 162–166.

49. Anderson M, Pasha T, Leighton J. Endoscopic perforation of the colon: lessons from a 10-year study. *Am J Gastroenterol* 2000; **95**: 3418–3422.

50. Waye J, Kahn O, Auerbach M. Complications of colonoscopy and flexible sigmoidoscopy. *Gastrointest Endosc Clin North Am* 1996; **6**: 343–377.

51. Karsenti D, Metman E, Viguier J *et al*. Transmission of hepatitis C virus by colonoscopy: study of 97 'presumed' risk patients. *Gastroenterol Clin Biol* 1999; **23**: 985–986.

52. Eckardt V, Kanzler G, Schmitt T, Eckardt A, Bernhard G. Complications and adverse effects of colonoscopy with selective sedation. *Gastrointest Endosc* 1999; **49**: 560–565.

Simon G. Darke

10

Management of recurrent varicose veins

DEFINITION AND INCIDENCE

Recurrent varicose veins are regarded here as those that follow surgery directed towards the sapheno-femoral or popliteal junction. This is in distinction to those occurring after injection sclerotherapy or simple multiple surgical avulsions. Within this definition remain vagaries depending on from whose perspective varicose veins are deemed to have 'recurred' – patient, surgeon, or independent observer. Additionally, recurrence may be influenced by the manner in which the patient has been followed up after primary surgery. In some countries, such as France for instance, this is prospective and systematic with pre-emptive intervention at the first sign of further problems. By such an approach, 'recurrence' is less likely to occur.

But these considerations aside, within the UK the results remain disappointing for clinician and patient alike. Whether followed up systematically after surgery[1–5] or new patients referred for further advice,[6,7] the incidence is ~15–20% within 3–5 years. This remains the case even if primary surgery is ostensibly optimised with pre-operative evaluation using duplex scanning and saphenous trunk stripping.[8,9]

These indifferent results have obvious resource implications and raise the question as to why recurrences occur.

Key point 1

- Recurrence in a proportion (~20%) of patients undergoing even well planned and executed primary varicose vein surgery is inevitable.

Mr Simon G. Darke MS FRCS, Consultant Surgeon, The Royal Bournemouth Hospital, Castle Lane East, Bournemouth BH7 7DW, UK

Table 1 Morphology of recurrent varicose veins

Limbs studied	95
Recurrent sapheno-femoral reflux	46
Recurrent sapheno-popliteal reflux	10
Multiple perforators	29
Emergence of sapheno-popliteal	9
Emergence of sapheno-femoral	1

MORPHOLOGY OF RECURRENCE

Consecutive patients referred for further treatment of recurrent varicose veins were comprehensively assessed with ascending and descending venography and ultrasonography.[7] By these means, it was possible to identify three main types of recurrence (Table 1).

1. Recurrence through a previously ligated saphenous junction (usually the sapheno-femoral, less often sapheno-popliteal).

2. Emergence through multiple perforating veins usually in thigh and calf (less frequently from the pelvis).

3. Emergence (persistence) through a previously unoperated saphenous system (usually the short saphenous).

Although this last group, as such, might not be considered true recurrence, it is included for completeness.

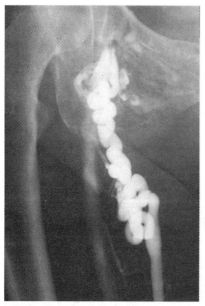

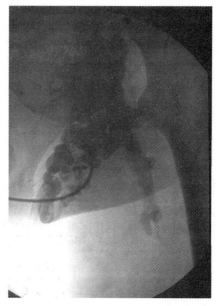

Fig. 1 Sapheno-femoral neovascularisation with persistent long saphenous trunk. Reproduced from Darke[7] with permission from WB Saunders.

Fig. 2 Extensive groin neovascularisation with no LSV trunk.

Table 2 Morphology of recurrent sapheno-femoral reflux

Total recurrent sapheno-femoral reflux	47
Neovascularisation	28
Missed/untied tributary	4
Incompetent SFV with thigh per.	9
Combined	4

RECURRENT SAPHENO-FEMORAL REFLUX

The results (Table 2) show that recurrence through the sapheno-femoral junction is the major contributor to the problem. In turn, this raises the question as to why this should be so. By means of descending venography, it was possible to identify three main types of recurrent sapheno-femoral reflux.

1. The development of new reconstituted veins by means of a process of neovascularisation. This has typical features of multiple serpentine vessels usually, but not always, linking to a persistent or accessory saphenous trunk (Figs 1 & 2). This important aspect is considered in more detail below.

2. A missed tributary at the time of the original surgery (Fig. 3).

3. Reflux down an incompetent superficial femoral vein and thigh perforator (Fig. 4). Explicitly, this is in the 'multiple perforator' group, but is included here because it is indistinguishable on continuous wave Doppler at the time of initial clinical evaluation (see below).

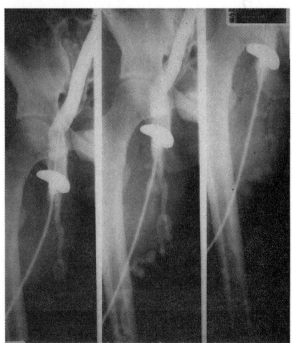

Fig. 3 Recurrent groin recurrence – untied tributary. Reproduced from Darke[7] with permission from WB Saunders.

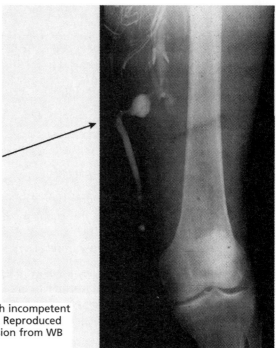

Fig. 4 Recurrence through incompetent SFV and thigh perforator. Reproduced from Darke[7] with permission from WB Saunders.

NEOVASCULARISATION

This concept remains controversial because it challenges the long-held assertion that the principal cause of groin recurrence is technical error. Some would argue that neovascularisation occurs only rarely, if at all, and that the principal reason for recurrence through the sapheno-femoral junction is due to untied tributaries or branches at the time of the original surgery. If this is correct, then meticulous dissection at the sapheno-femoral junction at the time of primary surgery should largely eradicate the problem of groin recurrence, which manifestly is not the case. On the other hand, if neovascularisation is the cause, then it may be that no matter how painstaking the primary procedure, some recurrences are inevitable. Furthermore, as discussed below, no matter how thoroughly the femoral vein is further explored for recurrence, there remains the risk that it will happen yet again. So the distinction is of more than simply academic significance.

Historical observations and the evidence for neovascularisation

The observation that the sapheno-femoral junction might reconstitute itself is not new and was first made by Langenbeck, arguably the father of venous

---

Key point 2

- The capacity to recur seems to be idiosyncratic and predisposes to further recurrence.

surgery. In 1861, he wrote:

> In one case of very large varix of the great saphena in a young man I had extirpated an enlarged vein in the length of three inches and ligated the upper and lower ends. One year later I found, in the region of the scar tissue of the extirpation, a new vein channel of the thickness of the quill of a crow's feather, which again joined the both ends of the full functioning remaining saphena.[10]

Thirty years later, Perthes reported a case on whom he had operated 5 years previously:

> A small packet at the site of ligature was extirpated and showed on examination several vessels extended downward from the dilated central end of the saphena. This ended for the most part in a type of blind sac; but one, the thickest, circled closely the site of ligation and communicated with the also dilated peripheral end of the saphena. It was therefore the renewal of the old observation of Langenbeck, who observed that the trunk of the vena saphena magna regenerated itself after a varix extirpation.[11]

Surgery at the time, of course, was confined to relatively crude saphenous ligation below the groin. Subsequently, Homans introduced accurate and anatomical dissection of the sapheno-femoral junction with explicit ligation of all local tributaries.[12] With this came the alternative view that recurrence was largely due to missed veins, which prevailed for many years.[5,13,14]

More recently, the concept of neovascularisation was re-introduced by Sheppard in 1978.[6] He argued that experienced surgeons knew the original surgery had been complete which was evident at 're-do' surgery by the scarring. He attributed 90% of recurrent varicose veins to further sapheno-femoral incompetence where flush ligation had been performed previously, many personally. He also postulated the phenomenon of re-recurrence supported by histological data. This phenomenon, of yet further recurrence, has since been reported by others[7] and is discussed further below under how it might be avoided at the time of 're-do' surgery.

Starnes, in 1984, supported these views based on venography, which was stated to show: 'a type of recurrence which can occur even after skilful high ligation, and ascribing all thigh recurrences to a missed venous branch at the time of high ligation is too simple an explanation'.[15]

Subsequently, Glass has contributed clinical and animal reports that have shed further light,[16–19] including 10 patients in whom he ligated and excised a segment of incompetent long saphenous to promote healing of ulceration. At a varying time after initial ligation, further excision of the entire saphenous system was undertaken including the area previously ligated. Histological data on these serial specimens showed that 2 weeks after transection the gap filled with thrombus into which small blood vessels grew. Over ensuing weeks these aligned. Within a year, they coalesced and enlarged, sometimes into a single trunk with muscle and elastin in their walls resembling mature veins.[16]

More recent prospective studies with duplex scanning have demonstrated the development of serpentine neovascularised recurrences following primary surgery shown to be technically comprehensive at postoperative imaging.[20,21] Similar studies further underscore these duplex-based data which will be described below in experience of various operative techniques to reduce re-recurrence.

So the concept of 'neovascularisation' has been with us for many years, although dormant for nearly a century. The more recent evidence, based on clinical observation, histological studies, animal experimentation and now compelling prospective duplex studies would seem to put the issue beyond dispute. It is strange, though commendable, that surgeons are more ready to attribute blame to technical inadequacy than nature's caprice.

It has to be conceded that an element of both forms of recurrence occur; indeed, in some patients there may be a combination of the two. If a tributary or saphenous stump is left at the junction, which expands and becomes tortuous and links by neovascularisation with distal varicosities, then an element of both has occurred.

> **Key point 3**
> - Three main morphological types of recurrence can be identified: (i) recurrent sapheno-femoral (popliteal) incompetence; (ii) multiple perforators; and (iii) emergence through a new saphenous system (not strictly recurrence).

CLINICAL EXAMINATION

HISTORY

As has been stated, the development of recurrences seems to signal that this may happen again. Important features in this respect are early age of onset of the original varicose veins suggestive of a strong inherent tendency, as is a family history. Rapid recurrence, particularly after ostensibly comprehensive original surgery, is similarly a sign of such a predisposition. These factors have to be born in mind when considering further intervention and counselling the patient.

Because of the potential complexities with further intervention and the significant possibilities of further recurrence, a clear understanding of what is worrying the patient should be established. Often, all that is required is re-assurance. Concerns may be purely cosmetic. It is the author's impression that aching and discomfort seem to be relatively less common than in primary varicose veins perhaps because saphenous reflux if re-established is in attenuated form. Skin changes and ulceration when present do not seem to benefit from surgery to recurrences.[22] So the indications for further intervention may be relative and limited.

> **Key point 4**
> - Of these, sapheno-femoral recurrence is the most prevalent and important and is principally due to the process of neovascularisation (as opposed to missed branches due to error at the time of primary surgery).

EXAMINATION

Useful information on clinical examination can be determined from continuous wave Doppler (CWD). It can be employed by adapting the principles for primary varicose veins, which have been described in detail elsewhere.[23] Briefly, the presence of recurrent sapheno-femoral reflux is demonstrated by a positive cough signal on insonating over a convenient distal varicosity. As mentioned above, however, this will not distinguish reflux down an incompetent superficial femoral vein and thigh perforator into the insonated varix.

New or recurrent reflux at the popliteal fossa also needs to be checked by the standard calf squeeze release. In the absence of any demonstrable reflux from either of these sites, the likely morphology is one of simple multiple perforators.

INVESTIGATION

More detailed investigations are usually necessary if further intervention is contemplated especially in the presence of recurrent saphenous reflux. If this is not present and a simple tidy up by avulsions for isolated perforators is contemplated, further imaging is usually still necessary otherwise this runs the risk of leaving behind an undetected and significant residual saphenous trunk (see below).

In the majority of cases, adequate information can be acquired with duplex ultrasound scanning, but in complex or difficult cases particularly regarding unusual deep connections such as the pelvis or the deep femoral vein, there

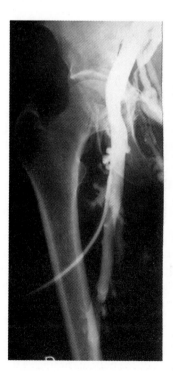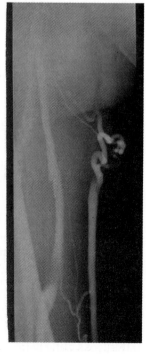

Fig. 5 Pelvic recurrence re-filling a persistent long saphenous trunk.

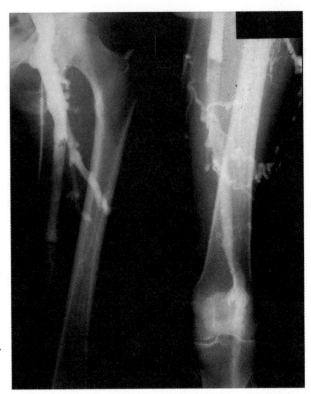

Fig. 6 Recurrence from distal deep femoral vein. Reproduced from Darke[7] with permission from WB Saunders.

may still be a need for varicography or venography (Figs 5 & 6). The relative use of these two generally complementary tools may be dictated by availability of local expertise.

The essential aspects, which need to be determined, are: (i) the type of recurrence that exists as defined above; (ii) if there is recurrent reflux from the sapheno-femoral or popliteal junction, the size and complexity of this needs to be estimated (see below); and (iii) presence and size of any residual or accessory saphenous trunks.

Armed with this information, a management strategy can be devised. Surgery should be tailored and its extent proportional to the patient's needs, anticipated benefit and risk. It should take into account the risks of further recurrence.

OPERATIVE STRATEGIES

RE-EXPLORATION OF THE SAPHENO-FEMORAL JUNCTION

It will be apparent from the above that in practical terms this represents the principal technical target when operating for recurrent varicose veins. It can be a challenging procedure and is not for the inexperienced, unsupervised trainee surgeon. For anyone, an assistant, sucker and vascular instruments may be advisable.

Incision

The key is to find the common femoral vein above the reconstituted junction. If this looks difficult (as in the obese patient) or where the tortuous recurrences

Key point 5

- Re-intervention is worthwhile, but should be planned and requires pre-operative imaging. Religation of saphenous recurrence, residual saphenous trunk stripping and multiple avulsions, in varying combinations are the principal tools.

are billowing up high into the groin, it may be better to make a new, relatively vertical incision sited just medial to the femoral artery pulsation. In less complex cases, it is possible through the old wound, but this can be more difficult especially if it takes you straight into the fragile subcutaneous varices.

Dissecting the reformed junction
The femoral vein can best be found as it exits from under the inguinal ligament, which is usually relatively virgin territory. Follow the vein down whence the re-established junction will start to come into view. Dissect down each side of this and then establish the lower border dissecting it free from what is now the superficial femoral vein below it. Place a vascular clamp onto its origin from the femoral vein and dissect it off. The femoral vein may need direct suturing with 5/0 or 6/0 vascular suture. The femoral vein should be completely clean of any tributaries.

Any residual saphenous trunk should now be removed (see below). If not evident, then the distal complex of varicosities should be oversewn.

Preventing further recurrence
What are the risks of all this happening again and can any additional manoeuvre be employed to prevent further neovascularisation? Sheppard was the first to address these issues, recognising the significant risks of further recurrence, and suggested that a flap of reflected pectineus muscle fascia might be mobilised and rotated to cover the denuded common femoral vein to act as a physical barrier.[6] This is easily performed because this fascia is now exposed medially and a rectangle of suitable size is readily mobilised to this effect. In a study to test the effectiveness of this procedure, 34 patients undergoing re-exploration of the groin for symptomatic recurrence were randomised to receive a pectineus patch/no patch after the femoral vein had been comprehensively isolated from all neovascularised recurrences. Patients were followed up by duplex ultrasound examination a minimum of 18 months later. The results showed that there were no apparent advantages of the patch and most patients were already showing further recurrence at that stage (11/17 patch, 13/17 no patch).[24] From this two important conclusions can be drawn. In time, most of these patients in whom neovascularisation has already occurred will do so again. Secondly, there seems little to gain in using a mechanical barrier with autogenous material.

What about the possibility of prosthetic material used in a similar manner? Initial experience with polytetrafluoroethylene (PTFE) on a mixture of primary and recurrent varicose veins showed similarly little benefit and once again a tendency for those that had already recurred to do so yet again.[25] However,

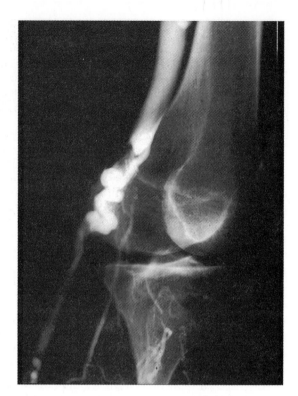

Fig. 7 Recurrent short saphenous with typical neovascularisation. Reproduced from Darke[29] with permission from Springer.

from the same department, Bhatti and colleagues subsequently studied the outcome of patching with PTFE on patients with established neovascularised recurrence similar to the group described above. However, there was no control group. Although recurrences did occur and some big, the overall incidence was only 12%. This seems to be less than the patients treated with the pectineus patch,[26] but the criteria for recurrence (length of follow-up and other factors) make comparisons of uncertain significance This is worthy of a formalised controlled trial. At the moment, therefore, there is no proven means of preventing further neovascularisation.

Recurrent sapheno-popliteal incompetence

As a broad statement, anything that can be said about the sapheno-femoral junction applies equally to this site. Strikingly similar images of neovascularisation occur (Fig. 7) and the problem is probably exacerbated by the particular technical difficulties in identifying and ligating the sapheno-popliteal junction, and the reluctance to strip the short saphenous trunk because of concerns of injury to the sural nerve at the time of primary surgery.[22,26–28] Re-exploration of this junction can be even more difficult and hazardous due to the close proximity of other vital structures. Nonetheless, technically satisfactory results can be achieved with careful dissection.

Merits of groin re-exploration

In a young, fit patient with symptoms with large recurrences and a persistent saphenous trunk (Fig. 1), there would seem to be little doubt that re-exploration

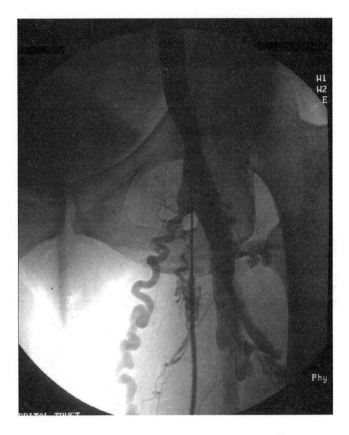

Fig. 8 Minor vessel neovascularisation; re-exploration seldom justified.

is likely to be worthwhile. But this of course is not always the case. Sometimes, the neovascularised recurrences are trivial (Fig. 8) and the extent of surgery required to expose them disproportionate to impact of re-ligation. This is why pre-operative duplex evaluation of the size and extent of the recurrences is so important. Similarly, in older patients, bearing in mind the risks of yet further recurrence, re-exploration may simply not be justified.

Removing the residual saphenous trunk

By and large, if re-intervention is contemplated and a significantly large and incompetent residual or accessory saphenous trunk has been identified on the pre-operative duplex, then it should be stripped. These were found to be present in over half of all forms of recurrence.[7] It may be worthwhile marking this distally immediately prior to surgery with Doppler because it less easy to cannulate and strip from above down in the re-explored groin because it terminates in the multiple serpiginous neovascularised vessels. Where a decision has been made to leave the groin (see above), a useful and easy compromise is to pass the stripper from below up, jamming it in the groin below the tortuous neovascularised varicosities, making a small incision and pulling it out. This can be a useful compromise (Fig. 9) Other segments of

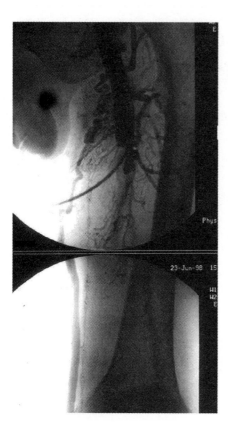

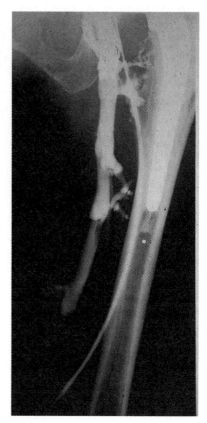

Fig. 9 Minor neovascularisation but persistent long saphenous trunk. Ideal for limited LSV strip.

Fig. 10 Multiple thigh perforators. Generally too inaccessible to justify flush deep ligation. Reproduced from Darke[29] with permission from Springer.

residual or accessory vein in the thigh can be similarly managed.

If the short saphenous trunk is to be stripped, it might best be done by the inversion technique because this may cause less risk to the sural nerve.

Sometimes the below-knee, long saphenous trunk may be a focus for recurrences and worthy of removal.

Multiple perforator recurrence

Perforators are usually multiple, relatively small and inaccessible (Fig. 10). It is seldom judicious to explore and flush ligate these at their origins from the deep system. The dissection required is usually disproportionate to any benefits. These patients can be treated by simple multiple avulsions, although by and large this is principally a cosmetic exercise and further recurrence is likely in view of the track record and the pragmatic decision to leave the deep origins essentially intact. Residual saphenous trunks may be a factor and should be removed as described above.

Key points for clinical practice

- Recurrence in a proportion (~20%) of patients undergoing even well planned and executed primary varicose vein surgery is inevitable.

- Recurrence The capacity to recur seems to be idiosyncratic and predisposes to further recurrence.

- Recurrence Three main morphological types of recurrence can be identified: (i) recurrent sapheno-femoral (popliteal) incompetence; (ii) multiple perforators; and (iii) emergence through a new saphenous system (not strictly recurrence).

- Recurrence Of these, sapheno-femoral recurrence is the most prevalent and important and is principally due to the process of neovascularisation (as opposed to missed branches due to error at the time of primary surgery).

- Recurrence Re-intervention is worthwhile, but should be planned and requires pre-operative imaging. Religation of saphenous recurrence, residual saphenous trunk stripping and multiple avulsions, in varying combinations are the principal tools.

- Recurrence The nature of the surgery should be kept proportionate to the patient's problems and to what it is likely to achieve, both immediately and in the long-term.

References

1. Hobbs JT. Surgery and sclerotherapy in the treatment of varicose veins. *Arch Surg* 1974; **109**: 793–796.
2. Jakobsen BH. The value of different forms of treatment for varicose veins. *Br J Surg* 1979; **66**: 182–184.
3. Royle JP. Recurrent varicose veins. *World Surg* 1986; **10**: 944–953.
4. Berridge DC, Makin GS. Day case surgery: a viable alternative for surgical treatment of varicose veins. *Phlebology* 1987; **2**: 103–108.
5. Lofgren EP. Treatment of long saphenous varicosities and their recurrence. A long term follow up. In: Bergan JJ, Yao JST. (eds) *Surgery of the Veins*. London: Grune & Stratton, 1985; 285–300.
6. Sheppard M. A procedure for the prevention of recurrent sapheno-femoral incompetence. *Aust NZ J Surg* 1978; **48**: 322–326.
7. Darke SG. The morphology of recurrent varicose veins. *Eur J Vasc Surg* 1992; **6**: 512–517.
8. Rutgers PH, Kitslaar PJ. Randomised trial of stripping versus high ligation combined with sclerotherapy in the treatment of the incompetent greater saphenous vein. *Am J Surg* 1994; **168**: 311–315.
9. Dwerryhouse S, Davies B, Harradine K, Earnshaw JJ. Stripping the long saphenous vein reduces the rate of reoperation for recurrent varicose veins: five year results of a randomised trial. *J Vasc Surg* 1999; **29**: 589–592.
10. Von Langenbeck B. Beirtrage zur chirurgischen Pathologie der Venen. *Arch Klin Chir* 1861; **1**: 1–80.
11. Perthes G. Ueber die Operatio Unterschenkel varicen nac: Trendelenburg. *Dtsch Med Wochenshr* 1895; **21**: 255–257.
12. Homans J. The operative treatment of varicose veins and ulcers, based upon a classification of these lesions. *Surg Gynecol Obstet* 1916; **22**: 143–158.

13. Edwards EA. Anatomical factors of ligation of the great saphenous veins. *Surg Gynecol Obstet* 1934; **59**: 916–928.

14. Dodd H, Cockett FB. *The Pathology and Surgery of Veins of the Lower Limb*. Edinburgh: E & S Livingstone, 1956.

15. Starnes HF, Vallance R, Hamilton DNH. Recurrent varicose veins. A radiological approach to investigation. *Clin Radiol* 1984; **35**: 95–99.

16. Glass GM. Neovascularisation in recurrence of the varicose great saphenous vein following transection. *Phlebology* 1987; **2**: 81–91.

17. Glass GM. Neovascularisation in restoration of continuity of the not femoral vein following surgical interruption. *Phlebology* 1987; **2**: 1–6.

18. Glass GM. Neovascularisation in recurrent varices of the great saphenous vein in the groin, phlebography. *Angiology* 1988; **39**: 577–582.

19. Glass GM. Prevention of recurrent sapheno-femoral incompetence after surgery for varicose veins. *Br J Surg* 1989; **76**: 1210.

20. Sarin S, Scurr JH, Coleridge-Smith PD. Stripping of the long saphenous vein in the treatment of primary varicose veins. *Br J Surg* 1994; **81**: 1455–1458.

21. Jones L, Braithwaite BD, Selwyn D, Cooke S, Earnshaw JJ. Neovascularisation is the principal cause of varicose vein recurrence. Results of a randomised trial of stripping the long saphenous vein. *Eur J Vasc Endovasc Surg* 1996; **12**: 442–445.

22. Darke SG. Recurrent varicose veins and short saphenous insufficiency: evaluation and treatment. In: Bergan JJ, Yao JST. (eds) *Venous Disorders*. Philadelphia, PA: WB Saunders, 1991; 217–232.

22. Darke SG, Vetrivel S, Foy DMA, Smith S, Baker S. A comparison of duplex scanning and continuous wave Doppler in the assessment of primary and uncomplicated varicose veins. *Eur J Vasc Endovasc Surg* 1997; **14**: 457–461.

23. Gibbs PJ, Foy DMA, Darke SG. Reoperation for recurrent saphenofemoral incompetence: a prospective randomised trial using a reflected flap of pectineus fascia. *Eur J Vasc Endovasc Surg* 1999; **18**: 494–498.

24. Earnshaw JJ, Davies B, Harradine K, Heather BP. Preliminary results of PTFE patch saphenoplasty to prevent neovascularisation leading to recurrent varicose veins. *Phlebology* 1998; **13**: 10–13.

25. Bhatti TS, Whitman B, Harradine K, Cooke G, Heather BP, Earnshaw JJ. Causes of re-recurrence after polytetrafluoroethylene patch saphenoplasty for recurrent varicose veins. *Br J Surg* 2000; **87**: 1356–1360.

26. Dodd H The varicose tributaries of the popliteal vein. *Br J Surg* 1965; **52**: 350–354.

27. Tong Y, Royle J. Recurrent varicose veins after short saphenous surgery: a duplex ultrasound study. *Cardiovasc Surg* 1996; **4**: 364.

28. Moosman DA, Hartwell SW. The surgical significance of the subfascial course of the lesser saphenous vein. *Surg Gynecol Obstet* 1964; **113**: 761–766.

29. Darke SG. Recurrent varices. In: Ballard JL, Bergan JJ. (eds) *Chronic Venous Insufficiency: Diagnosis and Treatment*. London: Springer, 2000; 86–90

Constantinos Kyriakides John H.N. Wolfe

11

Management of mycotic aortic aneurysms

Mycotic aortic aneurysms present a surgical challenge and are associated with a high morbidity and mortality. They constitute an uncommon heterogeneous pathological entity with a reported incidence of 1–3% of all abdominal aortic aneurysms.[1] In 1885, William Osler described a 30-year-old man who died after a period of diarrhoea, chills, headache, cough and fever. Post mortem examination revealed an aortic valve consumed with vegetations and, in the aortic arch, four aneurysms had developed as a consequence of endocarditis. These represented a case of mycotic endarteritis and the largest of these aneurysms had perforated and ruptured into the pericardium. Thus, the term mycotic aneurysm was introduced which is somewhat misleading as the majority of aortic infections nowadays are bacterial; consequently, some authors prefer to use the term 'infected aneurysm'.[2,3]

AETIOLOGY

The aetiology remains unclear although it is thought that bacteraemia and embolisation of infectious material into diseased atherosclerotic aortic wall may result in mycotic aneurysm formation. Rarely, bacteria through the vasa vasorum may colonise the intact vascular wall creating a suppurative process that leads to saccular aneurysm formation. In addition, an extravascular focus such as vertebral osteomyelitis may penetrate the aortic wall directly or through lymphatic tissue leading to necrosis and false aneurysm formation. Also, false aneurysm formation may occur as a result of direct arterial trauma with a contaminated instrument.[4–8]

Mr Constantinos Kyriakides MD FRCS, Senior Clinical Vascular Fellow, Regional Vascular Unit, St Mary's Hospital, Praed Street, London W2 1NY, UK

Mr John H.N. Wolfe MS FRCS, Consultant Vascular Surgeon, Regional Vascular Unit, St Mary's Hospital, Praed Street, London W2 1NY, UK (for correspondence)

Over the past 50 years, there has been a change in the aetiology of mycotic aneurysms. Since the introduction of antibiotics, endocarditis as a source of bacteraemia has become rare, and several risk factors for mycotic aneurysms, especially in the elderly, are currently more common. These include diagnostic and therapeutic arterial catheterisations, previous operations in remote sites, and suppressed immunocompetence secondary to chronic neoplastic disease, administration of cytotoxic agents and corticosteroids.[9]

The predominant micro-organisms associated with mycotic aortic aneurysms are *Staphylococcus* spp. (30%), *Streptococcus* spp. (10%), and *Salmonella* spp. (10%).[10] Fungal infections are rare and usually associated with immunosuppressive states, diabetes mellitus, and the use of contaminated needles by drug abusers.[8] In South Africa, HIV is now the commonest cause.[11]

Key point 1

- Mycotic aortic aneurysms have a tendency for rapid expansion and early rupture.

PRESENTATION AND DIAGNOSIS

In comparison to non-infected aortic aneurysms, mycotic aneurysms are more likely to be symptomatic with up to three-quarters of patients presenting with abdominal, back, or thoracic back pain, depending whether they are infra- or supra-diaphragmatic (Fig. 1). The majority present with pyrexia, a raised white cell count, and up to 50% may have positive blood cultures.[3]

Radiographic studies are of great value in the diagnosis and planning of the operation. CT imaging may reveal a number of features which, along with the

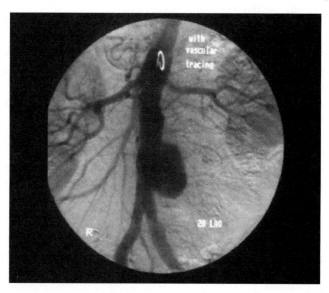

Fig. 1 Angiogram showing a localised saccular aneurysm (blow-out) of the aortic wall – typical appearance of a mycotic aneurysm.

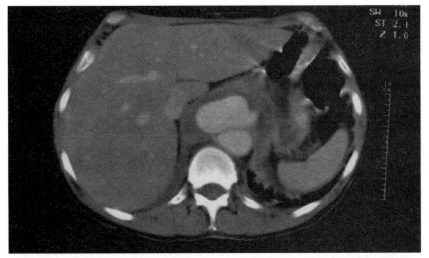

Fig. 2 Double lumen appearance of a saccular mycotic aneurysm of the supra-renal aorta.

Key point 2

- Clinical features usually include pyrexia, abdominal, back or chest pain.

Key point 3

- Blood cultures are positive in 50% of cases.

---

clinical findings, should point to the diagnosis of a mycotic aneurysm (Fig. 2). These include: (i) rapid expansion of a known aneurysm or a newly developed aneurysm; (ii) gas in the aortic wall; (iii) extravasation of contrast in the peri-aortic tissues; (iv) a saccular aneurysm; or (v) a soft tissue mass surrounding the aorta often accompanied by calcified atherosclerotic plaque.[6,12] MRI can also be of use in a similar fashion as CT.[13] Aortography may reveal a saccular, eccentric, or multilobulated appearance in an otherwise normal aorta.

Intra-operative findings may include evidence of gross contamination and sepsis with abscess formation. These should be distinguished from asymptomatic aneurysms in which bacteria are found incidentally in up to 15% of cases on routine thrombus culture.[3]

Key point 4

- CT, MRI and aortography are the radiological investigations of choice.

OPERATIVE MANAGEMENT

Because mycotic aortic aneurysms have a tendency for rapid expansion, this can often lead to rupture before operative intervention.[2] Once the diagnosis of a mycotic aortic aneurysm is made, antibiotic therapy and urgent surgical resection is indicated.

Controversy exists as to the best operative option for infrarenal mycotic aortic aneurysms. Some authors advocate proximal and distal arterial ligation, aneurysm resection with thorough debridement of surrounding infected tissues and extra-anatomic bypass in the form of either an axillo-bifemoral or two axillo-unifemoral grafts.[14–18] The risks of this approach include aortic stump rupture and a higher risk of thrombosis of the extra-anatomical bypass graft compared to an in-line graft.[19–21]

Alternatively, others have published on the use of in-line or *in situ* graft placement following thorough debridement of the infected field.[22–25] This can be achieved by using either standard prosthetic Dacron grafts or arterial homografts. Review of the literature in the use of Dacron grafts in *in situ* prosthetic reconstructions shows rather poor results, with an approximately 25% early mortality and a similar incidence of aortic septic complications and vascular re-interventions.[1,26]. Moreover, it has been suggested that some 20% of survivors following *in situ* reconstruction need a subsequent extra-anatomic bypass graft owing to infection of the initial graft.[27] In order to reduce the risk of infection of *in situ* grafts, it is recommended that they are soaked in rifampicin which has a considerable anti-staphylococcal activity and has been shown to bind significantly to gelatine-sealed Dacron grafts.[21,28,29]. Furthermore, the intra-operative application of gentamicin-releasing carriers has been reported as an adjunct to locally control sepsis and reduce the risk of graft infection.[30] Neither of these antibiotic treatments are proven. As an alternative to tubular graft replacement, a Dacron patch plasty can be performed if the lesion is well circumscribed and the adjacent aorta is not dilated, but the risk of further infection needs to be considered.[5] Therefore we do not advocate this.

Some authors have taken a selective approach whereby *in situ* reconstruction was performed in cases of low-grade infection as indicated by a well-circumscribed inflammatory process with the absence of pus. This is typical of salmonella infection; under these circumstances, we place a Dacron *in situ* graft. Conversely, if severe purulent infection is seen, an extra-anatomical bypass is considered.[3] Fichelle *et al.* operated on 25 infected infrarenal aortic aneurysms; *in situ* reconstruction of the aorta took place in 21 patients and only three deaths were related to the initial surgery (14%). In addition, all surviving patients were regularly followed up and none showed any sign of late septic recurrence. In the group of four patients who underwent extra-anatomic bypass, two died in the postoperative period and one underwent re-operation 2 years after the initial surgery. The authors concluded that complete resection, debridement of infected tissues, omental flap coverage, and long-term antibiotic therapy can achieve favourable results using in-line prosthetic graft reconstruction of infrarenal mycotic aortic aneurysms.[26] Similarly, in our series of four infrarenal and four juxta-renal, mycotic aortic aneurysms, six were repaired with *in situ* prostheses following extensive local debridement and two required axillo-femoral prosthetic grafts. There was one early death secondary to multi-organ failure amongst those patients that had an axillo-femoral graft and one late death from unrelated causes

> **Key point 5**
>
> - Extensive surgical debridement of infected tissues and the placement of an omental pedicle where appropriate, constitute standard surgical principles.

(median duration of follow-up was 38 months). Therefore, we concluded that, in the absence of uncontrolled sepsis, *in situ* repair of mycotic aortic aneurysms using prosthetic grafts can achieve durable results.

In recent years, because of the controversy surrounding *in situ* prosthetic grafts, there has been a renewed interest in the use of cryopreserved arterial homografts for the treatment of mycotic aortic aneurysms.[25,31] Arterial allografts have been in use for many years, but early reports were disappointing because of graft rejection secondary to unsuitable cryopreservation methods. In spite of this, in 1970 Szilagyi *et al.* published favourable results in 132 patients with arterial homografts.[32] At 5-years following surgery, 76 patients were alive and of these 53 had patent grafts (70%). At 15-years after surgery, 18 patients were still alive with patent grafts, with 22 patients having died with patent grafts. However, 14 patients had developed aneurysms – a well-documented complication of allografts in vascular surgery. More recently, Kieffer *et al.* reported their experience with arterial allografts in 43 patients with infected aortic grafts.[33] They reported a 12% operative mortality although none were homograft related. Three patients had homograft-related complications including septic rupture, occlusion and graft enteric fistula. During follow-up, two patients developed aneurysmal dilatation of their homografts at 38 and 42 months.[33] It is important to note that Szilagyi and Kieffer used non-cryopreserved aortic homografts in their series. It is thought that cryopreserved homografts are at a lesser risk of rupture or thrombosis.[22] In addition, cryopreservation seems to reduce the antigenic properties of homografts and makes them more resistant to bacterial colonisation.[34,35]

Infection involving the suprarenal and thoraco-abdominal aorta poses distinct challenges in management because visceral re-vascularisation is required so that there is no definitive way to perform a truly remote bypass. In each case, the visceral grafts must come in proximity to the infected supra-renal aorta. Thus, in these situations, graft placement is either in-line or in near anatomic location. Fortunately, these are rare cases in Britain. Since 1962, fewer than 50 patients have been reported in the English language literature. In addition, a variety of reconstructive techniques have been used; therefore, making firm conclusions as to the advantages of one technique over another is difficult.[36]

The majority of patients were treated by resection of the visceral aorta, graft interposition, and reperfusion of the visceral vessels by either 'side-arm' grafts

> **Key point 6**
>
> - Infrarenal mycotic aortic aneurysms are best dealt with aneurysmectomy and extra-anatomic bypass, particularly in the presence of severe sepsis.

or direct re-attachment to the aortic graft.[5,36] The authors who report this technique have suggested that *in situ* grafting is the treatment of choice for central mycotic aneurysms with some advising life-long oral antibiotic suppressive therapy.[5] Over an 11-year period, we have operated on seven mycotic thoraco-abdominal aneurysms. Based on the Crawford classification, three were type IV, three type III and one type II. All were repaired with in-line Dacron grafts. Two of the type IV died within 30 days of surgery. The median follow-up for the rest was 38 months. One of the type III repairs re-presented with graft infection after 2 years and died as a result. Although the numbers are small, a 20% re-intervention rate amongst survivors is what is generally reported in the literature.[1,26,27]

Others have reported resection of a supra-celiac aneurysm with closure of the aortic stump and reconstruction with an axillo-bifemoral graft that perfused the distal aorta and visceral arteries retrogradely.[37] The concern with an extra-anatomical bypass is the inadequate flow to perfuse viscera and legs. There is also a much higher risk of thrombosis with devastating consequences to the visceral arterial blood supply.[38]

More recently, Semba *et al.* reported a series of three high operative risk patients with mycotic thoracic aneurysms treated by endovascular stent grafts with no follow-up evidence of graft infection over a 4–24 month period.[39] Two of these patients presented with a contained leak. The authors concluded that stent graft placement allows for immediate patching of the leak and can be used as a stand-alone technique or allow for temporising measures prior to elective debridement and repair when the patient is stabilised.[39] Although stent graft technology appears promising, there are several shortcomings of the current technique. The devices need to be prepared ahead of time with construction and sterilisation of a single stent graft requiring 2–3 days. In addition, stent grafts of varying dimensions need to be available for emergency use as up to 60% of mycotic thoracic aneurysms can present as ruptures.[5] Additional considerations would include the placement of homografts on these stents as opposed to polyester and the option to soak the stent graft in an antibiotic solution.

POSTOPERATIVE MANAGEMENT

Intensive antibiotic therapy is crucial for successful treatment of infected aortic aneurysms and should be started in the pre-operative period. Broad-spectrum antibiotics should be used until culture sensitivities from blood and or aortic tissue, are available and a specific antibiotic in identified.[28] The optimum duration of antibiotic therapy is still uncertain with recommendations ranging from 6 weeks to life-long treatment.[5,28,40] Most authors, including ourselves, would recommend a 3-month course of postoperative antibiotic therapy, at

Key point 8
- Long-term culture-specific antibiotic therapy is essential in the postoperative period.

which stage it can be discontinued provided there is no clinical, haematological or radiological evidence of on-going sepsis.[3] Some authors advocate regular follow-up in the form of C-reactive protein measurements and CT scans.[3]

CONCLUDING REMARKS

The term mycotic aneurysm is misleading, as the majority of aortic infections are bacterial and not fungal. As a result, some authors prefer to use the term 'infected aneurysm'. Four main aetiological factors have been identified: (i) bacterial endocarditis leading to embolisation of infected material in diseased aortic wall; (ii) bacteria may colonise the intact vascular wall leading to saccular aneurysm formation; (iii) infection of pre-existing aneurysms; and (iv) false aneurysm formation after arterial trauma. Mycotic aneurysms tend to be symptomatic and are associated with rapid expansion; thus, they are at a high risk of rupture. Prompt intervention in the form of antibiotic therapy and surgical repair is required. The fundamental surgical principle is that of thorough tissue debridement with omental flap coverage where possible. Controversy exists as to the best surgical management of patients with infrarenal mycotic aneurysms. Most would advocate oversewing of the aortic stamp and excision of the aneurysm sac followed by an extra-anatomical bypass. Some authors have advocated *in situ* replacement of the aorta with either a prosthetic graft or a homograft with variable success. Others have adopted a selective approach by performing *in situ* reconstruction in cases of low-grade infection. Suprarenal mycotic aneurysms including thoracic and thoraco-abdominal aneurysms usually require in-line repair. Long-term postoperative antibiotic therapy based on culture sensitivities is essential.

Key points for clinical practice

- Mycotic aortic aneurysms have a tendency for rapid expansion and early rupture.
- Clinical features usually include pyrexia, abdominal, back or chest pain.
- Blood cultures are positive in 50% of cases.
- CT, MRI and aortography are the radiological investigations of choice.
- Extensive surgical debridement of infected tissues and the placement of an omental pedicle where appropriate, constitute standard surgical principles.

Key points for clinical practice (continued)

- Infrarenal mycotic aortic aneurysms are best dealt with aneurysmectomy and extra-anatomic bypass, particularly in the presence of severe sepsis.

- Supra-renal and thoraco-abdominal mycotic aortic aneurysms are best dealt with *in situ* reconstruction.

- Long-term culture-specific antibiotic therapy is essential in the postoperative period.

References

1. Alonso M, Caeiro S, Cachaldora J, Segura R. Infected abdominal aortic aneurysm: *in situ* replacement with cryopreserved arterial homograft. *J Cardiovasc Surg (Torino)* 1997; **38**: 371–375.
2. Jarrett F, Darling RC, Mundth ED, Austen WG. Experience with infected aneurysms of the abdominal aorta. *Arch Surg* 1975; **110**: 1281–1286.
3. Muller BT, Wegener OR, Grabitz K, Pillny M, Thomas L, Sandmann W. Mycotic aneurysms of the thoracic and abdominal aorta and iliac arteries: experience with anatomic and extra-anatomic repair in 33 cases. *J Vasc Surg* 2001; **33**: 106–113.
4. Mendelowitz DS, Ramstedt R, Yao JS, Bergan JJ. Abdominal aortic salmonellosis. *Surgery* 1979; **85**: 514–519.
5. Chan FY, Crawford ES, Coselli JS, Safi HJ, Williams Jr TW. *In situ* prosthetic graft replacement for mycotic aneurysm of the aorta. *Ann Thorac Surg* 1989; **47**: 193–203.
6. Parellada JA, Palmer J, Monill JM, Zidan A, Gimenez AM, Moreno A. Mycotic aneurysm of the abdominal aorta: CT finding in three patients. *Abdom Imaging* 1997; **22**: 321–324.
7. Rubery PT, Smith MD, Cammisa FP, Silane M. Mycotic aortic aneurysm in patients who have lumbar vertebral osteomyelitis. A report of two cases. *J Bone Joint Surg Am* 1995; **77**: 1729–1732.
8. Mestres CA, Garcia I, Khabiri E, Pomar JL. Multiple mycotic aortic aneurysms in a drug addict. *Asian Cardiovasc Thorac Ann* 2002; **10**: 196.
9. Rabitsch W, Brugger SA, Trubel W, Keil F, Greinix HT, Kalhs P. *Streptococcus pneumoniae* mycotic aortic aneurysm after allogeneic bone marrow transplantation. *Transplantation* 2002; **74**: 1048–1050.
10. Oz MC, McNicholas KW, Serra AJ, Spagna PM, Lemole GM. Review of *Salmonella* mycotic aneurysms of the thoracic aorta. *J Cardiovasc Surg (Torino)* 1989; **30**: 99–103.
11. Woolgar JD, Robbs JV. Vascular surgical complications of the acquired immunodeficiency syndrome. *Eur J Vasc Endovasc Surg* 2002; **24**: 473–479.
12. Rutgers PH, Koumans RK, Puylaert JB, Kitslaar PJ. Rapid evolution of a mycotic aneurysm of the abdominal aorta due to *Salmonella*. *Neth J Surg* 1990; **42**: 155–156.
13. Moriarty JA, Edelman RR, Tumeh SS. CT and MRI of mycotic aneurysms of the abdominal aorta. *J Comput Assist Tomogr* 1992; **16**: 941–943.
14. Belz J, Gattermann M, Schroder HJ. [Extra-anatomic bypass as therapy of infected bacterial (mycotic) infrarenal aortic aneurysm. A comparative, literature supported analysis]. *Chirurg* 1989; **60**: 479–483.
15. Pasic M, Carrel T, Vogt M, von Segesser L, Turina M. Treatment of mycotic aneurysm of the aorta and its branches: the location determines the operative technique. *Eur J Vasc Surg* 1992; **6**: 419–423.
16. Pasic M, Carrel T, Tonz M, Vogt P, von Segesser L, Turina M. Mycotic aneurysm of the abdominal aorta: extra-anatomic versus *in situ* reconstruction. *Cardiovasc Surg* 1993; **1**: 48–52.
17. Pasic M, Olah A, Laske A *et al.* [Mycotic aneurysm of the infrarenal aorta: surgical possibilities and results]. *Helv Chir Acta* 1992; **58**: 809–812.

18. Tanaka K, Kawauchi M, Murota Y, Furuse A. 'No-touch' isolation procedure for ruptured mycotic abdominal aortic aneurysm. *Jpn Circ J* 2001; **65**: 1085–1086.

19. Johansen K, Devin J. Mycotic aortic aneurysms. A reappraisal. *Arch Surg* 1983; **118**: 583–588.

20. Olah A, Vogt M, Laske A, Carrell T, Bauer E, Turina M. Axillo-femoral bypass and simultaneous removal of the aorto-femoral vascular infection site: is the procedure safe? *Eur J Vasc Surg* 1992; **6**: 252–254.

21. Robinson JA, Johansen K. Aortic sepsis: is there a role for *in situ* graft reconstruction? *J Vasc Surg* 1991; **13**: 677–682; discussion 682–684.

22. Vogt PR, von Segesser LK, Goffin Y, Pasic M, Turina MI. Cryopreserved arterial homografts for *in situ* reconstruction of mycotic aneurysms and prosthetic graft infection. *Eur J Cardiothorac Surg* 1995; **9**: 502–506.

23. Vogt PR, von Segesser LK, Goffin Y *et al*. Eradication of aortic infections with the use of cryopreserved arterial homografts. *Ann Thorac Surg* 1996; **62**: 640–645.

24. Vogt PR, Brunner-La Rocca HP, Carrel T *et al*. Cryopreserved arterial allografts in the treatment of major vascular infection: a comparison with conventional surgical techniques. *J Thorac Cardiovasc Surg* 1998; **116**: 965–972.

25. Vogt PR, Brunner-LaRocca HP, Lachat M, Ruef C, Turina MI. Technical details with the use of cryopreserved arterial allografts for aortic infection: influence on early and midterm mortality. *J Vasc Surg* 2002; **35**: 80–86.

26. Fichelle JM, Tabet G, Cormier P *et al*. Infected infrarenal aortic aneurysms: when is *in situ* reconstruction safe? *J Vasc Surg* 1993; **17**: 635–645.

27. John R, Korula RJ, Lal N, Shukla V, Lalitha MK. Salmonellosis complicating aortic aneurysms. *Int Angiol* 1994; **13**: 177–180.

28. Hollier LH, Money SR, Creely B, Bower TC, Kazmier FJ. Direct replacement of mycotic thoracoabdominal aneurysms. *J Vasc Surg* 1993; **18**: 477–484; discussion 485.

29. Ting AC, Cheng SW. Repair of *Salmonella* mycotic aneurysm of the paravisceral abdominal aorta using *in situ* prosthetic graft. *J Cardiovasc Surg (Torino)* 1997; **38**: 665–668.

30. Pasic M, von Segesser L, Turina M. Implantation of antibiotic-releasing carriers and *in situ* reconstruction for treatment of mycotic aneurysm. *Arch Surg* 1992; **127**: 745–746.

31. Vogt P, Pasic M, von Segesser L, Carrel T, Turina M. Cryopreserved aortic homograft for mycotic aneurysm. *J Thorac Cardiovasc Surg* 1995; **109**: 589–591.

32. Szilagyi DE, Rodriguez FJ, Smith RF, Elliott JP. Late fate of arterial allografts. Observations 6 to 15 years after implantation. *Arch Surg* 1970; **101**: 721–733.

33. Kieffer E, Bahnini A, Koskas F, Ruotolo C, Le Blevec D, Plissonnier D. *In situ* allograft replacement of infected infrarenal aortic prosthetic grafts: results in forty-three patients. *J Vasc Surg* 1993; **17**: 349–355; discussion 355–356.

34. Koskas F, Plissonnier D, Bahnini A, Ruotolo C, Kieffer E. *In situ* arterial allografting for aortoiliac graft infection: a 6-year experience. *Cardiovasc Surg* 1996; **4**: 495–499.

35. Koskas F, Plissonnier D, Bahnini A, Ruotolo C, Kieffer E. [Vascular allografts. Application to the treatment of aorto-iliac prosthetic infections with in situ revascularization]. *Chirurgie* 1997; **122**: 13–17.

36. Atnip RG. Mycotic aneurysms of the suprarenal abdominal aorta: prolonged survival after *in situ* aortic and visceral reconstruction. *J Vasc Surg* 1989; **10**: 635–641.

37. Atlas SW, Vogelzang RL, Bressler EL, Gore RM, Bergan JJ. CT diagnosis of a mycotic aneurysm of the thoracoabdominal aorta. *J Comput Assist Tomogr* 1984; **8**: 1211–1212.

38. Reddy DJ, Lee RE, Oh HK. Suprarenal mycotic aortic aneurysm: surgical management and follow-up. *J Vasc Surg* 1986; **3**: 917–920.

39. Semba CP, Sakai T, Slonim SM *et al*. Mycotic aneurysms of the thoracic aorta: repair with use of endovascular stent-grafts. *J Vasc Interv Radiol* 1998; **9**: 33–40.

40. Brown SL, Busuttil RW, Baker JD, Machleder HI, Moore WS, Barker WF. Bacteriologic and surgical determinants of survival in patients with mycotic aneurysms. *J Vasc Surg* 1984; **1**: 541–547.

Karim Brophy Eddie Chaloner Matthew Mattson

12

Recent advances in vascular trauma

The artery may be hard to find. It may be displaced from its anatomical site and the tissues round it may be stained with blood. Hasty dissection and blind dives with forceps are to be deprecated. (...) The artery proximal to its site of injury should therefore be controlled before the bleeding point is sought.

W.H. Ogilvie, 1944

The principles of vascular trauma surgery have not changed in the past 60 years, and Ogilvie's dictum is as true today as it was then – when ligation of an injured artery was the only option available to the war surgeon.[1] However, diagnostic adjuncts, surgical techniques and equipment have improved dramatically over the intervening period, and the contemporary surgical team has a much wider set of options for haemorrhage control and repair of damaged blood vessels.

In particular, the past decade has shown a dramatic rise in the use of endoluminal techniques in elective vascular practice, including angiographic embolisation, balloon occlusion catheters, and endovascular stenting. This article critically appraises the role of these techniques and discusses their place in the management of vascular trauma.

There are several applications of endoluminal techniques in vascular trauma. In the acute phase, transcatheter techniques are most frequently used to gain control of arterial haemorrhage, sometimes as a temporary measure prior to moving the patient to the operating theatre for open repair. Some acute haemorrhage can be definitively treated by angiographic embolisation alone,

Karim Brophy BSc FRCA FRCS, Specialist Registrar, The Royal London Hospital, Whitechapel, London, UK

Eddie Chaloner FRCS, Consultant Vascular Surgeon, University College Hospitals NHS Trust, London, UK (for correspondence)

Matthew Mattson BSc FRCR, Consultant Radiologist, The Royal London Hospital, Whitechapel, London, UK

Key point 1

- Interventional radiological techniques are an adjunct to trauma surgery. They do not necessarily eliminate the requirement for operation. Time is of the essence in the treatment of the bleeding patient. Access to the X-ray department facilities must not be allowed to delay the attainment of haemostasis.

and endoluminal methods have an important part to play in the treatment of later complications of vascular trauma, such as arteriovenous fistulae and false aneurysms.

Endoluminal treatment is less compromised by the anatomical distortion caused by large haematomas, false aneurysms or AV fistulae encountered at open operation. In addition, transluminal techniques are ideally suited to injuries that are difficult to access and control by standard surgical means. Vascular injuries in the true pelvis and zones 1 and 3 of the neck may be extremely challenging to control surgically, but relatively simple via transcatheter techniques.

The endoluminal route is also of benefit in the patient with multiple injuries or major medical co-morbidity where the patient may not survive the physiological insult of open surgery. The minimally invasive nature of endovascular surgery reduces the haemodynamic, ventilatory and metabolic disturbances associated with open operations. For example, a patient with brain and pulmonary injuries may have a significantly reduced secondary insult from stenting of a thoracic aorta injury than if open thoracotomy and repair was contemplated.

Careful patient selection is vital, however. Many of the techniques and equipment are new and there are few long-term follow-up studies of endovascular devices. As the majority of trauma patients are young, the long-term durability of stents and stent grafts is a major concern.

It must also be remembered that achieving haemostasis in an unstable bleeding patient is a matter of urgency – for endovascular techniques to be successful in the treatment of the patient with a major vascular injury, the relevant personnel and equipment must be available around the clock. Ideally, transcatheter intervention should be carried out in the resuscitation room; but, if this is not feasible, transfer of the patient from the emergency department to the radiology suite should not result in undue delays to treatment. Similarly, all the necessary hardware (catheters, embolising coils, stent grafts, *etc.*) must be available 'on the shelf' if endoluminal intervention in vascular injury is to be successful. Staffing and equipping such a 24-h service is inevitably expensive, both from the point of view of personnel costs and the costs of the equipment.

TEMPORARY HAEMORRHAGE CONTROL

Interventional radiology techniques can be used as an adjunct to surgery by achieving temporary vascular control before the patient is transferred to the operating theatre for definitive repair of a vessel injury. This technique is particularly useful in gaining proximal control in inaccessible anatomical sites, such as the subclavian or common iliac arteries. An occlusion balloon catheter can be placed in the bleeding artery, proximal to or across the site of injury.[2] If necessary, a second balloon can be placed distally for complete isolation of the injury, although this is rarely required. In emergency situations, standard angioplasty balloons can be used if the soft, compliant occlusion balloons are not available.

Following balloon haemorrhage control, the patient can then be transferred to the operating theatre. During the operation, inflation of the angioplasty balloon can assist the surgeon by preventing uncontrolled bleeding from obscuring the operative field. Identifying of the site of injury can be very difficult due to surrounding haematoma and distortion of the tissues. Having a palpable balloon within the haematoma is extremely useful in guiding the surgical dissection.

CASE 1: TRAUMATIC AXILLARY ARTERIOVENOUS FISTULA

Figure 1 shows the left subclavian angiogram of a 20-year-old male stabbed in the left supraclavicular fossa. He had an expanding haematoma below the clavicle and a left-sided haemothorax, which drained 300 ml initially and then another 200 ml in the next 30 min. He was tachycardic, but maintained his blood pressure. Angiography showed a traumatic arterio-venous fistula involving the first part of the axillary artery.

An angioplasty balloon catheter was placed into the axillary artery across the site of the fistula and haemorrhage control achieved (Fig. 2). The patient was then transferred to the operating room where the injury was repaired through an infraclavicular incision. The angioplasty balloon was easily palpable within the surrounding haematoma and was useful in guiding dissection.

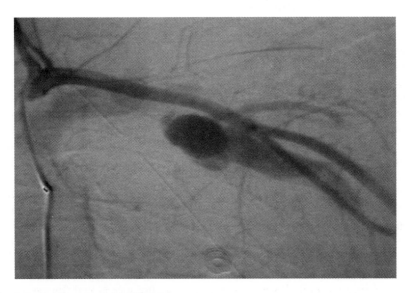

Fig. 1 Left axillary vessel A-V fistula.

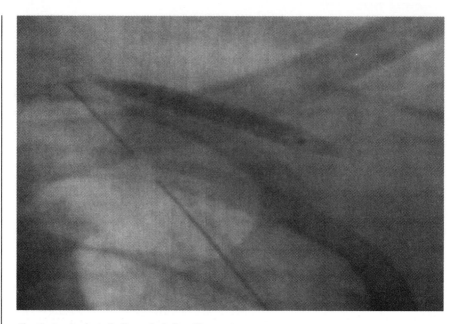

Fig. 2 Angioplasty balloon in left axillary artery.

Early proximal control of arterial haemorrhage by an intraluminal balloon may then help to reduce the extent of surgery and peri-operative blood loss. Access to interventional techniques for emergency haemorrhage control should become faster and easier as angiography capabilities are built into operating suites, and this may increase the range of injuries that become amenable to control with these techniques.

ANGIOGRAPHIC EMBOLISATION

Catheter-directed embolisation has been one of the therapeutic options available to the trauma surgeon for several years. The use of therapeutic angiography to embolise bleeding arteries of patients with pelvic fracture was described in the early 1970s. For several injury patterns, such as pelvic fracture, it is now the preferred method of haemorrhage control. The movement of haemodynamically unstable patients to a radiology area runs contrary to many surgeons' beliefs. However, when the angiography suite is a place of definitive haemorrhage control, then it should be accorded the same status for those injuries suitable for embolisation as the operating room is for surgically correctable haemorrhage.[4]

Embolisation of a bleeding artery is carried out by inserting small foreign bodies into the vessel proximal to the bleeding segment, with the intention that these will induce thrombosis. By reducing the arterial inflow pressure, it is hoped that the bleeding will cease spontaneously by activation of normal clotting mechanisms, and that bleeding from the venous side of the circulation will cease by a process of self-tamponade, once the arterial inflow is controlled. The advantage of embolisation over surgical techniques is that the vessel can be occluded as close as possible to the site of bleeding, thus reducing the risk

> **Key point 2**
>
> - Balloon occlusion catheters can be used to gain temporary control of bleeding vessels at the time of diagnostic angiography.
>
> - This technique can also aid the surgeon at subsequent open operation.

of collateral vessels opening up to supply the site of haemorrhage and also minimise the volume of tissue rendered ischaemic. Nevertheless, ischaemic necrosis of the tissue supplied by that vessel is a potential complication and may result in post-procedure necrosis or abscess formation.

A variety of wires, sponges and foams are used to embolise bleeding vessels. Gianturco coils are made of stainless steel wire fragments, surrounded by thrombogenic wool strands. Microcoils have been developed which are able to be deployed through microcatheters placed superselectively close to the bleeding point. Soluble gelatine sponge is an absorbable material available in sheet or powder form, which can be implanted into vessels as particulate matter. It is promoted as a temporary agent, with re-canalisation of the targeted vessel occurring at about 6 weeks, which may be an advantage in the trauma patient. Polyvinyl alcohol is a permanent solid agent used for therapeutic embolisation and has the advantage of expanding up to 15 times in length after contact with blood. Distal embolisation of these particulate compounds is a recognised complication of the technique.

PELVIC INJURY

Exsanguinating pelvic injury carries a high mortality unless treated appropriately and expeditiously. Surgical exploration of the pelvic retroperitoneum and attempted ligation of the internal iliac artery or its branches invariably has a poor outcome. Around 10% of all pelvic fractures have an associated arterial injury.[5] Some 20% of anterior-posterior compression and vertical shear injuries are associated with arterial haemorrhage, usually from the posterior division of the internal iliac. While only 2% of lateral compression injuries have an associated arterial injury, these are usually from the surgically inaccessible pudendal or obturator arteries.[6]

Patients in whom external stabilisation of the pelvic girdle does not produce haemodynamic stability should be transferred to the angiography suite for embolisation. Where there is concurrent intraperitoneal injury and laparotomy is unavoidable, the true pelvis can be packed and the patient subsequently transferred to the angiography suite for embolisation of pelvic vessels.[7,8] Identification of pelvic haemorrhage requires selective angiography of the anterior and posterior divisions of both internal iliac arteries in turn. Flush angiograms in the descending aorta or common iliacs may miss significant numbers of pelvic arterial bleeders. Once a bleeding point is identified, co-axial catheters may be used to allow superselective embolisation of the bleeding branch vessel and deployment of microcoils. If the bleeding point cannot be reached, an acceptable alternative is injection of soluble gelatin sponge into the feeding vessel in the hope that collateral vessel occlusion to non-target sites will be temporary with this agent.

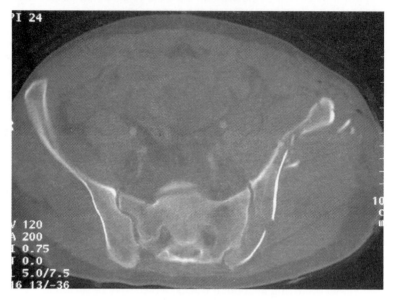

Fig. 3 Fractured left pelvis with buttock haematoma.

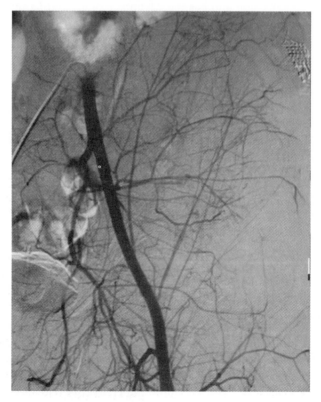

Fig. 4 Angiogram of left common iliac artery showing no obvious bleeding point.

CASE 2: PELVIC INJURY, ANGIOGRAPHY AND COIL EMBOLISATION

A 27-year-old man had a wall collapse on him and arrived tachycardic but maintaining his blood pressure. He had a lateral compression fracture of his pelvis on plain film and focused abdominal ultrasound examination was negative for free intraperitoneal fluid. Figure 3 shows his initial CT scan with contrast extravasation into the left buttock region. His tachycardia persisted and his blood pressure began to drop; therefore, the patient was transferred to the angiography suite. Figure 4 shows the initial common iliac angiogram that does not clearly indicate the arterial injury. Figure 5, however, is a selective study, which clearly shows contrast extravasation related to an injury to the superior gluteal artery. Figure 6 shows the leak controlled with coil embolisation. Haemodynamic stability was rapidly restored following the procedure and there were no complications related to re-bleeding or necrosis.

The advantages of angiographic embolisation of pelvic haemorrhage when compared to the complexity and poor outcome associated with open surgical intervention raise important questions about whether these injuries should be treated in centres where emergency interventional techniques are not available.

SPLEEN AND LIVER INJURY

Angiographic techniques are increasingly being used as an adjunct to non-operative management of damaged intra-abdominal solid organs. While non-

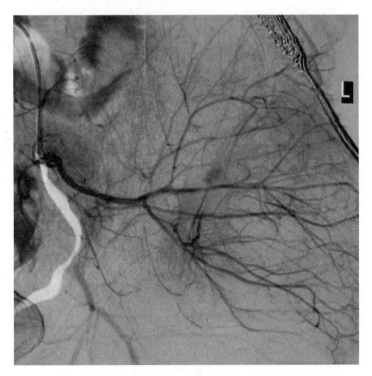

Fig. 5 Selective angiogram of internal iliac artery showing contrast leak into haematoma.

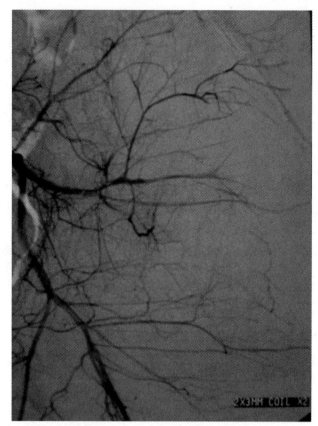

Fig. 6 Contrast leak controlled after embolisation.

operative management of splenic injury is now common practice, around 30% of patients will continue to bleed from the injured spleen and require a laparotomy. The use of angiographic techniques may be able to reduce this failure rate to around 3–8%.[9,10]

It is not yet clear which subset of patients with splenic injuries will benefit from angiographic embolisation although obvious contrast extravasation from the spleen on a CT scan will probably benefit.[11] The natural history of traumatic pseudo-aneurysms of the splenic artery is less well characterised, but embolisation may reduce the risk of rupture in this group.[12] Other patients that may have a higher failure rate of non-operative management are those with higher grades of injury (AAST grades 4 & 5) and the elderly.[13]

There are two basic techniques of splenic embolisation. The first is selective occlusion of segmental vessels using gel pledgets, microcoils, polyvinyl alcohol or thrombin. The second is the placement of coils in the splenic artery to reduce downstream pressure and allow normal haemostasis.[9] The latter technique has the theoretical advantage of conserving splenic parenchyma and later function.

CASE 3: PROXIMAL SPLENIC ARTERY COILING FOR SPLENIC INJURY

Figure 7 is an angiogram of a splenic injury diagnosed on CT scan, showing disruption of the upper pole of the spleen. The patient was haemodynamically

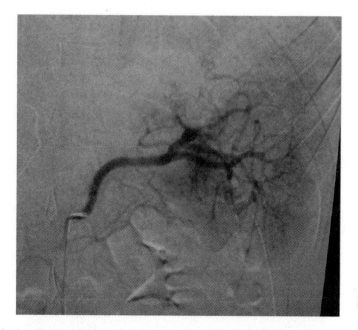

Fig. 7 Splenic artery angiogram showing contrast leak after splenic injury.

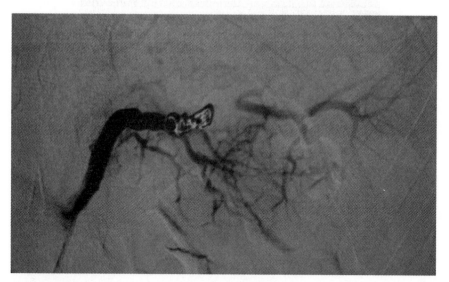

Fig. 8 Splenic angiogram after embolisation with coils.

stable, but there was active contrast extravasation identified on the CT scan. Coils were placed in the proximal splenic artery (Fig. 8). The patient remained stable and was managed non-operatively.

CASE 4: SUPERSELECTIVE EMBOLISATION OF SPLENIC INJURY

Figure 9 shows a selective angiogram of a splenic injury, with false aneurysm and contrast extravasation clearly visible. The patient was haemodynamically stable

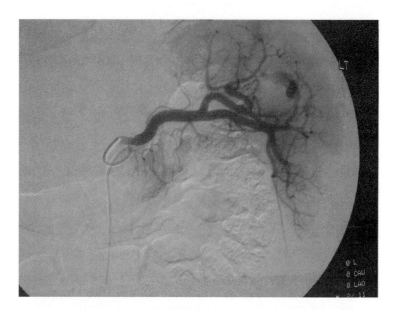

Fig. 9 Superselective splenic artery angiogram showing contrast leak.

and angiographic embolisation was performed as an adjunct to non-operative management. Figure 10 shows control of the injury with superselective gelatin pledget embolisation. The patient remained haemodynamically stable and was discharged home on day 5.

Angiographic embolisation has also been utilised in liver trauma to control free arterial haemorrhage or traumatic pseudo-aneurysms. Non-operative

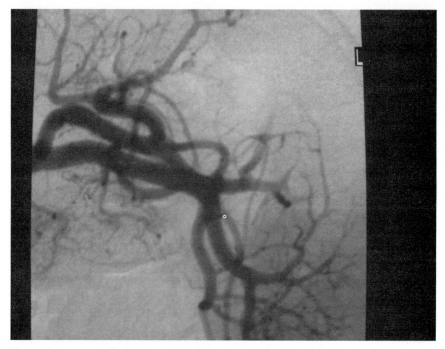

Fig. 10 Injury controlled using gel pledget embolisation.

management of liver injury is less likely to fail than splenic trauma. However, angiography may reduce the laparotomy rate in certain groups of patients, although which subgroups will benefit is less well established. Patients with contrast extravasation on CT scan, and with higher grades of liver injury may benefit from embolisation.[14] Very severe liver injuries are likely to require laparotomy, even after transcatheter embolisation.[15] Infarction is less likely with hepatic embolisation due to the dual blood supply of the hepatic parenchyma.

Angiography can be used as an adjunct to 'damage control surgery' in the abdomen. An injured spleen is usually removed during a damage control procedure, and an injured liver packed. Packing should control intrahepatic venous bleeding, but may not arrest arterial haemorrhage. Any patient with a liver injury who has undergone a 'damage control' procedure involving liver packing should probably undergo postoperative angiography and embolisation of active arterial haemorrhage.[16]

Key point 3

- Embolisation of bleeding vessels is particularly useful in inaccessible anatomical areas.
- Coils, foams and gels can be used alone or in combination to induce vessel thrombosis.
- Necrosis of tissue supplied by the embolised vessel is a risk, especially in solid organs, as is distal embolisation of coils and foams.

DIFFICULT SURGICAL ACCESS

Other areas where embolisation is now used in preference to surgery are in zone 3 penetrating injuries to the neck and facial fractures, where haemorrhage is from branches of the external carotid artery.[17,18] Similarly, haemorrhage from the vertebral artery may be extremely difficult to control surgically, but relatively easy endoluminally.[19,20] Lumbar artery injury is also well suited to embolisation.[21]

STENTS

Stents are hollow tubes composed of surgical steel alloy filaments woven into a flexible mesh cylinder. Stents may be either be uncovered or covered – covered stents are also known as stent grafts. Uncovered stents are used extensively in the management of atheromatous vessels, but their use in trauma is relatively limited. They can be used to re-establish patency of a vessel occluded by extrinsic compression and are useful in the management of intimal tears, compressing the tear and preventing the intramural leakage of blood.

Covered stent grafts that are impermeable to blood have a much greater application in vascular trauma. A stent graft can be placed across a vascular defect and exclude it from direct contact with the circulation. Stent grafts can, therefore, be used to treat vascular laceration and transection, arteriovenous fistula and false aneurysm formation. Caution must be exercised in the placement of a stent graft, as covering the ostia of branch vessels will lead to their occlusion.

Two types of stent and stent graft are available – self-expanding or balloon-expanded. Self-expanding stents expand as a constraining cover is removed. They are flexible and can be passed through tortuous blood vessels. However, their length after deployment is variable and depends on the diameter of the blood vessel into which the stent is placed. Balloon-expanded stents are deployed by inflating a balloon within the stent. Their length after deployment is not as variable, but they are more rigid and less able to traverse tortuous vessels.

AORTIC INJURY

Blunt trauma to the thoracic aorta is one anatomical area where operative management carries a particularly high mortality and morbidity. The deployment of a stent graft has significant potential advantages. Most blunt aortic injuries are at the level of the isthmus in the proximal descending aorta, just distal to the left subclavian artery. The use of an endoluminal graft in the descending aorta is not complicated by branching of visceral vessels, as is the case in the abdominal aorta. Paraplegia is a potential complication, due to occlusion of arteries to the spinal cord, although this appears to be rare with traumatic injuries. The few reported cases in the literature suggest encouraging results in terms of successful graft placement, documented CT

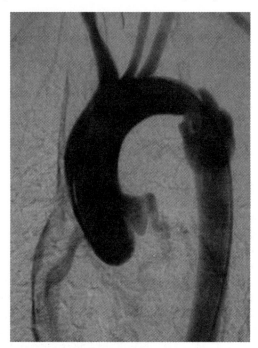

Fig. 11 Proximal descending aortic injury.

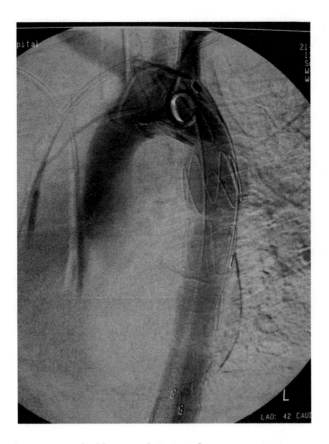

Fig. 12 Aortic tear treated with covered stent graft.

healing, absence of endoleak, minimal blood loss during the procedure and good short-term outcome.[22]

CASE 5: THORACIC STENT GRAFT FOR BLUNT AORTIC INJURY

A 20-year-old woman suffered severe multisystem trauma in a motor vehicle collision, including bilateral cerebral contusions, and bilateral rib fractures with lung contusions. She had evidence of aortic injury at the isthmus on CT scan and a decision was made to treat her with an endovascular stent graft, given her multiple other injuries and high risk of a thoracotomy and open repair. Figure 11 is an angiogram taken just prior to stent graft deployment showing the aortic injury in the proximal descending thoracic aorta. The false aneurysm is controlled with the thoracic stent graft (Fig. 12).

Covered stent grafts have also been used to treat false aneurysms, dissections and arteriovenous fistulae of the distal internal carotid artery.[23] Both blunt and penetrating injuries to the subclavian artery have been treated with covered stents, although the site of injury must be distal to the origin of the internal carotid artery to avoid covering the ostia with the covered portion of the stent.[24,25] There have also been several reports of renal artery stenting, mainly to cover intimal tears arising from blunt trauma.[26–28]

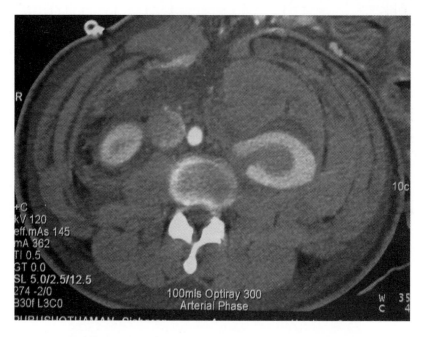

Fig. 13 CT scan of combined aortic and vena caval injury showing false aneurysm on the left (marked).

CASE 6: ABDOMINAL AORTIC STENT GRAFT

A 30-year-old man was stabbed in the right flank, and suffered injuries to his liver, duodenum and inferior vena cava (IVC). These injuries were repaired and the abdomen left open after a 35-unit blood transfusion. A subsequent CT scan showed that the extent of the injury had not been appreciated and, in fact, the injury had been through the IVC and aorta, with a large left-sided false aneurysm (Fig. 13). An angiogram confirmed the diagnosis (Fig. 14).

The patient underwent a second laparotomy, involving repair of the aorta and ligation of the IVC. The duodenal repair had broken down, was resected, repaired, and a pyloric exclusion performed. Unfortunately, this subsequently leaked, but was managed as a controlled fistula. On day 22 following surgery, the patient had a significant haemorrhage and became haemodynamically unstable, with fresh blood visible through the laparostomy dressing. The site of haemorrhage was unknown. An angiogram identified a breakdown of the aortic repair. A stent graft was placed across the aortic injury and haemorrhage control rapidly achieved. His follow-up has so far been uneventful.

The avoidance of complex operative surgical repair in the presence of large haematoma and potential uncontrollable haemorrhage makes the use of stent grafts in the definitive repair of vascular injury very appealing. However, the global experience at present consists mainly of isolated reported cases or small trials and the length of follow-up is short.[29] There is no long-term data on the durability of endoluminal treatment, and the young trauma patient may have to live with their stent for 50 or more years. The incidence of late complications such as graft infection, erosion, migration or thrombosis is unknown. Traumatic stent grafting should still be considered as under investigation,

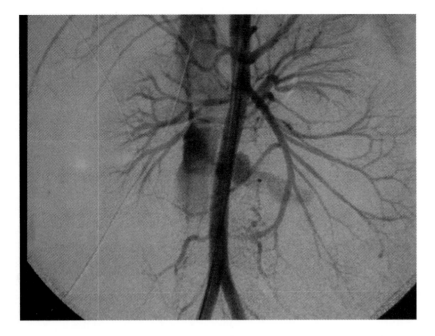

Fig. 14 Angiogram of aorto-caval and false aneurysm.

applied to carefully selected patients, and should be performed as part of a study rather than applied to patients on an *ad hoc* basis. In the absence of a current national trial, the minimum requirement is that results are submitted to a national registry.

SUMMARY

The development of endovascular techniques has widened the options available to the modern trauma surgeon for the management of vascular injury. Temporary haemorrhage control with balloon catheters is a valuable adjunct to surgery. Angiographic embolisation is now the procedure of choice for some injury patterns, and the role of stents and stent grafts is increasing as technology and the evidence-base improve.

Key point 4

- Bare stents can be used to treat intimal tears caused by blunt trauma. Covered stents are needed to treat penetrating injuries or arterio-venous fistulae. Stent grafts have the potential to be extremely useful in the management of penetrating vascular trauma. So far, only isolated cases or small series have been reported. The long-term consequences of implanting devices into young people are unclear.

Already, several trauma centres are designing resuscitation suites and operating suites with full angiographic capabilities. As these areas merge, and technology improves, exsanguinating haemorrhage that previously was difficult or impossible to control may be rapidly and effectively arrested.

As angiographic techniques become the standard of care for such injuries, units receiving such patients must have interventional radiology facilities available 24 hours-a-day. It may become difficult to support the management of acutely injured patients in units without such services. Already, it is difficult to countenance the management of exsanguinating pelvic haemorrhage in units without facilities for emergency angiographic embolisation. There will have to be some rationalisation of units receiving major trauma patients, and agreed protocols for the rapid transfer of injured patients between hospitals.

While these techniques are increasing their indications and frequency of application, there are few prospective, randomised studies to support their use. In many cases, such trials will be difficult or impossible to perform, and their use will have to be guided by large prospective cohort and comparative studies. Meanwhile, the enthusiasm for the use of stent grafts in the young trauma patient should be tempered until long-term follow-up studies are available. They represent a valuable alternative for patients with significant co-morbidity or multiple injuries that make open surgery hazardous.

Key points for clinical practice

- Interventional radiological techniques are an adjunct to trauma surgery. They do not necessarily eliminate the requirement for operation.

- Time is of the essence in the treatment of the bleeding patient. Access to the X-ray department facilities must not be allowed to delay the attainment of haemostasis.

- Balloon occlusion catheters can be used to gain temporary control of bleeding vessels at the time of diagnostic angiography. This technique can also aid the surgeon at subsequent open operation.

- Embolisation of bleeding vessels is particularly useful in inaccessible anatomical areas. Coils, foams and gels can be used alone or in combination to induce vessel thrombosis. Necrosis of tissue supplied by the embolised vessel is a risk, especially in solid organs, as is distal embolisation of coils and foams.

- Bare stents can be used to treat intimal tears caused by blunt trauma. Covered stents are needed to treat penetrating injuries or arterio-venous fistulae. Stent grafts have the potential to be extremely useful in the management of penetrating vascular trauma. So far, only isolated cases or small series have been reported. The long-term consequences of implanting devices into young people are unclear.

References

1. Ogilvie WH. *Forward Surgery in Modern War*. London: Butterworth, 1944.
2. Scalea TM, Scalfani SJ. Angiographically placed balloons for arterial control: a description of a technique. *J Trauma* 1991; **31**: 1671–1677.
3. Sobeh MS, Westacott S, Blakeney C, Ham RJ. Balloon angioplasty catheters for endovascular tamponade after vascular trauma. *Injury* 1993; **24**: 355–356.
4. Ben Menachem Y, Coldwell DM, Young JW, Burgess AR. Hemorrhage associated with pelvic fractures: causes, diagnosis, and emergent management. *AJR Am J Roentgenol* 1991; **157**: 1005–1014.
5. Burgess A, Eastridge BJ, Young JWR *et al*. Pelvic ring disruptions: effective classification system and treatment protocols. *J Trauma* 1990; **30**: 848–856.
6. O'Neill PA, Riina J, Sclafani S, Tornetta P. Angiographic findings in pelvic fractures. *Clin Orthop* 1996; **329**: 60–67.
7. *OTA-AAST Symposium on Exsanguinating Pelvic Injury*. Trauma.org 2000;5:11. Available: <http://www.trauma.org/ortho/pelvis.html>.
8. Bassam D, Cephas GA *et al*. A protocol for the initial management of unstable pelvic fractures. *Am Surg* 1998; **64**: 862–867.
9. Sclafani SJ, Shaftan GW, Scalea TM *et al*. Non-operative salvage of computed tomography-diagnosed splenic injury: utilization of angiography for triage and embolization for haemostasis. *J Trauma* 1995; **39**: 818–825.
10. Haan J, Scott J, Boyd-Kranis RL, Ho S, Kramer M, Scalea TM. Admission angiography for blunt splenic injury: advantages and pitfalls. *J Trauma* 2001; **51**: 1161–1165.
11. Shanmuganathan K, Mirvis SE, Boyd-Kranis R, Takada T, Scalea TM. Nonsurgical management of blunt splenic injury: use of CT criteria to select patients for splenic arteriography and potential endovascular therapy. *Radiology* 2000; **217**: 75–82.
12. Davies KA, Fabian TC, Croce MA *et al*. Improved success in non-operative management of blunt splenic injury: embolization of splenic artery pseudoaneurysms *J Trauma* 1998; **44**: 1008–1013.
13. *Eastern Association for the Surgery of Trauma Practice Management Guidelines: Non-Operative Management of Blunt Injury to the Liver and Spleen*. 2000. Available: <http://www.east.org/tpg.html>.
14. Poletti PA, Mirvis SE, Shanmuganathan K, Killeen KL, Coldwell D. CT criteria for management of blunt liver trauma: correlation with angiographic and surgical findings. *Radiology* 2000; **216**: 418–427.
15. Hagiwara A, Murata A, Matsuda T, Matsuda H, Shimazaki S. The efficacy and limitations of transarterial embolization for severe hepatic injury. *J Trauma* 2002; **52**: 1091–1096.
16. Carrillo EH, Spain DA, Wohltmann D *et al*. Interventional techniques are useful adjuncts in non-operative management of hepatic injuries. *J Trauma* 1999; **46**: 619–622.
17. Demetriades D, Chahwan S, Gomez H, Falabella A, Velmahos G, Yamashita D. Initial evaluation and management of gunshot wounds to the face. *J Trauma* 1998; **45**: 39–41.
18. Sclafani AP, Sclafani SJ. Angiography and transcatheter arterial embolization of vascular injuries of the face and neck. *Laryngoscope* 1996; **106**: 168–173.
19. Albuquerque FC, Javedan SP, McDougall CG. Endovascular management of penetrating vertebral artery injuries. *J Trauma* 2002; **53**: 574–580.
20. Demitriades D, Theodorou D, Ascenio J. Management options in vertebral artery injuries. *Br J Surg* 1996; **83**: 83–86.
21. Sclafani SJ, Florence LO, Phillips TF *et al*. Lumbar arterial injury: radiologic diagnosis and management. *Radiology* 1987; **165**: 709–714.
22. FujikawaT, Yukioka T, Ishimaru S. Endovascular stent grafting for the treatment of blunt thoracic aortic injury. *J Trauma* 2001; **50**: 223–229.
23. Gomez CR, May AK, Terry JB *et al*. Endovascular therapy of traumatic injuries of the extracranial cerebral arteries. *Crit Clin Care* 1999; **15**: 789–809.
24. D'Othee BJ, Rousseau H, Otal P *et al*. Noncovered stent placement in a blunt traumatic injury of the right subclavian artery. *Cardiovasc Intervent Radiol* 1999; **22**: 424–427.
25. Dutort DF, Strauss DC, Blaszczyk M *et al*. Endovascular treatment of penetrating thoracic outlet arterial injuries. *Eur J Vasc Endovasc Surg* 2000; **19**: 489–495.

26. Goodman DN, Saibil EA, Kodama RT. Traumatic intimal tear of the renal artery treated by insertion of a Palmaz stent. *Cardiovasc Intervent Radiol* 1998; **21**: 69–72.
27. Villas PA, Cohen G, Putnam III SG *et al*. Wallstent placement in a renal artery after blunt abdominal trauma. *J Trauma* 1999; **46**: 1137–1139.
28. Whigham Jr CJ, Bodenhamer JR, Miller JK. Use of the Palmaz stent in primary treatment of renal artery intimal injury secondary to blunt trauma. *J Vasc Interv Radiol* 1995; **6**: 175–178.
29. Weiss VJ, Chaikof EL. Endovascular treatment of vascular injuries. *Surg Clin North Am* 1999; **79**: 653–665.

Jayant S. Vaidya

Intra-operative radiotherapy for breast cancer

Over the last century, the treatment of breast cancer has evolved as the biology of the disease is better understood. In the mid-19th century, the humoral theory of breast cancer was overturned by a mechanistic model *viz.*, 'it arises in the breast and spreads centrifugally to regional lymph nodes and thence to rest of the body'. Charles Moore, (1821–1879) a surgeon from the Middlesex Hospital in London, among others, believed that the only way to cure breast cancer was very extensive surgery, in which the tumour was not violated.[1] The belief in this mechanistic model resulted in development of the Halsted radical mastectomy for the 'cure of the cancer of the breast', at the end of the 19th century.[2] Unfortunately, only 23% of patients treated by Halsted survived 10 years.[3] Even more radical surgery,[4] including the internal mammary lymph nodes, did not make a difference.[5,6] Prompted by the failures of radical operations to cure patients of breast cancer, Fisher[7] and others postulated that cancer spreads via blood stream even before its clinical detection, with the outcome determined by the biology of tumour–host interactions. This concept of 'biological predeterminism' suggested that:

1. Adjuvant systemic treatment of apparently localised tumours would be beneficial and may offer a chance of cure; this is now proven in the Oxford overview and, although the effect is only modest, the absolute number of lives saved is considerable, given that breast cancer is a common disease.

2. The extent of local treatment would not affect survival. Again, it was the genius of the Oxford overview[8,9] of 26,000 women from 36 trials resolved the controversy. In 1995, it concluded that postoperative radiotherapy had a substantial effect on reducing local recurrence rates (from 27.2% to 8.8% overall), but more radical local treatment, whether surgery or adjuvant

Jayant S. Vaidya MBBS MS DNB FRCS PhD, Honorary Lecturer and Specialist Registrar, Department of Surgery, Whittington Hospital, University College London, London W1W 7EJ, UK

radiotherapy, did not have any influence on appearance of distant disease and overall survival. At a 20-year follow-up,[9] it was found that radiotherapy reduced breast cancer mortality by 4–5% but other mortality, mainly cardiovascular was increased by an equivalent amount. This has resulted in acceptance of breast-conserving therapy as the standard of care.

One must realise that breast-conserving therapy in the form of wide local excision of the primary tumour, axillary surgery followed by a 6-week course of whole-breast radiotherapy including a tumour bed boost actually has the same radical intent as was achieved by the extirpative surgery of Halsted more than 100 years ago. In that respect, it is not really a change in the paradigm.

PROBLEMS WITH THE CURRENT STANDARD OF CARE

Nevertheless, properly delivered breast-conserving therapy (BCT) is now taken as equivalent to mastectomy and the current standard of care for early operable breast cancer is wide local excision and a 6-week course of whole-breast postoperative radiotherapy usually including a tumour bed boost. In spite of this concept being established for more than a decade, the rates of mastectomy in various populations are still very high, and this cannot be accounted for by a late stage of disease. Local culture and geography, surgeon's choice and patient preference, not necessarily in that order, all dictate which operation is chosen.

The disadvantages of the current practice of 6 weeks of postoperative radiotherapy after breast conservative surgery are:

1. The long course is a considerable strain on women especially when it comes after a 6-month course of chemotherapy.

2. Many women are forced to choose mastectomy because they live far away from a radiotherapy facility. This problem is not restricted to non-industrialised countries. In a study in the US, it was found that the farther the patient lives, the less is the likelihood that she will receive BCT and radiotherapy after breast conserving surgery (BCS). When the travel distance was less than 10 miles, 82% (*i.e.* 39% of total) of patients received radiotherapy after BCS; when it was 50–75 miles, 69% (22% of total) received it and when it was more than 100 miles, only 42% (14% of total) received it.[10]

3. Many women fail to complete the 6-week course and thus may be receiving sub-optimal treatment.

4. It takes up scarce resources of the radiotherapy centres and in many countries leads to long waiting lists.

5. Delay in delivery of radiotherapy either because of long waiting time or because chemotherapy is given first, may jeopardise its effectiveness and the window of opportunity to sterilise the target tissues of tumour cells/potential tumour cells may be lost.

6. It has been estimated that the externally delivered boost dose misses target volume in 24–88% of cases.[11,12] Thus a large proportion of local recurrences could be attributed to this 'geographical miss' alone.

> **Key point 1**
>
> - The usual 6-week course of postoperative radiotherapy after breast conserving surgery has several disadvantages that reduces its general applicability to a wide population, even amongst the most advanced health economies.

LOCAL RECURRENCE AFTER BREAST CONSERVING THERAPY AND RATIONALE BEHIND INTRA-OPERATIVE RADIOTHERAPY

Local recurrence of breast cancer can cause considerable psychological morbidity which may include a sense of failure. There are various theories to explain local recurrence. It may arise from tumour cells left behind or occur because of seeding of circulating metastatic cells in the surgical field rich in growth factors. The latter is supported by the fact that patients with early local recurrence have a relatively poor prognosis (RR, 0.34).[13] Recent data suggest that local recurrence may be facilitated by a local field defect. First, the morphologically normal cells surrounding breast cancer demonstrate a loss of heterozygosity, which is often identical to that of the primary tumour.[14] So these 'normal' cells are already on the brink of becoming cancer. In addition, aromatase activity in the index quadrant is higher than other quadrants[15] and via oestrogen has the potential to stimulate mutagenesis, growth and angiogenesis.[16,17] Young age appears to be a risk factor for local recurrence after breast conserving therapy[18] and radiotherapy seems to have a differential effect according to age.[19] Patients with ipsilateral breast tumour recurrence (IBTR) have an increased risk of carrying a mutant p53 gene (23% *versus* 1%) and young patients (< 40 years) with IBTR have a disproportionately increased risk (40%) of carrying a deleterious BRCA1/2 gene mutation.[20] This suggests that such local recurrence is probably related more to the background genetic instability rather than a different tumour biology at younger age. It appears that a dynamic interaction between the local factors (such as aromatase) present in the breast parenchyma, systemic hormonal milieu and genetic instability will determine the risk of local recurrence, in addition to the biology of the excised primary tumour.

Table 1 The site of local recurrence in large studies of breast conserving therapy

Study	Patients (*n*)	Proportion of recurrences in the index quadrant
Clark *et al.*[21] 1982	680	96%
Schnitt *et al.*[22] 1984	231	83%
Boyages *et al.*[23] 1990	783	81%
Kurtz *et al.*[24] 1990	1593	86%
Fisher *et al.*[13] 1992 (RT)	488	100%
Clark *et al.*[25] 1992 (RT arm)	416	(19/23) 83%
Clark *et al.*[25] 1992 (no RT arm)	421	(103/108) 86%
Veronesi *et al.*[26] 1993	570	90%
Total	5182	91%

The location of recurrence in the breast with respect to site of the primary tumour has been analysed in large series of breast conservation studies (Table 1). It is seen that 81–100% of early breast recurrences occur in the quadrant that harboured the primary tumour.[13,21–26] Bartelink[27] has reported that only 56% (47% in 'tumour bed' and 9% in scar) of local recurrences occurred in the original tumour bed. In addition, 27% recurred diffusely throughout the breast including the tumour bed – so that 29% recurred outside the index quadrant. However, these patients had intensive mammographic follow-up protocol which might have unearthed the subclinical occult tumours (see below) in other quadrants that may never have surfaced clinically.

It appears that local recurrence occurs in the index quadrant, whether or not radiotherapy is given.[21,25,28] That suggests that, whatever the cause of local recurrence, its location remains in the index quadrant and is not affected by radiotherapy. Second, we also know that local recurrence occurs in the index quadrant irrespective of clear margins. Of the breast conserving trials that have tested the effect of radiotherapy, the NSABP-B06,[29] Ontario,[30] Swedish,[31] and Scottish[32] trials had less extensive surgery compared with the Milan III trial.[26] The recurrence rate in the control arm of the Milan III trial, in which the tumours were smaller and excision was considerably wider, was low (8.8% *versus* 24–27% in other trials) even in the control group albeit at the cost of cosmesis. Nevertheless, radiotherapy reduced it even further and at the same proportional rate as in other trials. If local recurrence is caused by residual disease, then radiotherapy should have affected a much larger proportional reduction in those patients with positive margins or less extensive surgery. However, radiotherapy also reduces the rate of local recurrence in those patients with negative margins, which further suggests that local recurrence does not arise only from residual disease and that radiotherapy probably inhibits the growth of genetically unstable cells around the primary tumour. This is in contrast to the findings of whole-organ analysis of mastectomy specimens performed in three dimensions[33] which reveals that 63% of breasts harbour occult cancer foci and 80% of these are situated remote from the index quadrant. It, therefore, appears that these wide-spread and occult multifocal/multicentric cancers in other quadrants of the breast probably remain dormant for a long time and have a low risk of causing clinical tumours. This is corroborated by the high frequency (20% in young women [median age, 39 years] and 33% in women aged 50–55 years) of occult tumours found in 'normal' breasts when analysed in detail in autopsy studies.[34]

It is, therefore, hypothesized that radiotherapy to the tissues that surround the primary tumour is all that is probably necessary. Such an approach may solve many of the problems of postoperative radiotherapy mentioned earlier, and may increase the rates of breast-conserving surgery.

This approach of irradiating the index quadrant alone has been tested in the Christie Hospital trial[35] and, contrary to the popular myth, its findings are encouraging. A total of 708 patients were randomised to receive either the standard wide field (WF) radiotherapy or a limited field (LF) radiotherapy to the index quadrant. Overall, there was a higher recurrence rate in the latter (LF) arm. In the limited field arm, a constant size of radiotherapy field was used, irrespective of the tumour size, and this could have resulted in several instances of 'geographical misses'. More importantly, when the results were

> **Key point 2**
>
> - Since local recurrence after breast-conserving surgery occurs mainly in the area around the original primary tumour, it may be sufficient to target adjuvant radiotherapy to peri-tumoural tissues.

analysed according to the type of the primary tumour, it was found that limited field radiotherapy was inadequate only in infiltrating lobular cancers or cancers with extensive intraductal component (EIC). In the 504 cases of infiltrating duct carcinoma, there was no significant difference in the local recurrence rates of the two arms.

BRACHYTHERAPY

When patients with small infiltrating duct cancers with uninvolved nodes are treated with interstitial brachytherapy with radioactive wires, the recurrence rate is 0–4% at 2–5-year follow-up (see Table 2). It is important to note that the patients in these series have small tumours and have a low risk of local recurrence. In a recently published randomised trial,[36] this technique was found to be equivalent to whole-breast radiotherapy at 30-month follow-up. This is a very important result and is a proof of the principle of treating the

Table 2 Index field interstitial brachytherapy series – good prognosis patients at low risk of local recurrence

Institution	Radiotherapy technique	Median follow-up	Crude local recurrence rate (actual numbers)
Ninewells Hospital, Dundee, UK[37]	LDR	5.6	0% (0/11)
Ochsner Clinic, USA[38]	LDR/HDR	3.8	1.3% (2/150)
London Regional Cancer Center, Canada[39]	HDR	1.7	2.6% (1/39)
William Beaumont Hospital, USA[40]	LDR/HDR	3	0% (0/174)
Orebro Medical Centre, Sweden[41]	PDR	2.8	2.3% (1/43)
University of Kansas, USA[42]	LDR	4	0% (0/24)
National Institute of Oncology, Hungary[36]	HDR	4.5	4.4% (2/45)
Tufts University, USA[43]	HDR	2	0% (0/30)

LDR, low dose rate; HDR, high dose rate; PDR, pulsed dose rate; IORT, intra-operative (electrons) radiotherapy.

Table 3 Some characteristics of intra-operative radiotherapy systems

Device Company	Radiation type [*Wt of device]	Dose
INTRABEAM Photoelectron Corporation, Lexington, MA, USA	Soft X-rays at 50 kV [*1.8 kg]	Typical physical dose of 5 Gy at 1 cm or 10 Gy at 0.5 cm or 20 Gy next to the applicator over 25–30 min. Setting-up time ~10–12 min
MOBITRON Oncology Care Systems Group of Siemens Medical Systems, Intraop Medical Inc., Santa Clara, CA, USA	Electrons at 4–12 MeV [*1275 kg]	20 Gy physical dose in 3–5 min. Setting-up time ~20 min
NOVAC-7 Hitesys SpA, Italy	Electrons at 4–12 MeV [*650 kg]	20 Gy physical dose in 3–5 min. Setting-up time ~20 min

*Weight of treatment device (kg)

index quadrant. However, these studies employ standard high-dose rate brachytherapy delivered with a radioactive source (such as iridium, caesium wires, or radioactive pellets within a saline-filled balloon, *e.g.* Mammosite™) placed intra-operatively to cover a large field in the breast. These techniques need after-loading of the radioactive source in the wire or balloon templates. This typically is done in 5–7 fractions delivered in the postoperative period, over 4–5 days. This makes it fundamentally and conceptually different in terms of technique from the intra-operative radiotherapy which is delivered in one sitting at the time of primary surgery, although sharing the basic premise of treating only the index quadrant.

TECHNIQUES OF INTRA-OPERATIVE RADIOTHERAPY

We shall now consider the techniques of delivering intra-operative radiotherapy as a single fraction delivered in the operating theatre immediately after wide excision of the primary tumour. While brachytherapy using interstitial implants necessitated the treatment to be carried out in a specially shielded room, the other, older, intra-operative radiotherapy devices were technically cumbersome and often relied on transporting the patient from the operating theatre to the radiotherapy unit during surgery. Alternatively, operating theatres with built-in IORT systems were used in some centres. These technical and financial limitations to IORT delivery placed a substantial constraint on the wide-spread adoption of IORT in a variety of hospital settings. Recent advances in miniaturisation technology have enabled the development of mobile IORT devices. The first device to be used for IORT is the Intrabeam™ (Photoelectron Corporation, Lexington, MA, USA). The two

> **Key point 3**
>
> - Modern technology has allowed development of portable, powerful radiotherapy devices that can be used in standard unmodified operation theatres.

other systems are mobile linear accelerators – the Mobetron System (Oncology Care Systems Group of Siemens Medical Systems, Intraop Medical Inc., Santa Clara, CA, USA) and the Novac-7 System (Hitesys SpA, Italy). Some of the characteristics of these machines are given in Table 3.

RADIOBIOLOGY OF INTRA-OPERATIVE RADIOTHERAPY

Whether IORT has an identical biological effect on tissue compared with external beam radiotherapy is not known; but, because it is more conformational, the same physical dose of IORT is equivalent to a much higher dose of external beam radiotherapy. With regards to the specific mobile IORT systems currently being used in early breast cancer, the Intrabeam IORT system delivers a physical dose of 5.0 Gy administered at a distance of 1.0 cm from the breast tumour cavity for a period of 21 min that is equivalent to a biologically effective dose of 21.7 Gy. Using Novac-7 IORT technology, Veronesi *et al.*[26] have estimated that an external beam dose of 60 Gy delivered in 30 fractions at 2 Gy/fraction is equivalent to a single IORT fraction of 20–22 Gy (using an α/β ratio at 10 Gy, typical for tumours and acute reacting tissues). Using this same equation, but calculating the tolerance of late responding tissues (α/β ratio at 3 Gy) this equivalent value rises to at least 110 Gy. Radiobiological experiments[44] using cell cultures have suggested that the radiobiological effectiveness (RBE) of the Intrabeam system is 1.2–2.5. This was in agreement with microdosimetric analysis and modelling.[45] The PRS radiation is found to induce both necrotic and apoptotic cell death in addition to rapid cell death through non-apoptotic pathways.[46] Animal experiments have demonstrated that PRS can induce well-demarcated ablation in canine liver and kidney.[47–49] As a demonstration of its efficacy of ablating tumour tissue, 3 patients were treated with a PRS 400 (bare probe only, *i.e.* without the applicators, but with the same Intrabeam machine that is used for intra-operative radiotherapy). The tumour was localised on the Mammotest™, a digital, stereotactic, prone mammography table. The tumours (range, 1-2.5 cm) were ablated with a single dose of radiotherapy as demonstrated on biopsy and serial, contrast-enhanced MRI.[50]

There are no biological models or experimental evidence yet available to estimate the radiobiological effect of a single, large fraction of radiotherapy. The linear quadratic equations that are usually used for these estimates are

> **Key point 4**
>
> - Radiobiology of single-dose, intra-operative radiotherapy is still being studied and the optimum dose has not been established as yet.

reliable up to a single dose of 2–3 Gy, but not higher. It has been proposed (Prof. Frederik Wenz Mannheim, Germany; personal communication) that the low energy X-rays emitted by a system such as the Intrabeam™ may have special properties with respect to tumour and normal cells. Since the radiotherapy delivered by Intrabeam (called TARGIT for targeted intra-operative radiotherapy[51]) is over a period of 25–30 min and the normal tissue DNA repair mechanism takes only 10 min, there is ample time for normal tissues to repair whereas the tumour cells, being poor at DNA repair, would not survive. Thus the radiobiological effect of such a single fraction of radiotherapy may actually be paradoxically higher at greater depth.[44] Thus, the tissues immediately next to the applicator would have a high physical dose with low therapeutic ratio and those away from the applicator would have lower physical dose, but a high therapeutic ratio. This is an advantage of Intrabeam™ over the systems delivering electrons because the treatment time is short and the high (physical) dose region is small – it is expected that this would increase acute tumour effects while reducing long-term toxicity. The specific laboratory experiments to test this concept are already underway.

As yet, there is no firmly established, standardised IORT dose or dose rate for use in early breast cancer. IORT doses investigated for use in early breast cancer have ranged from 5 Gy to 22 Gy using a variety of different IORT systems.

EARLY RESULTS

Based on the hypothesis that index quadrant irradiation is sufficient and equipped with modern technology, in July 1998 we introduced the technique of intra-operative radiotherapy[52–54] that is delivered as a single-dose treatment using low energy X-rays, targeted to the peri-tumoural tissues from within the breast. In patients with small breast cancers (now the majority), this could be the sole treatment. In those with high risk of local recurrence, it would avoid any geographical miss and, in combination with external beam radiotherapy, may further reduce local recurrence.

The results of pilot studies using one such device that uses soft X-rays (Intrabeam™) are encouraging and a randomized trial (TARGIT)[51,55] is under way in the UK, Europe, USA and Australia. The Milan group is also testing the same approach,[56] using a mobile linear accelerator (Novac-7™) in a randomized trial (ELIOT). The completion of these trials is eagerly awaited. If proven effective, these novel approaches have the potential to save time and money, and enable many more women to conserve their breasts.

THE NOVAC-7 SYSTEM

Novac-7 (Hitesys SpA, Italy) is a mobile, dedicated, linear accelerator. Its radiating head can be moved by an articulated arm which can work in an existing operating room. It only delivers electron beams at four different nominal energies – 3, 5, 7, and 9 MeV radiation (Fig. 1).

Beams are collimated by means of a hard-docking system, consisting of cylindrical perspex applicators available in various diameters (4, 5, 6, 8, and 10 cm). The source-to-surface distance is 80–100 cm. For reasons of radiation

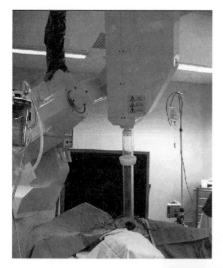

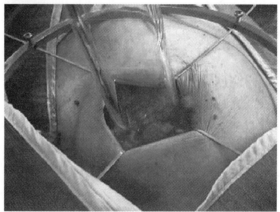

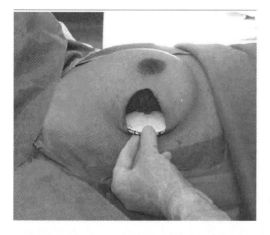

Fig. 1 The Novac-7 system – the arm of the mobile linear accelerator (A) is attached to a perspex cylinder that is introduced in the breast wound (B). The breast tissue is mobilized from the chest wall and overlying skin and apposed in the wound after placing a lead shield between the breast and pectoralis muscle (C). Figures taken from Veronesi et al.[56] with kind permission from Prof. Umberto Veronesi.

protection, a primary beam stopper (consisting of a lead shield, 15 cm thick) mounted on a trolley and three mobile barriers (100 cm length, 150 cm height and 1.5 cm lead thickness) are provided. Electron beams delivered by Novac-7 have very high dose/pulse values compared with those supplied by conventional medical linacs. Once the breast resection has been performed, the breast is mobilised off the pectoral muscle for 5–10 cm around the tumour bed and also separated from the skin for 3–5 cm in every direction. In order to minimise the irradiation of the thoracic wall, dedicated aluminum–lead disks (4 mm Al + 5 mm Pb) of various diameters (4–10 cm) are placed between the deep face of the residual breast and the pectoralis muscle. The breast is now sutured so as to obliterate the tumour bed and bring the target tissues together. The thickness of the target volume is measured by a needle and a ruler in at least three points and averaged. The skin margins are stretched out of the radiation using a home-made device consisting of a metallic ring furnished with four hooks. The cylindrical applicator (4–10 cm diameter) is now placed through the skin incision and in contact with the breast. The source cylinder is now 'docked' onto the upper end of the applicator. The optimal energy of the electron beam is selected on the basis of the previously measured target thickness. The primary beam stopper and the three mobile barriers are positioned, below and around the operating table, in order to provide good shielding from stray radiation, and all medical personnel leave the operating room. Once the radiotherapy is finished, the wound is closed in the usual manner.

THE INTRABEAM SYSTEM

In the Intrabeam, the X-ray tube (XRT) is powered by a 12 V supply, a miniature electron gun and electron accelerator (Figs 2 & 3). Radiation in the form of soft X-rays (low energy 50 kV) is emitted from the point source and is modulated by spherical applicators to give a uniform dose of radiotherapy in a spherical field in the tumour bed. There is quick attenuation of the radiation within tissues which reduces the damage to surrounding normal tissues and minimises the need for radiation protection by the operating personnel. Depending upon the size of the surgical cavity, various sizes of applicator spheres are available and, for each size, the radiation received is proportional to the time the machine is switched on and left *in situ*. The precise dose rate depends on the diameter of the applicator and the energy of the beam, both of which may be varied to optimise the radiation treatment. For example, a dose of about 5 Gy can be delivered in about 20 min at 1 cm from the margins of a 3.5 cm cavity after wide local excision of the tumour.

If necessary, the chest wall and skin can be protected (95% shielding) by radio-opaque, tungsten-filled polyurethane caps, which can be cut to size on the operation table – another advantage of using soft X-rays. With this elegant approach, the pliable breast tissue around the cavity of surgical excision wraps around the radiotherapy source (*i.e.* the target is 'conformed' to the source). This simple, effective technique avoids the unnecessarily complex and sophisticated techniques of interstitial implantation of radioactive wires or the even more complex techniques necessary for conformal radiotherapy by external beams with multi-leaf collimators from a linear accelerator. It eliminates 'geographical miss' and delivers radiotherapy at the earliest possible time after surgery. The quick attenuation of the radiation dose protects normal tissues and allows the treatment to be carried out in unmodified operating theatres. Thus, in theory, the biological effect and cosmetic outcome could be improved. The median follow-up time of the UK pilot feasibility study is now 36 months and there has been no

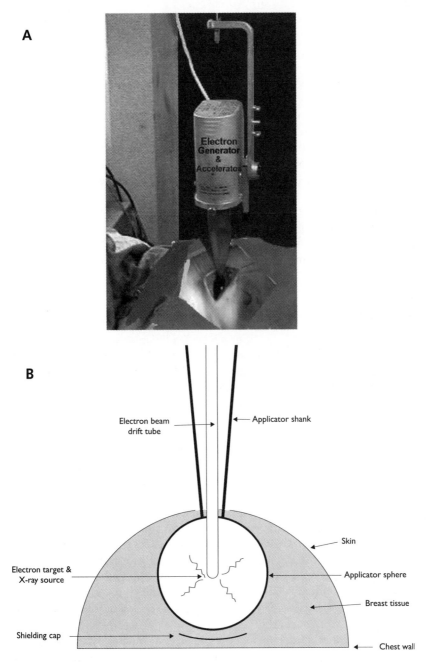

Fig. 2 (A) The Intrabeam system, with the X-ray source in the breast wound (tumour bed), and the electron generator and accelerator held by the gantry. The schematic diagram (B) shows how the target tissues are irradiated from within the breast and how the intrathoracic structures can be protected with a thin shield.

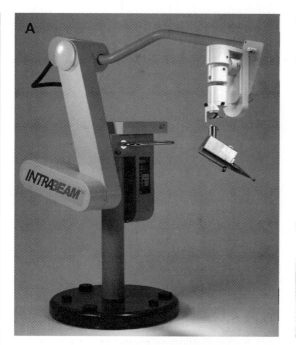
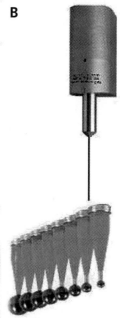

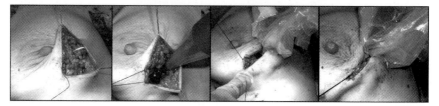

Fig. 3 The Intrabeam system (A), X-ray source and applicators (B). In (C), the figures demonstrate how the target breast tissue wraps around the applicator giving true conformal brachytherapy.

local recurrence. Including the US and Australian data,[55] a total of more than 100 patients have been treated with good short-term results.

The randomised trial TARGIT, which has collaboration of centres from the UK, Europe, USA, India and Australasia, is designed to test the hypothesis that the strategy of delivering targeted intra-operative radiotherapy in patients eligible for breast-conserving therapy with a facility to add whole breast radiotherapy in those patients who are at high risk of recurrence elsewhere in the breast (*e.g.* lobular cancers, EIC) is equivalent to the standard 6-week postoperative radiotherapy. In this pragmatic trial, each centre will have the ability to decide the level of uncertainty and, therefore, the trial will be stratified according to each centre's decision on which group of patients will receive whole breast radiotherapy in addition to the intra-operative dose. It is expected that the first results of this trial will be available in 2007.

Key point 5

- Results of pilot studies using modern intra-operative radiotherapy techniques are encouraging and several collaborating international groups are recruiting patients in randomised trials.

Key point 6

- Used as a boost, targeted intra-operative radiotherapy can avoid geographical miss and has the potential to reduce local recurrence. Used as a sole treatment for good prognosis breast cancers, it could replace the whole 6-week course of postoperative radiotherapy.

HEALTH ECONOMICS

Delivering intra-operative radiotherapy with Intrabeam™ prolongs the primary operation by 15–45 min and adds 1–2 h of radiotherapy physicists' time in preparation of the device. External beam radiotherapy, on the other hand, costs about 9 man-hours, 6 h of radiotherapy room time and 30–60 h of patient time. If the cost of conventional radiotherapy were £1200, considering only the 66% saving of man-hours the novel technique would save £900 per patient. So, assuming that 60% of the 27,000 breast cancer patients diagnosed every year in the UK are treated by conservative surgery and intra-operative radiotherapy, the novel technique would potentially save about £15 million (0.60 x 27,000 x 3750) per year for the NHS in the UK. This does not include the substantial saving of expensive resource time on linear accelerators and, most importantly, the saving of time, effort and inconvenience to patients. This is a very attractive aspect of novel technology that is, unlike most other 'new' treatments, actually less expensive than the current standard.

Key point 7

- Unlike most modern medical technology, some intra-operative systems may actually save money for the health system.

Key points for clinical practice

- The usual 6-week course of postoperative radiotherapy after breast conserving surgery has several disadvantages that reduces its general applicability to a wide population, even amongst the most advanced health economies.

References

1. Moore C. On the influence of inadequate operations on the theory of cancer. *R Med Chir Soc Lond* 1867; **1**: 244–280.
2. Halsted WS. The results of operations for the cure of cancer of the breast performed at The Johns Hopkins Hospital from June 1889 to January 1894. *Johns Hopkins Hospital Reports* 1894; **4**: 297–350.
3. Lewis D, Rienhoff Jr WF. A study of results of operations for the cure of cancer of the breast. *Ann Surg* 1932; **95**: 336.
4. Urban J. Management of operable breast cancer: the surgeon's view. *Cancer* 1978; **42**: 2066.
5. Lacour J, Le M, Rumeau C *et al.* [International therapeutic trial comparing the value of radical mastectomy (Halsted) and extended mastectomy (Halsted plus internal mammary node dissection) in the treatment of breast cancer. 5-year results]. *Chirurgie* 1976; **102**: 638–649.
6. Meier P, Ferguson DJ, Karrison T. A controlled trial of extended radical mastectomy. *Cancer* 1985; **55**: 880–891.
7. Fisher B. Laboratory and clinical research in breast cancer – a personal adventure: the David A. Karnofsky memorial lecture. *Cancer Res* 1980; **40**: 3863–3874.
8. Early Breast Cancer Trialists' Collaborative Group. Effects of radiotherapy and surgery in early breast cancer. An overview of the randomized trials. *N Engl J Med* 1995; **333**: 1444–1455.
9. Early Breast Cancer Trialists' Collaborative Group. Favourable and unfavourable effects on long-term survival of radiotherapy for early breast cancer: an overview of the randomised trials. [see comments]. *Lancet* 2000; **355**: 1757–1770.

10. Athas WF, Adams-Cameron M, Hunt WC, Amir-Fazli A, Key CR. Travel distance to radiation therapy and receipt of radiotherapy following breast-conserving surgery. *J Natl Cancer Inst* 2000; **92**: 269–271.

11. Sedlmayer F, Rahim HB, Kogelnik HD *et al*. Quality assurance in breast cancer brachytherapy: geographic miss in the interstitial boost treatment of the tumor bed. *Int J Radiat Oncol Biol Phys* 1996; **34**: 1133–1139.

12. Machtay M, Lanciano R, Hoffman J, Hanks GE. Inaccuracies in using the lumpectomy scar for planning electron boosts in primary breast carcinoma. *Int J Radiat Oncol Biol Phys* 1994; **30**: 43–48.

13. Fisher ER, Anderson S, Redmond C, Fisher B. Ipsilateral breast tumor recurrence and survival following lumpectomy and irradiation: pathological findings from NSABP protocol B-06. *Semin Surg Oncol* 1992; **8**: 161–166.

14. Deng G, Lu Y, Zlotnikov G, Thor AD, Smith HS. Loss of heterozygosity in normal tissue adjacent to breast carcinomas. *Science* 1996; **274**: 2057–2059.

15. O'Neill JS, Elton RA, Miller WR. Aromatase activity in adipose tissue from breast quadrants: a link with tumour site. *BMJ* 1988; **296**: 741–743.

16. Nakamura J, Savinov A, Lu Q, Brodie A. Estrogen regulates vascular endothelial growth/permeability factor expression in 7,12-dimethylbenz(a)anthracene-induced rat mammary tumors. *Endocrinology* 1996; **137**: 5589–5596.

17. Lu Q, Nakmura J, Savinov A *et al*. Expression of aromatase protein and messenger ribonucleic acid in tumor epithelial cells and evidence of functional significance of locally produced estrogen in human breast cancers. *Endocrinology* 1996; **137**: 3061–3068.

18. Harrold EV, Turner BC, Matloff ET *et al*. Local recurrence in the conservatively treated breast cancer patient: a correlation with age and family history [see comments]. *Cancer J Sci Am* 1998; **4**: 302–307.

19. Arriagada R, Le MG, Contesso G, Guinebretiere JM, Rochard F, Spielmann M. Predictive factors for local recurrence in 2006 patients with surgically resected small breast cancer. *Ann Oncol* 2002; **13**: 1404–1413.

20. Turner BC, Harrold E, Matloff E *et al*. BRCA1/BRCA2 germline mutations in locally recurrent breast cancer patients after lumpectomy and radiation therapy: implications for breast-conserving management in patients with BRCA1/BRCA2 mutations [see comments]. *J Clin Oncol* 1999; **17**: 3017–3024.

21. Clark RM, Wilkinson RH, Mahoney LJ, Reid JG, MacDonald WD. Breast cancer: a 21 year experience with conservative surgery and radiation. *Int J Radiat Oncol Biol Phys* 1982; **8**: 967–979.

22. Schnitt SJ, Connolly JL, Harris JR, Hellman S, Cohen RB. Pathologic predictors of early local recurrence in stage I and II breast cancer treated by primary radiation therapy. *Cancer* 1984; **53**: 1049–1057.

23. Boyages J, Recht A, Connolly JL *et al*. Early breast cancer: predictors of breast recurrence for patients treated with conservative surgery and radiation therapy. *Radiother Oncol* 1990; **19**: 29–41.

24. Kurtz JM, Jacquemier J, Torhorst J *et al*. Conservation therapy for breast cancers other than infiltrating ductal carcinoma. *Cancer* 1989; **63**: 1630–1635.

25. Clark RM, McCulloch PB, Levine MN *et al*. Randomized clinical trial to assess the effectiveness of breast irradiation following lumpectomy and axillary dissection for node-negative breast cancer. *J Natl Cancer Inst* 1992; **84**: 683–689.

26. Veronesi U, Luini A, Del Vecchio M *et al*. Radiotherapy after breast-preserving surgery in women with localized cancer of the breast [see comments]. *N Engl J Med* 1993; **328**: 1587–1591.

27. Bartelink H, Horiot JC, Poortmans P *et al*. Recurrence rates after treatment of breast cancer with standard radiotherapy with or without additional radiation. *N Engl J Med* 2001; **345**: 1378–1387.

28. McCulloch PG, MacIntyre A. Effects of surgery on the generation of lymphokine-activated killer cells in patients with breast cancer. *Br J Surg* 1993; **80**: 1005–1007.

29. Fisher B, Anderson S, Redmond CK, Wolmark N, Wickerham DL, Cronin WM. Re-analysis and results after 12 years of follow-up in a randomized clinical trial comparing total mastectomy with lumpectomy with or without irradiation in the treatment of breast cancer [see comments]. *N Engl J Med* 1995; **333**: 1456–1461.

30. Clark RM, Whelan T, Levine M *et al.* Randomized clinical trial of breast irradiation following lumpectomy and axillary dissection for node-negative breast cancer: an update. Ontario Clinical Oncology Group. *J Natl Cancer Inst* 1996; **88**: 1659–1664.

31. Liljegren G, Holmberg L, Bergh J *et al.* 10-Year results after sector resection with or without postoperative radiotherapy for stage I breast cancer: a randomized trial [see comments]. *J Clin Oncol* 1999; **17**: 2326–2333.

32. Forrest AP, Stewart HJ, Everington D *et al.* Randomised controlled trial of conservation therapy for breast cancer: 6-year analysis of the Scottish trial. Scottish Cancer Trials Breast Group [see comments]. *Lancet* 1996; **348**: 708–713.

33. Vaidya JS, Vyas JJ, Chinoy RF, Merchant N, Sharma OP, Mittra I. Multicentricity of breast cancer: whole-organ analysis and clinical implications. *Br J Cancer* 1996; **74**: 820–824.

34. Nielsen M, Thomsen JL, Primdahl S, Dyreborg U, Andersen JA. Breast cancer and atypia among young and middle-aged women: a study of 110 medicolegal autopsies. *Br J Cancer* 1987; **56**: 814–819.

35. Ribeiro GG, Magee B, Swindell R, Harris M, Banerjee SS. The Christie Hospital breast conservation trial: an update at 8 years from inception. *Clin Oncol (R Coll Radiol)* 1993; **5**: 278–283.

36. Polgar C, Sulyok Z, Fodor J *et al.* Sole brachytherapy of the tumor bed after conservative surgery for T1 breast cancer: five-year results of a phase I-II study and initial findings of a randomized phase III trial. *J Surg Oncol* 2002; **80**: 121–128.

37. Samuel LM, Dewar JA, Preece PE, Wood RAB. A pilot study of radical radiotherapy using a perioperative implant following wide local excision for carcinoma of the breast. *Breast* 1999; **8**: 95–97.

38. King TA, Bolton JS, Kuske RR, Fuhrman GM, Scroggins TG, Jiang XZ. Long-term results of wide-field brachytherapy as the sole method of radiation therapy after segmental mastectomy for T(is,1,2) breast cancer. *Am J Surg* 2000; **180**: 299–304.

39. Perera F, Engel J, Holliday R *et al.* Local resection and brachytherapy confined to the lumpectomy site for early breast cancer: a pilot study. *J Surg Oncol* 1997; **65**: 263–267.

40. Vicini FA, Baglan KL, Kestin LL *et al.* Accelerated treatment of breast cancer. *J Clin Oncol* 2001; **19**: 1993–2001.

41. Johansson B, Karlsson L, Liljegren G. PDR brachytherapy as the sole adjuvant radiotherapy after breast conserving surgery for T1-2 breast cancer. Program and abstracts, *10th International Brachytherapy Conference*, Madrid: Nucletron, 2000; 127.

42. Krishnan L, Jewell WR, Tawfik OW, Krishnan EC. Breast conservation therapy with tumor bed irradiation alone in a selected group of patients with stage I breast cancer. *Breast J* 2001; **7**: 91–96.

43. Wazer DE, Lowther D, Boyle T *et al.* Clinically evident fat necrosis in women treated with high-dose-rate brachytherapy alone for early-stage breast cancer. *Int J Radiat Oncol Biol Phys* 2001; **50**: 107–111.

44. Astor MB, Hilaris BS, Gruerio A, Varricchione T, Smith D. Preclinical studies with the photon radiosurgery system (PRS). *Int J Radiat Oncol Biol Phys* 2000; **47**: 809–813.

45. Brenner DJ, Leu CS, Beatty JF, Shefer RE. Clinical relative biological effectiveness of low-energy x-rays emitted by miniature x-ray devices. *Phys Med Biol* 1999; **44**: 323–333.

46. Kurita H, Ostertag CB, Baumer B, Kopitzki K, Warnke PC. Early effects of PRS-irradiation for 9L gliosarcoma: characterization of interphase cell death. *Minim Invasive Neurosurg* 2000; **43**: 197–200.

47. Chan DY, Koniaris L, Magee C *et al.* Feasibility of ablating normal renal parenchyma by interstitial photon radiation energy: study in a canine model. *J Endourol* 2000; **14**: 111–116.

48. Koniaris LG, Chan DY, Magee C *et al.* Focal hepatic ablation using interstitial photon radiation energy. *J Am Coll Surg* 2000; **191**: 164–174.

49. Solomon SB, Koniaris LG, Chan DY *et al.* Temporal CT changes after hepatic and renal interstitial radiotherapy in a canine model. *J Comput Assist Tomogr* 2001; **25**: 74–80.

50. Vaidya JS, Hall-Craggs M, Baum M *et al.* Percutaneous minimally invasive stereotactic primary radiotherapy for breast cancer. *Lancet Oncol* 2002; **3**: 252–253.

51. Vaidya JS, Baum M, Tobias JS, Houghton J. Targeted Intraoperative Radiothearpy (TARGIT)-trial protocol. *Lancet* 1999; <http: //www.thelancet.com/info/ info.isa?n1=authorinfo&n2=Protocol+review&uid=9920>.

52. Vaidya JS, Baum M, Tobias JS *et al*. Targeted intra-operative radiotherapy (Targit): an innovative method of treatment for early breast cancer. *Ann Oncol* 2001; **12**: 1075–1080.
53. Vaidya JS, Baum M, Tobias JS, Morgan S, D'Souza D. The novel technique of delivering targeted intraoperative radiotherapy (Targit) for early breast cancer. *Eur J Surg Oncol* 2002; **28**: 447–454.
54. Vaidya JS. *A Novel Approach for Local Treatment of Early Breast Cancer*. PhD Thesis, University of London 2002; 1–242.
55. Vaidya JS, Joseph D, Hilaris BS *et al*. Targeted intraoperative radiotherapy for breast cancer: an international trial. Abstract Book of *ESTRO-21, Prague 2002* 2002; **21**: 135.
56. Veronesi U, Orecchia R, Luini A *et al*. A preliminary report of intraoperative radiotherapy (IORT) in limited-stage breast cancers that are conservatively treated. *Eur J Cancer* 2001; **37**: 2178–2183.

Michael Baum Richard Sainsbury

14

Recent developments in the endocrine therapy of early breast cancer

Breast cancers, in company with prostate cancers, are unique in their sensitivity to endocrine manipulation. Consequently, the endocrine therapy of breast cancer has been a remarkable success story. Over the past 15 years, there has been a dramatic fall in mortality from the disease in both the UK[1] and in whites in the US. Most commentators attribute this to the direct or indirect effect of adjuvant hormonal manipulation. A large contribution to this success has been the cross-talk between clinical scientists and endocrinologists over the past 50 years. The laboratory research has typically been provoked following original observations made by clinicians. This may then suggest further clinical interventions with further 'biological fall-out'.

The cycle started with Beatson in 1896[2] and is currently resting with the 'Arimidex', Tamoxifen Alone or in Combination (ATAC) trial in 2002.[3]

Approximately 50 years after Beatson's landmark series of six cases of surgical castration for the treatment of advanced breast cancer (where he achieved a 30% response rate), Huggins and his colleagues first described surgical adrenalectomy as second-line endocrine therapy.[4] Both these remarkable studies were empirical observations, with either little or a misguided understanding of the biological rationale underlying the responses. This is, perhaps, the reason that the development of endocrine therapy for breast cancer has mostly been lead by surgeons in the UK.

The past 50 years have seen a concerted effort by endocrinologists and clinicians alike to understand and exploit these mechanisms for clinical benefit. A 'thread' that runs through this endeavour has been the search for the mechanism of response. The identification of the role of the oestrogen receptor (ER) in

Prof. Michael Baum MD ChM FRCS, The Portland Hospital, 212–214 Portland Street, London W1W 5QN, UK (for correspondence)

Mr Richard Sainsbury MBBS MD FRCS, Senior Lecturer in Surgery, University College London, UK

selecting the most appropriate patients for treatment was a fundamental step. The ER status of the primary tumour might be considered to be an inevitable limitation to endocrine therapy. However, such is the success of the endocrine approach to the treatment of breast cancer, one can predict that the next challenge endocrinologists will face is to determine the process leading to the loss of the ER mechanism. If this turns out to be an epigenetic phenomenon, then within a generation it might be possible to convert ER negative (ER⁻) tumours to an ER positive (ER⁺) phenotype – and that, one hopes, would be the beginning of the end of non-specific chemotherapy.

For the first 50 years after Beatson's original work on castration for metastatic breast cancer, little changed, although the discovery of the sex steroid hormones certainly provided a rational explanation for the therapeutic benefit of ovarian ablation. This rationale led Haddow and his colleagues to experiment with synthetic oestrogens,[5] and Adair and Herrman[6] to use androgens for advanced breast cancer. Huggins and colleagues[4] took a courageous leap forward with their description of bilateral adrenalectomy for metastatic breast and prostate cancer. In retrospect, the scientific rationale they described is bizarre, with justification based on animal experiments with a variety of tumours, only some of which might be considered to be hormone-sensitive. Because the role of the adrenal gland in the synthesis of oestrogen precursors had not yet been described, they thought that any responses seen in the experimental setting were related to a non-specific effect of the corticosteroid hormones. Huggins and colleagues described 18 cases of bilateral adrenalectomy, of which there were 7 with advanced breast cancer; 6 of the breast cancer cases were premenopausal and had undergone prior oophorectomy. There were two partial responses, one stable disease, and three cases progressed. This response rate is indeed what might be expected for second-line endocrine therapy of advanced disease. This paper was an adumbration of the future work on the extra-ovarian source of oestrogen synthesis, and the search for a safe and efficient way of down-regulating peripheral conversion of cholesterol to sex steroids via aromatase activity, which ultimately lead to the ATAC trial (*vide infra*).

As the source of oestrogens in premenopausal women is the ovaries and their function is influenced by hypothalamic–pituitary interaction, therapeutic strategies are complex with the options of targeting the ovaries directly (ovarian ablation by surgery or radiotherapy) or indirectly via hypophysectomy (obsolete) or the GnRH (gonadotrophin releasing hormone) agonist class of drugs. For post-menopausal women, the source of oestrogen is from the peripheral aromatization in the body fat depots of androgens synthesized in the adrenal gland. There are thus two surgical approaches, hypophysectomy or adrenalectomy (both obsolete) or a pharmacological approach with the third generation of aromatase inhibitors.

Here, recent developments for pre- and post-menopausal women will be considered separately. However, it is also worth recalling what has been

---

Key point 1

- Breast cancer is often responsive to endocrine manipulation, especially if hormone-receptor positive.

achieved so far with tamoxifen, which provides an equal protection from relapse in the adjuvant therapy of both pre- and post-menopausal women.

CURRENT STATUS OF ADJUVANT THERAPY WITH TAMOXIFEN

It is now known that the benefit of tamoxifen in adjuvant therapy after the surgical treatment of early breast cancer is greater than its benefit in advanced disease. The first trials for adjuvant therapy were started in the late 1970s, and the results reported during the next decade. In early studies, the control groups were given no adjuvant therapy, and the treated groups received tamoxifen for either 1 or 2 years.

The first trial to show a disease-free survival advantage with adjuvant tamoxifen therapy was the Nolvadex Adjuvant Trial Organisation (NATO) study, published in 1983.[7] More than 1100 women with early breast cancer were randomised to no further therapy after mastectomy (with optional postoperative radiotherapy), or tamoxifen treatment (20 mg daily for 2 years). Node-positive premenopausal women and both node-positive and node-negative post-menopausal women were included; most of the patients were post-menopausal, and fewer than half of all patients entered had histologically-proven involved nodes. There was a highly significant proportional reduction in both recurrence rate (36%) and mortality (29%) after a median follow-up of 66 months. An analysis of log hazard ratios at various intervals after initiation of treatment indicated that treatment beyond 2 years might be beneficial.

Soon after the NATO trial, other studies demonstrated similar benefits with tamoxifen given for 2 or 5 years after surgery, and the first overview of adjuvant tamoxifen therapy demonstrated convincingly that adjuvant tamoxifen was associated with relative-risk reductions for both relapse (25%) and death (17%) over a 10-year period. Significant effects were observed regardless of nodal status. Furthermore, the groups most likely to benefit were post-menopausal women with ER-positive tumours; however, post-menopausal women with ER-negative tumours and premenopausal women with ER-positive cancer also showed significant benefits. The most recent overview (1998) confirmed the results for ER-positive tumours, but stated: 'for women with tumours that have been reliably shown to be ER-negative, adjuvant tamoxifen remains a matter for research'. The, as yet unpublished, 2000 overview confirms that only ER-positive women should receive adjuvant tamoxifen.

The optimum duration of tamoxifen is still undetermined. Two years of therapy is clearly sub-optimal, but 5 years is probably close to the optimal duration; the current data certainly suggest this. Two large scale trials have been designed to address the issue: ATTOM (Adjuvant Tamoxifen Treatment Offer More?) and ATLAS (Adjuvant Tamoxifen – Longer Against Shorter).

Key point 2
- Tamoxifen has been the mainstay of treatment for over 25 years and is effective for pre- and post-menopausal women.

CHEMOTHERAPY *VERSUS* TAMOXIFEN IN PRE-MENOPAUSAL WOMEN

The 1992 overview[8] showed that women below 50 years of age having tamoxifen only had a 12% reduction in the risk of disease recurrence, but a non-significant 6% fall in mortality (less than that obtained with cytotoxic chemotherapy). This is in contrast to women over the age of 50 years, where the figures are 29% and 20%, respectively, which indicates that endocrine therapy is most effective in this older group of women. A question not answered in the overview is whether patients with ER-positive tumours gain more benefit from tamoxifen than chemotherapy. The NSABP (National Surgical Breast and Bowel Project) B-14[9] study investigated pre- and post-menopausal patients with node-negative, ER-positive early breast cancer. After 10 years of follow-up, the patients who received tamoxifen (compared to placebo) showed significant benefits in rates of disease-free survival, distant disease-free survival, and overall survival. The follow-up to this study (NSABP B-20)[10] investigated a similar group of patients, with treatment groups of tamoxifen alone or tamoxifen following chemotherapy. Women given tamoxifen after CMF (cyclophosphamide, methotrexate and 5-fluorouracil), regardless of age, had a significant benefit in disease-free survival. The evidence, therefore, suggests that tamoxifen is effective in women with ER positive tumours regardless of their menopausal status; however, a convincing comparison between tamoxifen alone and chemotherapy alone has not been carried out.

Tamoxifen appears to add to the response to treatment by chemotherapy.[11] In one study, the disease-free survival rate at 5 years was 90% in ER-positive patients treated with tamoxifen plus CMF, significantly better than the 84% found in those treated with tamoxifen alone.

Recurrence of disease during tamoxifen treatment is relatively common, but the reasons for this are not clear. Three possibilities include: (i) loss of ER status; (ii) selection of ER-negative clones; or (iii) reduction in circulating tamoxifen (or metabolite) concentrations. However, these do not explain acquired resistance in most cases. Other explanations have been investigated, including a reduced cellular concentration of tamoxifen, or a conversion to an inactive metabolite – the evidence is equivocal. Surprisingly, resistance to tamoxifen can occur even while tumours remain ER-positive and are functionally responsive to oestrogens.

One 'spin-off' of the overviews (of 37,000 women world-wide) is the ability to quantify the risk of side-effects with adjuvant tamoxifen treatment. Tamoxifen is a complicated drug and, in addition to its main antagonist effect, has some agonist properties which may be responsible for some of the potentially adverse affects – and, it must be said, some of the unexpected additional benefits.

Probably because of these partial agonist properties, tamoxifen appears to reduce the incidence of ischaemic heart disease (mainly through a beneficial effect on lipids), and seems to prevent the loss of bone mineral density in post-menopausal women (although not in premenopausal women). Tamoxifen has also been used in the treatment of mastalgia, but is unlicensed for this indication.

On the downside, tamoxifen has been implicated in an increased incidence of endometrial cancers. An ascertainment bias cannot be excluded, as patients receiving tamoxifen are screened more intensively for uterine abnormalities than those in the control groups. Transvaginal ultrasonography may detect what appears to be endometrial thickening, resulting in a hysteroscopy, which may reveal latent endometrial cancer.

In the past, there have been concerns about reports of crystalline retinal deposits and other ocular toxicities; however, recent data from several large trials indicate that the incidence of tamoxifen-related eye disease is very low. Finally, even though tamoxifen is a weak promoter of hepatocellular carcinoma in rats, no increase in the incidence of liver tumours has been reported in any of the clinical trials.

In 30 years, tamoxifen has emerged as an important weapon in the fight against breast cancer; its use has undoubtedly saved thousands of lives and it will be many years before its role will be surpassed. However, because of the side-effects mentioned above and the development of resistance, it is important to look at the newer endocrine therapies alone or in addition to tamoxifen for pre- and post-menopausal women, respectively.

GnRH AGONISTS IN PREMENOPAUSAL WOMEN

The world overview of adjuvant systemic therapy in early breast cancer of 1985 is one of the seminal events in the history of the endocrine management of breast cancer. For the first time, unequivocal and statistically robust data were presented to the medical community confirming that the appropriate use of adjuvant systemic therapy was associated with a significant and prolonged improvement in survival.[11] The follow-up overview analyses of 1990, 1995 and 2000 added to and strengthened the original observations.[8,12,13] Since 1985, mortality rates for breast cancer in the UK have fallen by approximately 30% from an all-time high in the late 1970s and this fall has been ascribed, in the main, to the wide-spread adoption of adjuvant systemic therapy.[1]

There were two anticipated and one surprise observations emerging from the 1985 overview. First, the advantage of combination chemotherapy amongst premenopausal women with little or no detectable effect in the older women. Second, the value of tamoxifen amongst post-menopausal women with no demonstrable effect amongst premenopausal women. However, the unexpected result was the meta-analyses of the mature data from a few relatively small trials of ovarian suppression (surgical castration or ovarian irradiation). The benefits of ovarian suppression were of the same order of magnitude as those achieved by cytotoxic chemotherapy.

The observations of 1985 effectively established a research agenda for the next 15 years, maturing at the time of the overview in Oxford of September 2000. This agenda included further trials on the role of cytotoxic chemotherapy

---

Key point 3

- Ovarian ablation by permanent means (surgery, radiotherapy) or reversibly by LHRH agonists is as effective as chemotherapy in pre-menopausal women with oestrogen-receptor positive tumours.

in post-menopausal women, trials of tamoxifen in premenopausal women, the selection of tamoxifen on the basis of oestrogen receptor status, and the benefits of combining chemotherapy and endocrine therapy.

DOES ADJUVANT CHEMOTHERAPY MEDIATE ITS EFFECT INDIRECTLY VIA CHEMICAL OVARIAN SUPPRESSION?

The original observation that ovarian suppression and chemotherapy each produced an improvement in disease-free survival for premenopausal women poses the question as to whether this effect was mediated indirectly by the same biochemical pathway. There are four sets of observations that support this hypothesis.

1. It is recognised that cytotoxic chemotherapy will induce amenorrhoea in a proportion of premenopausal women ranging from about 60% to close on 100% depending on age. The younger the woman, the more resistance to the castrating effect of cytotoxic drugs.[14]

2. The endocrinological profile of a woman exposed to cytotoxic chemotherapy is similar to that of a castrated woman. In other words, oestradiol levels fall and gonadotrophin levels rise.[15,16]

3. There is now an extensive literature showing that the induction of amenorrhoea by adjuvant cytotoxic chemotherapy is in itself a prognostic factor. Those women developing a permanent amenorrhoea fare better than those whose menstrual periods return during or after the completion of the course of treatment. This association is seen most clearly amongst women whose tumours express the oestrogen receptors.[17–19]

4. Finally, there are the trials which attempt to compare endocrine therapy and chemotherapy for premenopausal women stratified according to their oestrogen receptor status.

These trials will now be discussed in greater detail.

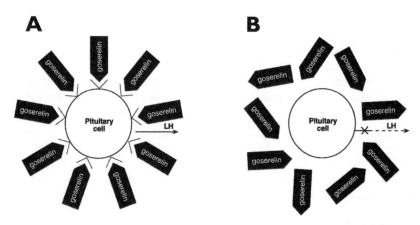

Fig. 1 Mode of action of goserelin. (A) Hypersecretion of luteinizing hormone (LH) following acute administration of goserelin; (B) hyposecretion of LH after chronic administration of goserelin.

Table 1 Relation between oestrogen receptor concentration and first event. Adapted with permission from Scottish Cancer Trials Breast Group. *Lancet* 1993; **341:** 1293–1298,[19] © The Lancet Ltd

Oestrogen receptor (fmol/mg protein)	Total	HR Ovarian ablation/CMF (95% CI)	
0–4	60	1.79 (0.82–3.89)	1.74 (0.95–3.19)
5–19	40	1.59 (0.59–4.27)	
20–99	116	0.70 (0.38–1.27)	0.65 (0.37–1.15)
≥ 100	22	0.45 (0.08–2.7)	

The Scottish trial

The Scottish breast cancer trial was the first to attempt a comparison of ovarian suppression and cytotoxic chemotherapy in early breast cancer.[19] In this study, ovarian suppression was achieved either by surgical castration or X-ray menopause. Patients of all pathological stage and oestrogen receptor status were recruited and randomised to ovarian suppression or six cycles of classical CMF. The trial was slow to recruit and the eventual numbers were modest. Nevertheless, these results provided sufficient information to support the next generation of studies. The results of the trial were more or less as anticipated in that there was an apparent equivalence amongst the unselected patients. However, when stratified according to oestrogen receptor status, those who were ER positive fared better with ovarian suppression whereas those who were ER negative faired better with cytotoxic chemotherapy (Table 1).

Trials involving GnRH analogues

A more recent portfolio of clinical trials for premenopausal women commenced recruiting in the mid-1980s following the availability of the GnRH agonists (primarily goserelin). This class of drug acts on the hypothalamus to produce a reversible ovarian suppression down-regulating gonadotrophin release via the process of tachyphylaxis acting on the LHRH receptors of a pituitary gland (Fig. 1).[20] Goserelin had already been demonstrated to be a safe and effective treatment for advanced or metastatic breast cancer in premenopausal women, providing an alternative to surgical castration or an X-ray menopause.[21,22] This drug, therefore, appeared to be an ideal candidate for use in the adjuvant treatment of early breast cancer particularly for the younger woman who wished to preserve fertility and also where there were long-term concerns about osteoporosis for a prematurely castrated woman. There are three trial categories: (i) equivalence trials of goserelin *versus* standard chemotherapy; (ii) trials comparing combination endocrine therapy with goserelin and tamoxifen *versus* standard chemotherapy; and (iii) trials exploring the additive effect of endocrine therapy for women undergoing standard cytotoxic therapy as first choice.

The ZEBRA trial

The ZEBRA trial is an international collaborative group designed and powered to demonstrate equivalence between goserelin and adjuvant chemotherapy

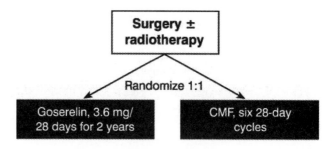

Fig. 2 Protocol for the ZEBRA trial of goserelin *versus* CMF (cyclophosphamide, methotrexate, 5-fluorouracil) treatment.

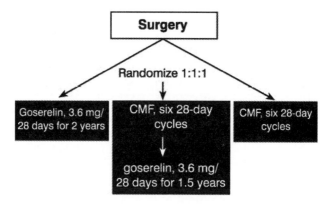

Fig. 3 IBCSG VIII protocol of goserelin *versus* CMF (cyclophosphamide, methotrexate, 5-fluorouracil) *versus* the combination. A fourth arm of no treatment was discontinued 2 years after recruitment.

(Fig. 2).[23] Following surgery, patients were randomised to 2 years of goserelin or six cycles of chemotherapy using CMF. Close on 2000 patients were recruited – ER-positive, ER-negative, and ER-unknown. Where the women were known to be oestrogen receptor positive, the results demonstrated an 'equivalence' within a predetermined and statistically acceptable narrow confidence interval. This 'equivalence' is not an intuitively obvious outcome if one assumes that cytotoxic chemotherapy can achieve its effect directly by cell-kill and indirectly by ovarian suppression. However, this could be explained by a significant proportion of the patients receiving CMF failing to achieve permanent amenorrhoea.

The IBCSG (International Breast Cancer Study Group) VIII trial which has yet to be reported (Fig. 3) has two arms identical to the ZEBRA analyses and will help to confirm whether these two approaches are equivalent for oestrogen receptor positive patients.

TRIALS OF COMBINATION ENDOCRINE THERAPY VERSUS CHEMOTHERAPY

There are two recently reported trials comparing ovarian suppression and tamoxifen with conventional CMF, namely GROCTA02 (Fig. 4)[24] and the Austrian Breast Cancer Study Group (ABCSG) trial (Fig. 5).[25] The Italian breast

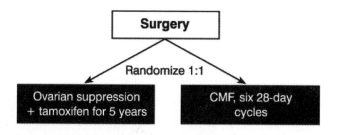

Fig. 4 Protocol for the GROCTA trial of ovarian suppression plus tamoxifen (5 years) *versus* CMF (cyclophosphamide, methotrexate, 5-fluorouracil) treatment. Ovarian suppression was achieved either by oophorectomy (*n* = 6), ovarian irradiation (*n* = 31) or 2 years goserelin treatment (*n* = 87).

cancer adjuvant group (GROCTA) compared ovarian ablation (which included oophorectomy and ovarian irradiation, although 70% of the patients had goserelin) plus 5 years of tamoxifen *versus* CMF. They included 244 premenopausal women who were ER positive and node-positive or node-negative with a median follow-up of nearly 5 years. The Austrian study compared goserelin for 3 years and tamoxifen for 5 years *versus* six cycles of CMF. Over 1000 premenopausal patients were recruited, all of whom were hormone-receptor positive but either node-positive or node-negative with a median follow-up of about 4 years. Both studies demonstrated the benefit of combining ovarian suppression and tamoxifen *versus* CMF alone.

In the Austrian study, patients treated with combination endocrine treatment had a significantly improved recurrence-free survival compared with CMF ($P < 0.02$) while in the Italian study there was no difference between tamoxifen plus ovarian suppression and CMF with respect to either disease-free or overall survival. Again, these results are not surprising if one bears in mind that CMF fails to achieve complete amenorrhoea in all women and the more recent evidence that the addition of tamoxifen to cytotoxic chemotherapy improves outcome over chemotherapy alone. This particular issue has been addressed directly by the INT 0101\E5188 intergroup study.

INT 0101\E5188 (Intergroup Study ECOG\SWOG\CALGB Trial)[26]
The design of this trial is illustrated in Figure 6. After local therapy, patients are randomised between six cycles of CAF (cyclophosphamide, adriamycin and 5-fluorouracil), six cycles of CAF followed by 5 years of goserelin and six cycles

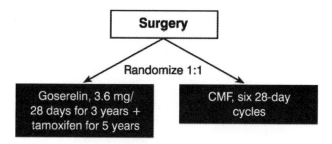

Fig. 5 Protocol for the ABCSG trial of goserelin (3 years) plus tamoxifen (5 years) *versus* CMF (cyclophosphamide, methotrexate, 5-fluorouracil) treatment.

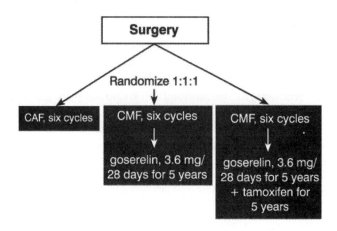

Fig. 6 ECOG/SWOG protocol of CAF (cyclophosphamide, adriamycin, 5-fluorouracil) *versus* CAF plus goserelin *versus* CAF plus goserelin plus tamoxifen.

of CAF followed by goserelin and tamoxifen each for 5 years. Over 1500 premenopausal patients were recruited, all of whom were ER- and or PR-positive with involved axillary lymph nodes, and the median follow-up is now 6 years. The latest results show a significant improvement in 5-year disease-free survival for the addition of goserelin and tamoxifen to chemotherapy compared with the addition of goserelin alone; there was also a small numerical, but non-significant, benefit for adding goserelin alone to chemotherapy.

ZIPP combined analysis[27]

Shortly after the 1985 world overview, four collaborative groups met in order to design a prospective, multicentre clinical trial to explore the options of adjuvant systemic therapy for premenopausal women. The groups concerned were the British Cancer Research Campaign Breast Cancer Trials Group, the Stockholm Breast Cancer Trials Group, a group from South-East Sweden and an Italian collaborative group, GIVIO. The intention was that each group

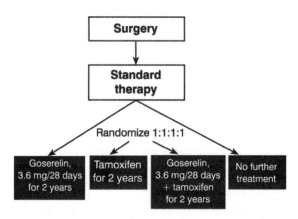

Fig. 7 Protocol for the ZIPP analysis of goserelin (2 years) *versus* tamoxifen (2 years) *versus* goserelin + tamoxifen (2 years) *versus* no further treatment.

would run a trial of similar design with the idea of a meta-analysis as the data matured. The design of the trial is complex and it is illustrated in Figure 7. Following adequate local therapy, a decision was made relating to adjuvant chemotherapy. In the majority of cases, this was determined by the lymph node status. The patients were then randomised four ways in order to develop a 2 x 2 factorial design. The randomisation options were goserelin for 2 years, tamoxifen for 2 years, goserelin and tamoxifen both for 2 years or no adjuvant endocrine therapy. In all, 2631 patients were recruited for the combined analyses. All were less than 50 years old and were both oestrogen-receptor positive and negative or node-positive and node-negative. Of the patients, 43% had adjuvant chemotherapy as an elective option prior to randomisation to the endocrine treatment. The median follow-up for the latest analyses is approximately 5 years.

The complexity of the ZIPP trial analyses demonstrates the hazard of attempting to answer all the questions whilst running the risk of answering none. However, taking these results and adding them to the sum of experience to the trials reported above, the message that appears is clear – in unselected patients there is a significant advantage in prescribing goserelin for disease-free survival which reaches borderline significance for overall survival.

CLINICAL GUIDELINES

From this wealth of emerging new data, it is possible to distil some rational clinical guidelines for everyday practice.

1. The GnRH analogues have no role to play in oestrogen-receptor negative patients (with one exception *vide infra*), but must be considered to have a role in premenopausal women where the tumours are oestrogen-receptor positive.

2. Patients receiving adjuvant chemotherapy who fail to achieve amenorrhoea should be offered ovarian suppression either with GnRH analogues or, perhaps if close to the natural menopause, with laparoscopic ovarian ablation.

3. It is important to involve the patient in the decision-making process.

4. Many patients are terrified by the short-term toxicity of chemotherapy and also need to be informed of the long-term consequences of a permanent chemical castration including osteoporosis and other side-effects such as cognitive impairment.[28]

5. It is evident that for oestrogen-receptor positive patients, 2 years of goserelin is equivalent to CMF, but offers a woman the potential of return of normal ovarian function, fertility and protection from the long-term consequences of osteoporosis.

6. Tamoxifen has an added advantage over chemotherapy alone and it appears that tamoxifen added to goserelin is an advantage over goserelin alone and equivalent to chemotherapy plus tamoxifen. However, much of the difficulty in deciding on these therapeutic options are more cultural/sociological than scientific.

It is essential that both practicing clinicians and their well-informed patients realise that this is a time of uncertainty and revolution concerning the role of ovarian suppression in the management of early breast cancer. However, with the maturation of the trials already described together with the long-awaited publication of the IBCSG VIII trial, these will be clarified.

The consensus statement prepared after the last St Gallen meeting (2000)[29] proposed that node-negative women with oestrogen-receptor positive tumours at moderate risk for survival as well as those with node-positive disease should be offered ovarian ablation therapy instead of, or in addition to, chemotherapy.

AROMATASE INHIBITORS AND POST-MENOPAUSAL WOMEN

Although adrenalectomy may have been effective in the management of breast cancer, many patients with metastatic disease are poor operative risks. A medical ablation of adrenal function would have wider application. Aminoglutethemide, the first of such drugs, blocks adrenal conversion of steroids to oestrogens relatively high in the biosynthetic pathway. 'Medical adrenalectomy' induced by the interruption of steroidogenesis at the level of the conversion of cholesterol to pregnenolone can achieve an objective response (OR) in metastatic breast cancer amongst women without ovarian function, to a similar extent as a surgical adrenalectomy. Medical adrenalectomy may, therefore, be more widely applicable to women who are a poor operative risk.

THE NEW GENERATION OF ORAL AROMATASE INHIBITORS

The majority of endocrine therapies for breast cancer involve inhibition of some aspect of the oestrogen system (*i.e.* the synthesis of oestrogen or the binding of oestrogen to its receptor). The aromatase inhibitors act by blocking aromatase, the enzyme that catalyzes the final and rate-limiting step in the synthesis of oestrogens. Aromatase is an enzyme complex consisting of a cytochrome P450 haemoprotein and NADPH-cytochrome P450 reductase. The expression of aromatase is controlled by several different promoters; consequently, expression is tissue-specific. In premenopausal women, the most significant activity of aromatase is in the ovaries. Ovarian expression of aromatase is regulated by the gonadotropins luteinizing hormone (LH) and follicle-stimulating hormone (FSH). Aromatase is also expressed, although at lower levels, in non-ovarian tissues, such as muscle and fat, in both premenopausal and post-menopausal women. These non-ovarian tissues become the dominant sources of oestrogen in post-menopausal women and, in these tissues, expression of aromatase is not regulated by LH or FSH. Early aromatase inhibitors (notably aminoglutethimide) had limited selectivity for aromatase over these other converting enzymes. Thus, treatment of patients with these early inhibitors required co-administration of corticosteroids and was associated with substantial side-effects. The modern aromatase inhibitors have much higher specificity and the non-selective agents remain of interest only from a historical perspective.

Currently, the available aromatase inhibitors fall into two classes: (i) the class I inhibitors, which bind aromatase irreversibly and have a steroidal structure; and (ii) the class II agents, which bind aromatase in a reversible manner and are non-steroidal. The first highly selective aromatase inhibitors (AIs) to become available were the class II inhibitors – anastrozole and letrozole (a third agent, vorazole, was used in the early trials, but never developed for the market place). Agents in this class are believed to inhibit the enzyme by interacting with the haem iron The first class I aromatase inhibitor was formestane, which is available in several countries outside of the US. The related compound, exemestane, is now approved in the US for second-line therapy of advanced breast cancer in post-menopausal women. These steroidal AIs bind to the substrate-binding site of the aromatase enzyme. Once bound, a reactive group on the drug forms a covalent bond with the enzyme. This covalent modification renders the substrate-binding site unavailable, thereby inactivating the enzyme. This class of compound, because of the specificity of its mode of action, is remarkably non-toxic and, therefore, lends itself to the management of the early disease.

Key point 4

- The third generation aromatase inhibitors are more effective than tamoxifen in patients with advanced disease.

ADJUVANT AROMATASE INHIBITORS AND THE ATAC ('ARIMIDEX', TAMOXIFEN ALONE OR IN COMBINATION) TRIAL

For the reasons explained above, the third generation of oral AIs lend themselves ideally as candidates to either enhance the activity of tamoxifen or replace it entirely in the adjuvant setting. A number of trials are exploring the role of both the steroidal and non-steroidal agents, used either head-to-head, sequentially or in combination with tamoxifen. The first to complete recruitment and to have been presented in public is the ATAC trial, but for completeness, Table 2 lists on-going studies.

The ATAC trial[3] is the largest adjuvant breast cancer study ever conducted in post-menopausal breast cancer patients with early breast cancer, and provides the first report of a new-generation aromatase inhibitor compared with tamoxifen. A unique feature of this trial was the inclusion of the combination arm, which enabled the investigation of any possible additive effects through the use of two drugs with different modes of action. It is

---

Key point 5

- The ATAC trial has shown that anastrazole is superior to tamoxifen (or the combination of both drugs) for disease-free survival and has a superior safety profile although the long-term effects on bone still require elucidation.

Table 2 On-going adjuvant aromatase inhibitor trials

Trial name	Patient status	Trial description
Anastrozole		
ABCSG AU08	Post-menopausal	Phase III: 3 years of anastrozole *versus* 3 years tamoxifen, after initial 2 years of tamoxifen
GR0001	Post-menopausal	Phase III: 3 years of anastrozole *versus* 3 years tamoxifen, after initial 2 years of tamoxifen
IT02	Post-menopausal	Phase III: 3 years of anastrozole *versus* 3 years tamoxifen, after initial 2 years of tamoxifen
ABCSG AU06	Post-menopausal	Phase III: 5 years of tamoxifen *versus* 2 years of tamoxifen and aminoglute-thimide plus 3 years of tamoxifen. Both arms followed by 3 years of anastrozole
Ham-AT	Post-menopausal	6 months of anastrozole alone, tamoxifen alone or anastrozole plus tamoxifen
ABCSG AU12	Premenopausal	3 years anastrozole plus goserelin *versus* 3 years of tamoxifen plus goserelin. Patients receive additional zolerdronate
Letrozole		
BIG 01-98	Post-menopausal	Phase III: Tamoxifen (5 years) *versus* tamoxifen (2 years) followed by letrozole (3 years) *versus* letrozole (5 years) *versus* letrozole (2 years) followed by tamoxifen (3 years)
NCIC MA.17	Post-menopausal	Phase III: tamoxifen (5 years) followed by placebo or letrozole (5 years)
Exemestane		
BIG 02-97	Post-menopausal	Tamoxifen (5 years) *versus* tamoxifen (2 years) followed by exemestane (3 years)
NSABPB33	Post-menopausal	Tamoxifen (5 years) followed by exemestane or no therapy (2 years)

possible that anastrozole, by depleting the oestrogen receptor of its natural ligand whilst allowing tamoxifen to exert its beneficial effect via alternative biological mechanisms, could act synergistically in treating early breast cancer.

Post-menopausal patients with operable invasive breast cancer, who had completed their primary treatment and who were candidates to receive adjuvant hormonal therapy, were randomized into the ATAC trial. The primary objectives of the trial were to compare tamoxifen and anastrozole and to compare tamoxifen and the combination of anastrozole plus tamoxifen as adjuvant treatment in terms of time-to-recurrence of breast cancer and tolerability. The secondary objectives were time to distant recurrence, survival, and incidence of new breast primaries.

A total of 9366 patients were recruited into this multicentre international study between July 1996 and 2000, and were randomized into one of the three treatment arms (anastrozole 1 mg, tamoxifen 20 mg, and anastrozole plus tamoxifen

Table 3 Distribution of events in the ATAC trial

	First events			
	Anastrozole (n = 3125)	Tamoxifen (n = 3116)	Combination (n = 3125)	In total (n = 9366)
Local recurrence	67	83	81	231
Distant recurrence*	158	182	204	544
Contralateral breast cancer	14	33	28	75
Invasive	9	30	23	62
Ductal carcinoma *in situ*	5	3	5	13
Deaths before recurrence	78	81	70	229
Total	317 (10.1%)	379 (12.2%)	383 (12.3%)	1079 (11.5%)
	Events at any time			
Distant recurrence*	180	203	232	615
Deaths after recurrence	122	122	145	389
All deaths	200	203	215	618

*Including five deaths (2, 1, 2, deaths on anastrozole, tamoxifen, and the combination, respectively), which were attributed to breast cancer without prior information about recurrence.

combination). Patients were assessed at entry, 3 months, and 6 months, and thereafter at 6-monthly intervals up to 5 years, and annually up to 10 years. The treatment groups were well balanced with respect to demographic and pretreatment characteristics.

A total of 1079 first events were recorded (Table 3), of which 850 (79%) were recurrences or new contralateral tumours and 229 (21%) were deaths without recurrence. In total, there were 618 deaths (200 in the anastrozole group, 203 in the tamoxifen group, and 215 in the combination group), of which 389 were deaths after a recurrence.

Disease-free survival was significantly prolonged for anastrozole-alone patients compared with those who received either tamoxifen alone (HR = 0.83, [95% CI, 0.71–0.96], P = 0.013) or the combination (HR = 0.81, [95% CI, 0.70–0.94], P = 0.006). The combination was not significantly different from tamoxifen alone (HR = 1.02, [95% CI, 0.89–1.18], P = 0.8).

There was no major difference in the number of patients dying from any cause prior to a breast cancer recurrence (78 in the anastrozole arm, 81 in the tamoxifen arm, and 70 in the combination arm). When these patients were censored at the time of death, the hazard ratio for time to recurrence (including new tumours) was further reduced in the anastrozole arm compared to tamoxifen (HR = 0.79, [95% CI, 0.67–0.94], P = 0.008). In comparison with the combination treatment, anastrozole also showed a greater benefit for this endpoint (HR = 0.75, [95% CI, 0.63–0.89], P = 0.0007). However, no difference was observed between the tamoxifen-alone arm and the combination arm (HR = 1.06, [95% CI, 0.90–1.24], P = 0.5).

Of the potential predictive factors for interactions of anastrozole or tamoxifen, hormone receptor status was close to significance with the comparison of effects of treatments in the receptor-positive subgroup being predefined in the protocol. The potential chemotherapy interaction, which was close to significance, was unexpected and not fully understood. This requires further events and longer follow-up before any meaningful conclusions can be drawn on the relative efficacy of anastrozole and tamoxifen after primary chemotherapy treatment. However, it can be argued that after chemotherapy, anastrozole and tamoxifen have equivalent effects. As it is known that tamoxifen adds to the advantages of adjuvant chemotherapy from the world overview, it is fair to assume that anastrazole will have benefits of a similar order of magnitude.

In the receptor-positive population, time-to-recurrence (breast cancer events) was improved in the anastrozole group (HR = 0.73, [95% CI, 0.59–0.90], P = 0.003). There was no significant difference between the tamoxifen and the combination arm (HR = 1.09, [95% CI, 0.90–1.32], P = 0.4). No difference was found between the two treatments for receptor-negative patients (HR = 1.13, [95% CI, 0.79–1.61], P = 0.5). When all events are included (disease-free survival) the hazard ratio in receptor-positive patients for anastrozole *versus* tamoxifen was 0.78 (95% CI, 0.65–0.93, P = 0.005).

A striking reduction in contralateral breast primaries as a first event was found in the anastrozole arm; when compared with tamoxifen, the odds were reduced by 58% (OR = 0.42, [95% CI, 0.22–0.79], P = 0.007). The incidence of contralateral breast primaries observed with tamoxifen was similar when compared with the combination arm (OR = 0.84, [95% CI, 0.51–1.40], P = 0.5).

Most of the contralateral breast cancers were invasive (83%) and, when the analysis is restricted to these events, the difference is somewhat larger (9 in the anastrozole arm *versus* 30 in the tamoxifen arm *versus* 23 in the combination arm (OR [anastrozole *versus* tamoxifen] = 0.30, [95% CI, 0.14–0.63], P = 0.001). Findings for the hormone-receptor positive subgroup were consistent with the overall results (OR [anastrozole *versus* tamoxifen]= 0.29, [95% CI, 0.13–0.64], P = 0.002).

The occurrence of predefined side-effects is of interest. In all cases, there was no distinguishable difference between tamoxifen and the combination. However, there were statistically significant and medically relevant reductions in the anastrozole *versus* tamoxifen groups for hot flushes, vaginal discharge, vaginal bleeding, ischaemic cerebrovascular events and venous thrombo-embolic events (including deep vein thromboses) and endometrial cancer. By contrast, musculoskeletal disorders and fractures were significantly increased. The greatest increase in fractures on anastrozole treatment appeared to be in the spine, but no increase of hip fractures was seen. Other non-prespecified side-effects (notably fibroids and other endometrial findings) were substantially reduced on anastrozole. Weight gain was very similar in the three treatment arms, with the average weight gain being 1.65 kg or 2.5% over 2 years in each group.

CONCLUSIONS

How can newly diagnosed patients be best advised? Certainly, there is a choice of adjuvant endocrine therapy for post-menopausal HR+ patients. For example, if tamoxifen is specifically contra-indicated (*e.g.* because of a previous history of thrombo-embolic disease), then anastrozole could be considered; but, beyond that, it is too early for a proper risk–benefit analysis to be calculated. In fact, the balance of benefits *versus* harm may allow a selective approach based on age prognostic factors and biological predictive measurements.

The third generation of specific aromatase inhibitors has made a very exciting contribution to the management of hormone responsive breast cancer. Their role in advanced breast cancer has overtaken that of tamoxifen which should be relegated to a second-line treatment. As far as the primary disease is concerned, the ATAC data suggest that there is an alternative to tamoxifen in selected post-menopausal women with HR⁺ disease. With more mature follow-up, it might even show that, after a passage of nearly 20 years, tamoxifen has lost its 'pole-position' in the adjuvant stakes as well.

Key points for clinical practice

- Breast cancer is often responsive to endocrine manipulation, especially if hormone-receptor positive.

- Tamoxifen has been the mainstay of treatment for over 25 years and is effective for pre- and post-menopausal women.

- Ovarian ablation by permanent means (surgery, radiotherapy) or reversibly by LHRH agonists is as effective as chemotherapy in pre-menopausal women with oestrogen-receptor positive tumours.

- The third generation aromatase inhibitors are more effective than tamoxifen in patients with advanced disease.

- The ATAC trial has shown that anastrazole is superior to tamoxifen (or the combination of both drugs) for disease-free survival and has a superior safety profile although the long-term effects on bone still require elucidation.

References

1. Quinn M, Allen E. Changes in incidence of and mortality from breast cancer in England and Wales since introduction of screening. *BMJ* 1995; **311**: 1391–1395.
2. Beatson GT. On the treatment of inoperable cases of carcinoma of the mamma: suggestions for a new method of treatment, with illustrative cases. *Lancet* 11 July 1896; 104–107.
3. The ATAC (Arimidex, Tamoxifen Alone or in Combination) Trialist Group. Anastrozole alone or in combination for adjuvant treatment of postmenopausal women with early breast cancer: first results of the ATAC randomised trial. *Lancet* 2002; **359**: 2131–2139.
4. Huggins C, Bergenstal DM. Inhibition of human mammary and prostatic cancer by adrenalectomy. *Cancer Res* 1952; **12**: 134–141.
5. Haddow A, Watkinson JM, Patterson E, Koller PC. Influence of synthetic oestrogens upon advanced malignant disease. *BMJ* 1944; **2**: 393–398.
6. Adair FE, Herrman JB. The use of testosterone proprionate in the treatment of advanced carcinoma of the breast. *Ann Surg* 1946; **123**: 1023–1035.
7. Baum M, Brinkley DM, Dossett JA et al. Controlled trial of tamoxifen as adjuvant agent in management of early breast cancer. Interim analysis at four years by the Nolvadex Adjuvant Trial Organisation. *Lancet* 1983; **2**: 257–261.
8. Early Breast Cancer Trialists' Collaborative Group. Systemic treatment of early breast cancer by hormonal, cytotoxic, or immune therapy. *Lancet* 1992; **339**: 1–15, 71–85.

9. Fisher B, Redmond C, Brown A et al. Adjuvant chemotherapy with and without tamoxifen in the treatment of primary breast cancer: 5-year results from the National Surgical Adjuvant Breast and Bowel project Trial. *J Clin Oncol* 1986; **4**: 459–471.

10. Fisher B, Digman J, Wolmark N et al. Tamoxifen and chemotherapy for lymph node negative, estrogen receptor-positive breast cancer. *J Natl Cancer Inst* 1997; **89**: 1673–1682.

11. Early Breast Cancer Trialists' Collaborative Group (EBCTG). Effects of tamoxifen and cytotoxic therapy on mortality in early breast cancer. An overview of 61 randomized trials among 28,896 women. *N Engl J Med* 1988; **319**: 1681–1692.

12. Early Breast Cancer Trialists' Collaborative Group. Tamoxifen for early breast cancer: an overview of the randomised trials. *Lancet* 1998; **351**: 1451–1467.

13. Early Breast Cancer Trialists' Collaborative Group. Polychemotherapy for early breast cancer: an overview of the randomised trials. *Lancet* 1998; **352**: 930–942.

14. Bines J, Oleske DM, Cobleigh MA. Ovarian function in premenopausal women treated with adjuvant chemotherapy for breast cancer. *J Clin Oncol* 1996; **14**: 1718–1729.

15. Mehta RR, Beattie CW, Das Gupta TK. Endocrine profile in breast cancer patients receiving chemotherapy. *Breast Cancer Res Treat* 1992; **20**: 125–132.

16. Poikonen P, Saarto T, Elomaa I et al. Prognostic effect of amenorrhoea and elevated serum gonadotropin levels induced by adjuvant chemotherapy in premenopausal node-positive breast cancer patients. *Eur J Cancer* 2000; **36**: 43–48.

17. Del Mastro L, Venturini M, Sertoli MR et al. Amenorrhoea induced by adjuvant chemotherapy in early breast cancer patients: prognostic role and clinical implications. *Breast Cancer Res Treat* 1997; **43**: 183–190.

18. Pagani O, O'Neill A, Castiglione M et al. Prognostic impact of amenorrhoea after adjuvant chemotherapy in premenopausal breast cancer patients with axillary node involvement: results of the International Breast Cancer Study Group (IBCSG) trial VI. *Eur J Cancer* 1998; **34**: 632–640.

19. Scottish Cancer Trials Breast Group and ICRF Breast Unit, Guy's Hospital, London. Adjuvant ovarian ablation versus CMF chemotherapy in premenopausal women with pathological stage II breast carcinoma: the Scottish trial. *Lancet* 1993; **341**: 1293–1298.

20. Jonat W. Luteinizing hormone-releasing hormone analogues – the rationale for adjuvant use in premenopausal women with early breast cancer. *Br J Cancer* 1998; **78** (Suppl. 4): 5–8.

21. Taylor CW, Green S, Dalton WS et al. Multicenter randomized clinical trial of goserelin versus surgical ovariectomy in premenopausal patients with receptor-positive metastatic breast cancer: an Intergroup study. *J Clin Oncol* 1998; **16**: 994–999.

22. Boccardo F, Rubagotti A, Perrotta A et al. Ovarian ablation versus goserelin with or without tamoxifen in pre-perimenopausal patients with advanced breast cancer: results of a multicentric Italian study. *Ann Oncol* 1994; **5**: 337–342.

23. Kaufmann M. 'Zoladex' (goserelin) vs CMF as adjuvant therapy in pre/perimenopausal, node-positive, early breast cancer: preliminary efficacy results from the ZEBRA study [abstract]. *Breast* 2001; **10** (Suppl. 1): S30.

24. Boccardo F, Rubagotti A, Amoroso D et al. Cyclophosphamide, methotrexate, and fluorouracil versus tamoxifen plus ovarian suppression as adjuvant treatment of estrogen receptor-positive pre-/perimenopausal breast cancer patients: results of the Italian Breast Cancer Adjuvant Study Group 02 randomized trial. *J Clin Oncol* 2000; **18**: 2718–2727.

25. Jakesz R, Hausmaninger H, Samonigg H et al. Complete endocrine blockade with tamoxifen and goserelin is superior to CMF in the adjuvant treatment of premenopausal, lymph node-positive and -negative patients with hormone-responsive breast cancer [abstract]. *Breast* 2001; **10** (Suppl. 1): S10.

26. Davidson NE, O'Neill A, Vukov A. Effect of chemohormonal therapy in premenopausal, node-positive, receptor-positive breast cancer: an Eastern Cooperative Oncology Group Phase III Intergroup Trial (E5188, INT-0101). *Breast* 1999; **8**: 232–233.

27. Baum M, Houghton J, Odling-Smee W et al. Adjuvant 'Zoladex' in premenopausal patients with early breast cancer: results from the ZIPP trial [abstract]. *Breast* 2001; **10** (Suppl. 1): S32–S33.

28. Brezden CB, Phillips KA, Abdolell M et al. Cognitive function in breast cancer patients receiving adjuvant chemotherapy. *J Clin Oncol* 2000; **18**: 2695–2701.

29. Goldhirsch A, Glick JH, Gelber RD, Coates AS, Senn H-J. Meeting highlights: International Consensus Panel on the Treatment of Primary Breast Cancer. *J Clin Oncol* 2001; **19**: 3817–3827.

Richard J. Sutton Sanjeev Sarin

Comparative surgical audit

We live in challenging and changing times. No longer can we, as surgeons, work and operate with the autonomy to which we have historically been accustomed. The healthcare profession as a whole, but especially surgeons, are increasingly accountable for their actions to local multidisciplinary teams, to their own professional organisations through re-validation, to health authority managers, the government, the media and to the population whom we serve. This issue has been brought sharply into focus by recent, high-profile surgical scandals that have been perceived to demonstrate a failure of professional self-regulation. The need for accountability, the desire of professional bodies to maintain standards and the wish of patients for ever more information is leading to increasingly sophisticated information appearing in the public domain.

In this culture of increased scrutiny, surgeons must be able to demonstrate clearly and accurately how they perform through comparative audit of mortality and morbidity rates. League tables with comparisons between different hospitals and individual surgeons are being adopted and published.[1] Such information is often contentious, especially when the data from which it is drawn are frequently incomplete or inaccurate and the methods of analysis are not standardised but open to debate and interpretation.[2] Nevertheless, however inaccurate this information is, it will be consumed with great interest by governing bodies and the wider public.

AUDIT OF STRUCTURE AND PROCESS

Donabedian developed the classic triad for measuring quality of healthcare: structure, process and outcome.[3] **Structural data** are characteristics of healthcare

Mr Richard J. Sutton FRCS, Specialist Registrar, Department of Surgery, Watford General Hospital, Vicarage Road, Watford, Hertfordshire WD18 0HB, UK

Mr Sanjeev Sarin MS FRCS, Consultant Surgeon, Department of Surgery, Watford General Hospital, Vicarage Road, Watford, Hertfordshire WD18 0HB, UK (for correspondence)

Key point 1

- Quality of healthcare may be evaluated by assessing the **structures** designed to provide it, the **process** of delivering it or measuring the **outcome** of delivery.

providers and hospitals, such as number and speciality of doctors and of facilities and equipment available. **Process data** result from the interaction between providers of healthcare and patients, such as the tests ordered and the number of patients treated. **Outcome** is defined by the subsequent health status of the patient and is dependent upon the structure and process of the healthcare delivered.

Surgeons rely heavily upon outcome data. However, it is clearly important to evaluate both process and structure. Collation of these delivery aspects is, in most respects, easier and more immediate than for outcome. The danger lies in the interpretation of the data collected as there may be contentious, or perhaps erroneous, assumptions derived from them; incorrect importance may be placed on an aspect of structure or process and of its relationship to outcome. Decisions made by departments or regulatory organisations derived from measuring process lead to predetermined **care pathways**. Whilst this should lead to the standardisation of patient care irrespective of surgeon or institution, it has the effect of removing clinical freedom and can be used to force change, however inappropriate. Many patients, especially those on the extreme margins of risk (high or low) do not fall into nicely defined categories and may be inappropriately treated by managed care pathways.

One particular aspect of evaluation of process is that of measurement of workload and the assumption that increased volume of index procedures relates to improved outcome, *i.e.* that a surgeon who performs many index operations will automatically achieve better results than those undertaking a few. This is an important argument behind the drive to increased surgical sub-specialisation and one that has been hotly debated.[4] Reduced amount of time in training increasingly means that newly qualified surgeons (with a correspondingly reduced surgical repertoire) have to sell themselves as super-specialists. The quest to increase numbers of particular cases performed means that even within units there is further specialisation, *e.g.* one urologist does all the renal whilst the other the bladder tumours. Although this may be superficially re-assuring, meaningful interpretation is impossible, especially when the workload of the unit may not have changed. The one consistent theme in the medical literature is that the overall workload through any one

Key point 2

- The correlation of workload as an indicator of outcome is more valid when considering the workload of a unit rather than for an individual surgeon.

particular unit appears to relate most strongly to outcome, not individual surgeon volume.[4] Secondly, whilst raw numbers may be easier to collect, they do not address whether outcomes for the high volume, poor repertoire surgeon are satisfactory or not.

AUDIT OF OUTCOME

The measurement of outcome is both simultaneously more important and more difficult. Commonly used measures of outcome are morbidity and mortality, which are discussed below followed by the principles of risk-adjusted analysis and risk scoring and how these relate to comparative surgical audit.

Key point 3

- Measurement of morbidity and mortality are the most commonly used primary end-points for assessing outcome.

Morbidity is a valuable end-point for assessing surgical performance and has implications for both a patient's quality-of-life as well as consumption of healthcare resources. It is of most importance to those operations and specialities that inherently have a low mortality rate. However, meaningful comparative audit of morbidity is much more problematic to achieve than for mortality because of the difficulties associated with collection of accurately reported data and with definitions of what actually constitutes a complication. Clearly, it is feasible to audit a single, defined complication for any given index procedure, such as the incidence of recurrent laryngeal nerve palsy in thyroid surgery. Even with such a succinct remit, accurate data collection and, therefore, comparison between surgeons or units will be limited by inaccuracies in reporting such as observer bias, unless independent or blinded. It follows that a single scoring system used to compare morbidity for a broad range of operations and patient populations will be even more limited and inaccurate. This has clearly been demonstrated by the most extensive comparative surgical audit yet undertaken – the National Veterans Affairs Surgical Risk Study.[5]

Mortality is a more finite and indisputable end-point than morbidity and has thus been used to much greater extent and success in comparative surgical audit. However, aspects of this seemingly clear end-point are debated as whether to measure in-hospital mortality or 30-day mortality. Most series have measured in-

---

Key point 4

- Analysis of morbidity is much more difficult and inaccurate than for mortality, but is vital for those specialties and procedures that have an inherently low mortality rate.

---

hospital mortality,[6–9] but recent work suggests this may underestimate true mortality by up to 20% when compared to 30-day mortality rates.[10]

RISK-ADJUSTED ANALYSIS

Simple collection of crude numbers of the dead or injured alone is insufficient to reflect quality of care as, to compare morbidity or mortality directly, the original populations should be identical. True comparisons can only be made if risk adjustment is used to allow for the differences in case-mix between units and surgeons. This is termed **risk-adjusted analysis**. In general, it is based upon the principle of identifying variables that the investigator suspects may affect outcome, such as the mode of presentation, physiological parameters, and the nature, extent and difficulty of surgery.

Traditionally, the 'adjustments' are performed using multivariate logistic regression analysis. This technique identifies those variables that independently and significantly affect the outcome, and generates an equation which predicts the likelihood of the outcome occurring in any given patient. The accuracy of the prediction is then tested against a further set of patients. Classification tables, receiver operating characteristic (ROC) curves and calibration curves are used to assess 'goodness-of-fit'. Clearly, studies with large numbers of patients assessing large numbers of variables are likely to give more accurate predictions. However, it is the authors' experience that the larger the data set required, the less accurate and reliable the data. This view may reflect the current trend to minimize the number of variables collected.

Key point 5

- Risk-adjusted analysis is essential to interpret the crude figures of morbidity and mortality and to correct them for case-mix.

An alternative approach to risk stratification is to use a Bayesian model.[11] Bayes' theorem is a basic formula in probability theory first described in the 18th century. Rather than producing a rigid equation, this method allows the probability of an event to be revised as additional relevant information is obtained (*e.g.* another variable). The Bayes' model is then tested in much the same way by using ROC curves and calibration curves. The intuitive appeal of this methodology is that the system can 'learn' and that data already collected are not wasted as new information becomes available.

Key point 6

- Risk stratification can be achieved via the traditional but static multivariate logistic regression analysis or by the more fluid Bayesian model.

Table 1 Risk scoring systems used to predict complicated outcome

ASA score (American Society of Anesthesiology)
APACHE (acute physiology and chronic health evaluation), II & III
Ranson's score (acute pancreatitis)
SAPS (Simplified Acute Physiology Score)
Cardiac Index
Revised Trauma Score

RISK SCORING SYSTEMS

Risk scoring systems used to predict complicated outcome or mortality are not a new phenomenon and there are many examples (Table 1). However, they were not designed specifically for the purposes of comparative surgical audit. The best and most widely used example is the classification of pre-operative physical status described by the American Society of Anesthesiologists (ASA score) in 1963. Patients are allocated to one of five categories based on general medical history and examination without requiring any specific investigations (Table 2). 'E' can be added to denote emergency surgery and signify a worse prognosis. Whilst the score is simple and already in almost universal use, there is potential for inter-observer subjective error. It is effective at predicting mortality when used alone[12] or when combined with other parameters[9,13] as postoperative mortality rates rise steadily with the ASA grade.

The Acute Physiology and Chronic Health Evaluation (APACHE) scoring system has been used extensively in the intensive care setting. Its aim is to allow for the classification of patients on the basis of the severity of illness to facilitate comparison of outcome, the evaluation of new therapies and as an indicator of daily progress. The original APACHE system was complex, requiring the use of 34 physiological variables, taking the worst value obtained in the first 24 h of admission to intensive care, combined with a simple evaluation of chronic health (similar to ASA). More recently, the APACHE system has been modified and simplified to create APACHE II[14] and APACHE III,[15] although these still require 12 or 18 physiological variables, respectively.

The APACHE mortality prediction model uses the APACHE score combined with factors for the diagnostic category and whether or not an emergency operation was performed to give a calculated risk of mortality. Using this model, APACHE II has been validated both in general[14,16–18] and surgical[19–23] intensive care patients with some success, although results have not always been

Table 2 American Society of Anesthesiologists classification

I	Normal healthy patient
II	Mild systemic disease
III	Severe systemic disease, not incapacitating
IV	Incapacitating systemic disease that is a threat to life
V	Moribund, not expected to survive 24 h with or without an operation

Table 3 Methods of risk-adjusted analysis in comparative surgical audit

POSSUM (Physiology and Operative Severity Score for enUmeration of
     Morbidity and Mortality)

Surgical Risk Scale

E-PASS (Estimation of Physiologic Ability and Surgical Stress)

National Veterans Affairs Surgical Risk Study

Speciality Registries

accurate.[24,25] Clearly, it does have a role to play in the evaluation of surgical patients in an intensive care setting, especially those with intra-abdominal sepsis,[20] but its more general role for risk-adjusted analysis in comparative surgical audit for a broader range of surgical patients is limited by its complexity and by the requirement to collate variables over 24 h.

RISK-ADJUSTED ANALYSIS, RISK SCORING SYSTEMS AND COMPARATIVE SURGICAL AUDIT

Ideally, a risk assessment score for comparative surgical audit should be quick and easy to use at the bed-side. The parameters collected should be small in number, be available for every patient undergoing any operation, be in common use across the healthcare system and leave little room for observer bias. The score should then be easy to calculate from the data collected. Also, it should be possible to integrate the scoring system into pre-existing audit programmes with a minimum of disruption.

A number of methods have been proposed for standardising patient data to permit direct, meaningful comparisons of patient outcome irrespective of differences in population for the sole purpose of comparative surgical audit (Table 3). All of the proposed methods include operative details, thereby excluding all those patients with surgical conditions who do not undergo a surgical procedure during admission.[6]

POSSUM

The Physiological and Operative Severity Score for the enUmeration of Mortality and morbidity was described by Copeland *et al.* in 1991.[26] It is currently the most tested system for assessing outcomes by risk-adjusted analysis in the UK.

POSSUM is a two-part scoring system that includes a physiological assessment and a measure of operative severity (Table 4). There are 12 physiological variables, each divided into 4 grades with an exponentially increasing score. The authors state that the physiological variables are those that are present at the time of surgery[27] and include symptoms and signs, results of simple biochemical and haematological investigations, as well as electrocardiographic changes. If a particular variable is not available, a score of 1 is allocated. Some variables may be assessed by means of clinical symptoms or signs or by means of changes on the chest radiograph. The minimum score is 12, with a maximum of 88. The operative severity part of the score includes 6 variables, each divided into 4 grades with an exponentially increasing score.

Table 4 POSSUM: physiological and operative parameters

Physiological parameters	Operative parameters
Age	Operative severity
Cardiac history	Multiple procedure
Respiratory history	Total blood loss
Blood pressure	Peritoneal soiling
Pulse rate	Presence of malignancy
Glasgow Coma Score	Mode of surgery
Haemoglobin	
White blood cell count	
Serum urea	
Serum sodium	
Serum potassium	
Electrocardiogram	

Once these scores are known, it is possible to estimate the predicted risk of mortality and morbidity using a complex equation.

Whilst POSSUM has performed favourably in mortality and morbidity risk prediction and comparative surgical audit,[26,28] it does have its limitations. Most notably, it consistently overestimates mortality for low risk procedures.[7,8,29,30] The Portsmouth Predictor Equation (p-POSSUM) was specifically designed to correct this fault by modifying the statistical analysis of the data collected, although this too overestimates mortality for all risk groups except in the highest (90–100%).[31] This inability to predict risk accurately in low-risk surgery is a major handicap, as the vast majority of general surgical procedures undertaken in the Western world fall into this category. The absolute minimum risk of mortality using POSSUM is 1.08%[8] and for p-POSSUM is 0.2%.[7] Even the latter is too high, as the risk of mortality for a fit patient undergoing minor or intermediate surgery approaches zero.[32,33]

The second criticism is that the formula for establishing a POSSUM score is complex and still a matter of some debate.[8,31,34] The relative performance of POSSUM and p-POSSUM depends upon the method of analysis, which maybe 'linear' or 'exponential'. It has been found that the most accurate prediction of mortality is achieved with linear analysis of p-POSSUM or exponential analysis of POSSUM, though exponential analysis is unwieldy.[31]

Thirdly, whilst the data required for POSSUM are simple, they are not available for every patient. In our experience, over 70% of patients undergoing a general surgical procedure could not be allocated a POSSUM score,[35] principally because the investigations necessary for a POSSUM score were not required for most patients.

Another factor is timing. In the original study, POSSUM patients were scored immediately prior to surgery,[26] allowing for post admission resuscitation. However, with p-POSSUM, scoring was done on admission.[7,8] Recent snapshot surveys based on the POSSUM dataset have been unclear about the time of scoring, and some groups have erroneously applied the p-POSSUM equation (derived from data collected on admission) to the data scored pre-operatively.

Since pre-operative intervention affects outcome,[36,37] ambiguity of this kind will distort the results. Even if the time of scoring were standardised to be pre-operative, a surgical firm that aggressively pre-optimised patients would not be shown to be providing better care, only to be operating on fitter patients than the average!

The final criticism is that the operative parameters collected to calculate POSSUM may contrive to obscure poor surgical standards. A high total blood loss or the need for multiple procedures would automatically give a high POSSUM score and expected mortality or morbidity. However, they might result from poor surgical technique rather than from the intrinsic difficulty of the case. Whilst POSSUM would predict mortality accurately in these cases, the clumsy surgeon would be exonerated because of the 'difficulty' of the case. With regard to these parameters, as well as to the presence of malignancy (which is also incorporated into the operative severity score), there is concern that these data are not appropriate or relevant outside of general and gastrointestinal surgery. Other areas of specialisation, such as vascular surgery[38] and orthopaedics,[27] have formulated their own POSSUM operative scoring systems and are even proposing procedure-specific equations, thus potentially diluting its overall applicability and ability to provide meaningful comparison across the range of surgical specialities.

The Surgical Risk Scale

In response to the above concerns, an alternative system was described recently in the UK, called the Surgical Risk Scale (SRS).[6] It was based on the principle that patient outcome can be predicted by the mode of presentation, co-morbidity and the magnitude of the surgical procedure. Thus, it incorporates the CEPOD grade (Confidential Enquiry into Peri-operative Deaths), the ASA grade, and the BUPA operative grade. These are easily collectable data, which require no special investigations and are totally independent of surgeon-related variables.

The CEPOD and BUPA categories were allocated a linear ordinal scale (Table 5) and the SRS was designed by adding together the values of the three variables, generating a scale ranging from 3 to a maximum of 14. It was prospectively analysed on over 7000 general surgical patients, in both emergency and elective settings, demonstrating that it is an effective tool for predicting mortality. In-hospital mortality was used as the end-point, rather than the more accurate 30-day mortality. Nevertheless, it was found to be least as accurate as other scoring systems[8,9,26,39] and is less complicated.

One of the principal advantages of the SRS is that it is independent of the surgeon, so that differences in surgical care and outcome can be highlighted. Surgeon-dependent variables are excluded, such as blood loss and peritoneal soiling. The score is calculated per procedure, rather than for the admission. Thus, a surgeon who undertakes one correct operation will be treated equally with the surgeon who undertakes multiple operations for the same problem. It should be remembered that POSSUM allocates extra points for multiple procedures. The SRS does not contain specific operative details so that it may apply equally well to all areas of general surgery and to other surgical specialities, such as orthopaedics and gynaecology. The score is not only easy to calculate, but also allows for clear visualisation of the result as there are only

Table 5 The Surgical Risk Scale

CEPOD	Description	Score
Elective	Routine, booked non-urgent case (*e.g.* inguinal hernia)	1
Scheduled	Booked admission (*e.g.* Ca colon or AAA)	2
Urgent	Cases requiring treatment with 24–48 h of admission	3
Emergency	Cases requiring immediate treatment (*e.g.* ruptured AAA)	4

BUPA	Description	Score
Minor	Removal of sebaceous cyst, gastroscopy	1
Intermediate	Unilateral hernia repair, colonoscopy	2
Major	Appendicectomy, open cholecystectomy	3
Major plus	Laparoscopic cholecystectomy, gastrectomy	4
Complex major	Anterior resection, aneurysm repair, oesophagectomy	5

ASA	Description	Score
1	No systemic disease	1
2	Mild systemic disease	2
3	Systemic disease affecting activity	3
4	Serious systemic disease	4
5	Moribund, not expected to survive	5

12 possible scores. This may enhance the ability of the surgeon to form a more objective and accurate pre-operative assessment of risk, which could then improve the information given to the patient and relatives.

E-PASS

In Japan, an alternative risk-scoring system has been developed called Estimation of Physiologic Ability and Stress (E-PASS) and has been prospectively evaluated in a multicentre study of a consecutive series of 902 patients undergoing elective gastrointestinal surgery.[40] It was found to predict accurately in-hospital morbidity and mortality.[40] The system comprises a pre-operative risk score, a surgical stress score and a comprehensive risk score that is calculated from both the former two scores. No special investigations are required. The authors suggest that its role may not only be limited to comparative surgical audit, but can also be used to help select the most appropriate surgical procedure for individual patients.

However, E-PASS has only been evaluated in a very select group of patients: those undergoing elective gastrointestinal surgery. Emergency cases were excluded, as were those with systemic immune response syndrome. The minimum risk of mortality is again too high (0.13%) and, as specific operative details are included within the score, it is not truly independent of the surgeon. Lastly, the system for calculating a comprehensive risk score is somewhat complex.

National Veterans Affairs Surgical Risk Study

In the US, the Department of Veterans Affairs has undertaken an exhaustive, prospective audit of all major operations undertaken in all surgical specialities in 123 affiliated hospitals between 1991 and 1997, which included over 400,000 operations.[41] This required a large team of staff dedicated solely to audit and a integrated, complex computer network (VISTA). An initial dataset was created between 1991 and 1993 of 87,000 patients in 44 hospitals of 30-day mortality and 21 postoperative adverse events (morbidity), along with length of stay, nature of surgery and a range of pre-operative physiological measures. Multivariate logistic regression analysis revealed that patient risk factors predictive of mortality included serum albumin, ASA class, emergency surgery and 31 additional pre-operative variables.[42] Risk factors predictive of postoperative morbidity were serum albumin, ASA class, complexity of surgery and 17 other pre-operative risk variables.[5] Overall, serum albumin was found to be the most significant predictive variable,[5,42] which corresponds well with other work.[43,44]

After the initial trial period, the audit process was expanded to involve 123 centres. The defined factors most predictive of risk are entered for each patient into the computer system. Comparative surgical audit by means of risk-adjusted analysis is undertaken for mortality and morbidity for all non-cardiac surgical specialities between the centres at regular intervals and the results are fed back to the individual hospitals. During the time period that the programme has been in operation, mortality and morbidity rates have fallen significantly and the authors attribute some of this reduction to modification of surgical practices in the light of information provided by the audit process.[41] It is of interest to note that the authors found analysis of morbidity more difficult and inaccurate.[5] There was no correlation of morbidity to mortality across the centres. That is to say, a hospital with a high risk-adjusted mortality rate would not necessarily show a high risk-adjusted morbidity rate, contrary to expectation. The authors felt that reporting inaccuracies were probably to blame for this discrepancy.

Key point 7

- The most tested systems for comparative surgical audit are POSSUM and SRS in the UK, and The National Veterans Affairs Surgical Risk Study in the US.

Clearly, the National Veterans Affairs Surgical Risk Study is a very impressive achievement. However, it may not be applicable for use in other healthcare systems. The amount of data collected and assimilated is huge, many pre-operative risk factors are required to be documented and a large team of staff are needed to process and maintain the data-base. The direct total cost of the programme is about US$4 million annually, or approximately US$38 for each major procedure assessed (at 1998 prices).[41] In addition, although a large number of operations has been audited only a rather select population has been assessed. The patients using these centres are predominantly old, socially and economically disadvantaged, and almost exclusively male. A further criticism of the study is that pre-operative variables predictive of risk were not collected on admission, but immediately prior to surgery. Lastly, each surgical speciality has a different risk model, so comparison across specialities is not possible.

Speciality registries

In the UK, a number of surgical sub-speciality organizations have set up registries to which individual surgeons can submit their data. A number of reports are available of which the National Audit of Bowel Obstruction due to Colorectal Cancer[45] and the National Vascular Database[46] are two relevant to general surgery. The ways in which an individual surgeon's data can be presented are outlined. In particular, the problem of a 'bad run' is dealt with by the introduction of the idea that a surgeon may be regarded as being in credit or debit as to how his actual peri-operative death rate compares with that expected.

Key point 8
- Use of index procedures is prone to error and manipulation.

As the number of operations increases a cumulative risk-adjusted outcome plot graphically demonstrates whether the outcomes are just drifting around what is expected or whether there is a genuine divergence. The level at which the deviation triggers an alarm has to be set by the relevant specialist organization. However, interpretation of the data requires great care as it is assumed that the risk models are robust and accurate. The Society of Cardio-thoracic Surgeons has developed and maintains the longest running database in the UK and the web site provides an excellent review of the issues involved in interpretation of such data (<www.ctsnet.org>). Moreover, these registries currently rely on participants enduring data collection at its extreme – for example, to submit a patient with an abdominal aortic aneurysm to the National Vascular Database requires the collection of at least 75 pieces of data and having to make over 200 yes/no decisions in filling a spreadsheet. The datasets for femoral reconstructions and carotid endarterectomy are no less voluminous. Secondly, within a subspecialty, the analysis is almost always based on very specific procedures or a specific diagnosis. The advantage, of course, is that there is less variability about what is being analysed. The disadvantage, however, of using 'index' procedures is that they are prone to manipulation with the danger that only the fittest with the greatest chance of survival will get the operation, and thereby enter the registry.

Key point 9
- The goal of a unified, single scoring system applicable across a range of surgical specialties may be unattainable.

Key point 10

- Accurate prospective collection of limited amount of relevant data is likely to be more fruitful than a 'more is better' approach.

CONCLUSIONS

Comparative surgical audit of outcome is essential and is almost certain to become mandatory. It must be adjusted for case-mix to have any validity. The prediction of mortality following a surgical procedure is now very accurate and statistical techniques that 'learn' with time hold even more promise. How this improved accuracy relates to surgical performance is less obvious and, as most surgery is now of the low risk variety, mortality alone cannot be relied upon wholly. Low-risk specialities may have to rely on the less satisfactory measures of process, morbidity or patient questionnaires.

Key points for clinical practice

- Quality of healthcare may be evaluated by assessing the **structures** designed to provide it, the **process** of delivering it or measuring the **outcome** of delivery.

- The correlation of workload as an indicator of outcome is more valid when considering the workload of a unit rather than for an individual surgeon.

- Measurement of morbidity and mortality are the most commonly used primary end-points for assessing outcome.

- Analysis of morbidity is much more difficult and inaccurate than for mortality, but is vital for those specialties and procedures that have an inherently low mortality rate.

- Risk-adjusted analysis is essential to interpret the crude figures of morbidity and mortality and to correct them for case-mix.

- Risk stratification can be achieved via the traditional but static multivariate logistic regression analysis or by the more fluid Bayesian model.

- The most tested systems for comparative surgical audit are POSSUM and SRS in the UK, and The National Veterans Affairs Surgical Risk Study in the US.

- Use of index procedures is prone to error and manipulation.

- The goal of a unified, single scoring system applicable across a range of surgical specialties may be unattainable.

- Accurate prospective collection of limited amount of relevant data is likely to be more fruitful than a 'more is better' approach.

The holy grail of a single unified way of measuring 'performance' of surgeons is far from achieved and the ideal of a single, simple, scoring system for both mortality and morbidity that is applicable across a range of surgical specialities may be unattainable. Whether we should be aiming for a 'generalist' technique (such as Possum or SRS) or for more specific procedure/speciality-based systems (such as the Vascular Surgical Society database) is not clear. There is no doubt that the entire premise relies on the timely, prospective collection of accurate data, which is the single biggest hurdle at present.

References

1. <www.drfoster.co.uk/hospital-guide/nhs/hospitalperformance>.
2. Little R. A doctor's guide to Dr Foster. *BMJ* 2002; **324**: 522.
3. Donabedian A. Effectiveness of quality assurance. *Int J Qual Health Care* 1996; **8**: 401.
4. Soljak M. Volume of procedures and outcome of treatment. *BMJ* 2002; **325**: 787–788.
5. Daley J, Khuri SF, Henderson W et al. Risk adjustment of the postoperative morbidity rate for the comparative assessment of the quality of surgical care: results of the National Veterans Affairs Surgical Risk Study. *J Am Coll Surg* 1997; **185**: 328–340.
6. Sutton RJ, Bann S, Brooks MJ, Sarin S. The Surgical Risk Score as an improved method of risk-adjusted analysis in comparative surgical audit. *Br J Surg* 2002; **89**: 763–768.
7. Prytherech DR, Whiteley MS, Higgins B et al. POSSUM and Portsmouth POSSUM for predicting mortality. *Br J Surg* 1998; **85**: 1217–1220.
8. Whiteley MS, Prytherech DR, Higgins B et al. An evaluation of the POSSUM surgical scoring system. *Br J Surg* 1996; **83**: 812–815.
9. Klotz HP, Candinas D, Platz H et al. Pre-operative risk assessment in elective general surgery. *Br J Surg* 1996; **83**: 1788–1791.
10. Goldacre MJ, Griffith M, Gill L, Mackintosh A. In-hospital deaths as a fraction of all deaths within 30 days of hospital admission for surgery: analysis of routine statistics. *BMJ* 2002; **324**: 1069–1070.
11. Bland JM, Altman DG. Bayesians and frequentists. *BMJ* 1998; **317**: 1151–1160.
12. Vacanti CJ, Van Houton RJ, Hill RC. A statistical analysis of the relationship of physical status to post operative mortality in 63 388 cases. *Anesth Analg* 1970; **49**: 564–566.
13. Hall JC, Hall JL. ASA status and age predict adverse events after abdominal surgery. *J Qual Clin Pract* 1996; **16**: 103–108.
14. Knaus WA, Draper EA, Wagner DP, Zimmerman JE. APACHE II: a severity of disease classification system. *Crit Care Med* 1985; **9**: 818–829.
15. Knaus WA, Wagner DP, Draper EA et al. The APACHE III prognostic system. Risk prediction of hospital mortality for critically ill hospitalised adults. *Chest* 1991; **100**: 1619–1636.
16. Rowan KM, Kerr JH, Major E, MacPherson K, Short A, Vessey MP. Intensive Care Society's Acute Physiology And Chronic Health Evaluation (APACHE II) study in Britain and Ireland: a prospective, multicentre, cohort study comparing two methods for predicting outcome for adult intensive care patients. *Crit Care Med* 1994; **22**: 1392–1401.
17. Wong DT, Crofts SL, Gomez M, MacGuire GP, Byrick RJ. Evaluation of predictive ability of APACHE II system and hospital outcome in Canadian intensive care unit patients. *Crit Care Med* 1995; **23**: 1177–1183.
18. Beck DH, Smith GB, Taylor BL. The impact of low-risk intensive care unit admissions on mortality probabilities by SAPS II, APACHE II AND APACHE III. *Anaesthesia* 2002; **57**: 21–26.
19. Giangiuliani G, Mancini A, Gui D. Validation of a severity of illness score (APACHE II) in a surgical intensive care unit. *Intensive Care Med* 1989; **15**: 519–522.
20. Bohnen JMA, Mustard RA, Oxholm SE, Schouten BD. APACHE II score and abdominal sepsis. A prospective study. *Arch Surg* 1988; **123**: 225–229.
21. Poenaru D, Christou NV. Clinical outcome of seriously ill patients with intra-abdominal infection depends on both physiologic (APACHE II score) and immunologic (DTH score) alterations. *Ann Surg* 1991; **213**: 130–136.

22. Bosscha K, Reijnders K, Hulstaert PF, Algra A, van der Werken C. Prognostic scoring systems to predict outcomes in peritonitis and intra-abdominal sepsis. *Br J Surg* 1997; **84**: 1532–1534.

23. Berger MM, Marazzi A, Freeman J, Chiolero R. Evaluation of the consistency of Acute Physiology and Chronic Health Evaluation (APACHE II) scoring in a surgical intensive care unit. *Crit Care Med* 1992; **20**: 1681–1687.

24. Vassar MJ, Wilkerson CL, Duran PJ, Perry CA, Holcroft JW. Comparison of the APACHE II, TRISS and a proposed 24-hour ICU point system for prediction of outcome in ICU trauma patients. *J Trauma* 1992; **32**: 490–500.

25. Moreno R, Morais P. Outcome prediction of intensive care: results of a prospective, multicentre Portuguese study. *Intensive Care Med* 1997; **23**: 177–186.

26. Copeland GP, Jones D, Walters M. Possum: a scoring system for surgical audit. *Br J Surg* 1991; **78**; 355–360.

27. Copeland GP. The POSSUM system of surgical audit. *Arch Surg* 2002; **137**: 15–19.

28. Sommer F, Ehsan A, Caspers H-P, Klotz T, Engelmann U. Risk adjustment for evaluating the outcome of urological operative procedures. *J Urol* 2001; **166**: 968–972.

29. Sagar PM, Hartley MN, Mancey-Jones B *et al*. Comparative audit of colorectal resection with the POSSUM scoring system. *Br J Surg* 1994; **81**: 1492–1494.

30. Tekkis PP, Kocker HM, Bentley AJE *et al*. Operative mortality rates among surgeons. Comparison of POSSUM and p-POSSUM scoring systems in gastrointestinal surgery. *Dis Colon Rectum* 2000; **43**: 1528–1532.

31. Midwinter MJ, Tytherleigh M, Ashley S. Estimation of mortality and morbidity risk in vascular surgery using POSSUM and the Portsmouth predictor equation. *Br J Surg* 1999; **86**: 471–474.

32. Gough MH, Kettlewell MGW, Marks CG, Holmes SJK, Holderness J. Audit: an annual assessment of the work and performance of a surgical firm in a regional teaching hospital. *BMJ* 1980; **281**: 913–918.

33. Deans GT, Odling-Smee W, McKelvey STD, Parks GT, Roy DA. Auditing perioperative mortality. *Ann R Coll Surg Engl* 1987; **69**: 185–187.

34. Wijensinghe LD, Mahmood T, Scott DJA *et al*. Comparison of POSSUM and the Portsmouth Predictor equation for predicting death following vascular surgery. *Br J Surg* 1998; **85**: 209–212.

35. Bann SD, Sarin S. Comparative audit: the trouble with POSSUM. *J R Soc Med* 2001; **94**: 632–634.

36. Wilson J, Woods I, Fawcett J *et al*. Reducing the risk of major elective surgery: randomised control trial of pre-operative optimisation of oxygen delivery. *BMJ* 1999; **318**: 1099–1103.

37. McLloy B, Miller A, Copeland GP, Kiff R. Audit of emergency pre-operative resuscitation. *Br J Surg* 1994; **81**: 200–202.

38. Jones DR. Playing POSSUM with ruptured aneurysms. *Eur J Vasc Surg* 1991; **4**: 488.

39. Pillai SB, van Rij AM, Williams S *et al*. Complexity- and risk-adjusted model for measuring surgical outcome. *Br J Surg* 1999; **86**: 1567–1572.

40. Haga Y, Ikei S, Waada Y *et al*. Evaluation of an Estimation of Physiologic Ability and Surgical Stress (E-PASS) scoring system to predict postoperative risk: a multicentre prospective study. *Surg Today* 2001; **31**: 569–574.

41. Khuri SF, Daley J, Henderson W *et al*. The Department of Veterans Affairs' NSQIP. The first national, validated, outcome based, risk-adjusted and peer-controlled program for the measurement and enhancement of the quality of surgical care. *Ann Surg* 1998; **228**: 491–507.

42. Khuri SF, Daley J, Henderson W *et al*. Risk adjustment of the postoperative mortality rate for the comparative assessment of the quality of surgical care: results of the National Veterans Affairs Surgical Risk Study. *J Am Coll Surg* 1997; **185**: 315–327.

43. Corti MC, Guralnik JM, Salive ME, Sorkin JD. Serum albumin level and physical disability as predictors of mortality in older persons. *JAMA* 1994; **260**: 1036–1042.

44. Klonoff-Cohen H, Barrett-Connor EL, Edelstein SL. Albumin levels as a predictor of mortality in the healthy elderly. *J Clin Epidemiol* 1992; **45**: 207–212.

45. Stamatakis J, Kinsman R, Thompson M, Chave H. *National Audit of Bowel Obstruction due to Colorectal Cancer July 2000*. The Association of Coloproctology of Great Britain and Ireland, The Royal College of Surgeons, 35/43 Lincoln's Inn Fields, London WC2A 3PN, UK.

46. Earnshaw JJ, Kinsman R, Ridler B. *The National Vascular Database Report 2001*. The Vascular Surgical Society of Great Britain and Ireland, The Royal College of Surgeons, 35/43 Lincoln's Inn Fields, London WC2A 3PN, UK (available to download at <www.vssgbi.org>).

Michael Douek Irving Taylor

16

Recent randomised controlled trials in general surgery

A selection of important randomised controlled trials in general surgery published over the last year, are reviewed in this chapter. These trials focus on the management of surgical disease in the fields of general, breast, upper gastrointestinal, colorectal, hepatobiliary and pancreatic, endocrine and melanoma surgery.

GENERAL CONDITIONS

THROMBOPROPHYLAXIS IN GENERAL SURGICAL PATIENTS

Thromboprophylaxis with heparin is now accepted clinical practice for all patients undergoing major surgery, but the optimal duration of postoperative thromboprophylaxis is not known. At most hospitals, heparin is discontinued prior to discharge, although it is recognised that the risk of thrombo-embolism remains high for several weeks. Several randomised trials compared low molecular heparin prophylaxis for 1 week and 1 month. Longer heparin prophylaxis was shown to reduce significantly the incidence of deep venous thrombosis following orthopaedic surgery[1] and, more recently, also following cancer surgery.[2] The ENOXACAN II study[2] demonstrated that, after surgery for abdominal or pelvic cancer, prophylaxis with Enoxaparin for 1 month significantly reduced the incidence of venographically proven deep venous thrombosis.

Mr Michael Douek MD FRCS, Lecturer in Surgery, Royal Free and University College Medical School, University College London, Charles Bell House, 67–73 Riding House Street, London W1W 7EJ, UK (for correspondence)

Prof. Irving Taylor MD ChM FRCS, Professor of Surgery, Head of Department of Surgery, Royal Free and University College Medical School, University College London, Charles Bell House, 67–73 Riding House Street, London W1W 7EJ, UK

APPENDICITIS

A Cochrane review recently evaluated randomised controlled studies comparing laparoscopic with open appendicectomy.[3] A total of 39 studies compared laparoscopic appendicectomy (with or without diagnostic laparoscopy). In hospitals where laparoscopic expertise is available, laparoscopy has several advantages over open appendicectomy. Laparoscopy is associated with less postoperative pain on day 1, shorter hospital stay, and earlier return to normal activity. Disadvantages include a higher cost and longer duration of surgery. Wound infections are less likely following laparoscopic appendicectomy (OR, 0.47; 95% CI, 0.36–0.62), but the odds of an intra-abdominal abscess is increased nearly 3-fold (OR, 2.77; 95% CI, 1.61–4.77). In the presence of perforation, the risk of residual intra-abdominal sepsis is higher, and thus the open approach should be preferred.

Several studies demonstrated that ultrasound is useful in the diagnosis of acute appendicitis, although sensitivity is low. Kaiser *et al.*[4] randomised 600 children with a clinical suspicion of appendicitis to either ultrasound or ultrasound followed by abdominal computed tomography (CT). The ultrasound only and ultrasound/CT arms had a sensitivity of 86% *versus* 99%, specificity of 95% *versus* 89% and negative predictive value of 92% and 99% for the diagnosis of acute appendicitis, respectively. Thus, in equivocal cases, the addition of a CT scan can improve diagnostic accuracy.

INGUINAL HERNIAS

The EU Trialists' Collaboration, aimed at evaluating newer methods of groin hernia repair, published its most recent meta-analysis,[5] which includes trials up to June 2000. Repair of groin hernia with synthetic mesh reduces the risk of recurrence by about 50%, irrespective of the placement method. In addition, mesh repair appears to reduce the chance of developing persistent groin pain, particularly following laparoscopic repair. Despite the recognised advantages of laparoscopic repair including reduced postoperative pain and earlier hospital discharge, it was suggested that laparoscopic repair is not cost-effective for routine use. Another meta-analysis, limited to laparoscopic inguinal hernia trials,[6] concluded that mesh open-hernia repair provides equivalent outcomes to laparoscopic repair, but at a lower cost and without the potential risk of serious complications. However, long-term data from a randomised controlled trial comparing laparoscopic (TAPP) with open-hernia mesh repair (awaiting publication[7]) demonstrated clear clinical advantages of the laparoscopic approach in terms of reduced groin pain (2% *versus* 10%; $P = 0.006$) and paraesthesia (2.5% *versus* 22.5%; $P < 0.001$). Recurrence rates were similar in the two groups (1.6% *versus* 2.5%).

UMBILICAL HERNIAS

Repair by primary suture rather than using a mesh is the standard technique used to repair umbilical hernias. Arroyo *et al.*[8] randomised 200 elective patients to either primary suture or mesh repair. The vast majority (98%) of procedures were undertaken under local anaesthetic. Hernia recurrence rates were 10-fold

Key point 1

- After surgery for abdominal or pelvic cancer, prophylaxis with Enoxaparin for 1 month significantly reduces the incidence of venographically proven deep venous thrombosis.

Key point 2

- In hospitals where laparoscopic expertise is available, laparoscopy has several advantages over open appendicectomy. However, in the presence of perforation, the risk of residual intra-abdominal sepsis is higher with laparoscopy and thus the open approach should be preferred.

Key point 3

- Repair of groin hernia with synthetic mesh reduces the risk of recurrence by about 50%, irrespective of the placement method. Mesh repair reduces the chance of developing persistent groin pain.

higher with suture repair (11% *versus* 1%) at a mean follow-up of 64 months. No significant difference was seen in duration of operation, mean post-operative stay, mean pain scores, or early complication rate.

ENTERAL AND PARENTERAL POSTOPERATIVE NUTRITION

Early enteral feeding following major gastrointestinal surgery is usually avoided despite growing evidence of clear advantages. Lewis *et al.*[9] carried out a systematic review and meta-analysis of all studies comparing enteral feeding (oral, nasogastric or nasojejunal) *versus* 'nil-by-mouth'. Eleven studies with a total of 837 patients, were reviewed. Early feeding significantly reduced the risk of infection (RR, 0.72; 95% CI, 0.54–0.98) and mean length of hospital stay. Non-significant risk reductions were also observed in several other outcome measures including anastomotic dehiscence (RR, 0.53; $P = 0.08$), wound infection, pneumonia, intra-abdominal abscess and mortality. Clearly, the available data are insufficient to conclude that early enteral feeding should be the norm, at present.

BREAST SURGERY

BREAST SCREENING

A meta-analysis of all randomised controlled trials of breast screening[10] and a Cochrane review[11] by Olsen and Gotzsche, led to a stormy debate and controversy. The authors concluded that the currently available reliable evidence does not show a survival benefit of mass screening for breast cancer.

Of the 8 randomised controlled studies to date, 6 were found to be of poor quality or flawed and were thus excluded from the analysis. Another important finding (excluded from the Cochrane review, but published in *The Lancet* website) is that mass screening leads to increased use of more aggressive treatment, increasing the number of mastectomies by 20% and number of mastectomies or wide local excisions by 30%, in the screened group. More recently, Nystrom *et al.*[12] published their latest overview of all the Swedish randomised trials. Over 247,010 patients have been entered and followed up for a median time of 15.8 years. The benefit of breast cancer mortality began to emerge after 4 years, continued to increase until 10 years and was, thereafter, maintained in absolute terms. Statistically significant reductions in breast cancer mortality were observed in the 5-year age groups 55–59, 60–64 and 65–69 years (RR, 0.76, 0.68, 0.69, respectively). However, over 1,864,770 women-years were needed to achieve this result. Although the resulting reduction of mortality is now accepted, the clinical utility of screening is still questioned and a cost-effectiveness analysis by the National Institute for Clinical Excellence (NICE), will hopefully be undertaken.

SENTINEL LYMPH NODE BIOPSY

The accuracy of sentinel node (the first lymph node to contain metastatic cancer) status in predicting axillary node status is no longer under dispute. Several prospective, national, randomised, controlled trials are underway to assess the impact of sentinel node biopsy on axillary morbidity, recurrence rates, disease-free and overall survival. In the UK, the BASO (British Association of Surgical Oncology)/ALMANAC (Axillary Lymphatic Mapping Against Nodal Axillary Clearance) Trial is well underway.[13] Patients are randomised to sentinel node biopsy guided axillary treatment (surgery or radiotherapy) based on paraffin histology, or to conventional axillary treatment (axillary node sampling or clearance). The primary end-points are axillary morbidity, health economics and quality-of-life. In the US, the NSABP B-32 trial and American College of Surgeons Oncology Group (ACOSOG) Z0010/Z0011 trials are underway. In the ACOSOG Z0011 trial,[14] patients with clinical T1/T2 N0M0 breast cancer and a positive sentinel node are randomised to axillary node clearance or no axillary node clearance. The primary end-point is overall survival, and secondary end-points are surgical morbidity and distant disease-free survival.

Although initial results of these studies will become available in 2002–2004, there is a vast amount of evidence in support of sentinel node biopsy.[15] As a result, at many centres, sentinel node biopsy is now regarded as standard practice. However, it is more prudent to await the results of randomised controlled studies before abandoning routine axillary lymph node clearance, particularly in women with larger tumours.

RADIOTHERAPY

Breast radiotherapy is now regarded as standard treatment following breast conserving surgery. Bartelink *et al.*[16] evaluated the effect of a supplementary dose of radiotherapy to the tumour bed on the rate of local recurrence.

Following breast conserving surgery for early breast cancer resected with pathologically clear margins and axillary node clearance, 2657 patients were randomised to either standard radiotherapy (50 Gy to the whole breast in 2 Gy fractions over 5 weeks) or standard radiotherapy plus an additional localised dose of 16 Gy to the tumour bed given in 8 fractions, using an external electron beam. At 5.1 years median follow-up, the actuarial rates of local recurrence were 7.3% with standard treatment and 4.3% with the additional radiation (hazard rate, 0.59; $P < 0.001$), independent of whether the patients received adjuvant chemotherapy. Patients under 50 years of age, particularly those 40 years old or younger, benefited most. Distant disease-free survival and overall survival, were similar in the two treatment groups with 5-year rates of 87% and 91%, respectively.

ENDOCRINE THERAPY

Tamoxifen remains the most important adjuvant endocrine treatment for breast cancer, but its supremacy has recently been challenged by the results of the ATAC (Arimidex, Tamoxifen and Combined) Trial, from the UK. This international multicentre trial[17] had 3 arms: anastrazole, tamoxifen or the combination of the 2 agents. A total of 9366 post-menopausal women with invasive operable breast cancer were randomised, exceeding recruitment expectations and making this study the largest adjuvant chemotherapy trial ever completed. Interim results at 2.5 years follow-up, demonstrated that anastrazole monotherapy is superior to tamoxifen and also to the combination. Disease-free survival was 89.4% with anastrazole, 87.4% with tamoxifen (hazard ration, 0.83; $P = 0.013$) and 87.2% with the combination. Anastrazole reduced the relative risk of recurrence by 22% ($P = 0.005$) and the risk of a second primary by 58% ($P = 0.007$). It was also better tolerated than tamoxifen in terms of rate of endometrial cancer ($P = 0.02$), vaginal bleeding ($P < 0.0001$), vaginal discharge ($P < 0.0001$), cerebrovascular accidents ($P = 0.0006$), venous thrombo-embolic events ($P = 0.0006$) and hot flushes ($P < 0.0001$). Tamoxifen was significantly better tolerated than anastrazole with respect to musculoskeletal disorders ($P < 0.0001$) and fractures ($P < 0.0001$). Although these results are encouraging, they should be interpreted with caution until results at 5-year follow-up become available in 2003/2004. As a result of this short follow-up period, the American Society of Clinical Oncology (ASCO), has not yet embraced anastrazole as the new standard and tamoxifen remains the standard for adjuvant endocrine therapy of breast cancer.[18]

CHEMOTHERAPY

A Cochrane systematic review undertaken by the Early Breast Cancer Trialists' Collaborative Group[19] confirmed the strong evidence from randomised controlled trials supporting the use of systemic adjuvant chemotherapy in the management of early breast cancer. In women with early breast cancer (stage I/II), adjuvant polychemotherapy (*e.g.* with CMF or an anthracycline-containing regimen) produces an absolute improvement of about 7–11% in 10-year survival for women aged under 50 years at presentation, and of about 2–3% for those aged 50–69 years.

There is now also evidence in favour of a single course of peri-operative chemotherapy in patients with early breast cancer. In the European Organization for Research and Treatment of Cancer (EORTC) Trial 10854, 2795 patients were randomised to either one dose of an anthracycline-containing regimen given within 36 h of surgery or surgery alone. At a median follow-up of 11 years, both progression-free survival and locoregional control were significantly improved in the treatment arm, particularly in node-negative patients.

The EORTC trial 10902, compared pre-operative or neo-adjuvant chemotherapy, with postoperative chemotherapy.[20] A total of 698 patients with no evidence of metastatic spread (T1c to T4b, N0 or N1), were randomised to 4 cycles of FEC (5-fluorouracil, epirubicin and cyclophosphamide) either pre- or postoperatively. In the postoperative group, the initial dose was administered within 36 h after surgery. At a median of 4.7 years follow-up, there was no significant difference in overall survival, progression-free survival or time to locoregional recurrence. However, neo-adjuvant chemotherapy increased the number of patients suitable for breast conserving surgery. A total of 57 patients were down-staged (23%) but 14 patients (18%) underwent mastectomy rather than the planned breast conserving surgery. Interestingly, 13 patients (4.5%) who received neo-adjuvant chemotherapy, were found to have a complete histological response.

Key point 4

- The latest overview of all the Swedish screening trials demonstrated a survival benefit of mass screening for breast cancer. However, the number of mastectomies is increased by 20% and wide local excisions by 30%, in the screened group.

Key point 5

- Following breast conserving surgery for early breast cancer, standard adjuvant postoperative radiotherapy with additional dose to the tumour bed reduces the risk of local recurrence, especially in women under 50 years of age.

Key point 6

- Early results of the UK ATAC trial (anastrazole, tamoxifen or the combination), demonstrated that anastrazole monotherapy was superior to tamoxifen and also to the combination. However, a 5-year course of adjuvant tamoxifen remains the standard therapy for women with hormone receptor-positive breast cancer.

UPPER GASTROINTESTINAL SURGERY

PREVENTION OF ERCP-INDUCED PANCREATITIS

Sublingual prophylactic treatment with glyceryl trinitrate (GTN), at a dose of 2 mg administered 5 min prior to ERCP, has been shown to reduce the occurrence of pancreatitis at 24 h but not the extent of hyperamylasaemia or the severity of pancreatitis.[21] Shori et al.[22] found that GTN administered prior to ERCP, improves cannulation success rates. Of 254 patients randomised to GTN or no GTN prior to ERCP, cannulation failure rates were 7.0% in the GTN group and 15.8% in the no-GTN group ($P < 0.0002$).

LAPAROSCOPIC CHOLECYSTECTOMY *VERSUS* MINI-LAPAROTOMY

Mini-laparotomy has been suggested as a cost-effective alternative to laparoscopic cholecystectomy, but studies to date suggest that the laparoscopic approach is superior. Ros et al.[23] randomised 724 patients with symptomatic gallstones (acute or elective) to either mini-laparotomy or laparoscopic cholecystectomy. Mean operating time was significantly longer in the laparoscopic group. Although mean hospital stay was similar (2 days), median sick leave and time to return to normal activity were shorter in the laparoscopic group. There was no difference in postoperative complications between the groups. Although most patients were operated on by surgeons with an operative experience exceeding 25 cases, this was not a prerequisite and the number of cases undertaken by experienced surgeons was not comparable. Laparoscopic cholecystectomy should, therefore, be the preferred approach until further comparative research is undertaken to evaluate the reproducibility and extent of surgical training required for mini-laparotomy.

OESOPHAGEAL CARCINOMA

Neo-adjuvant (primary) chemotherapy in patients with operable oesophageal carcinoma should be considered in patients with resectable oesophageal cancer. In a meta-analysis of all randomised controlled trials comparing neo-adjuvant chemotherapy and surgery with surgery alone,[24] neo-adjuvant chemotherapy was associated with a lower rate of oesophageal resection, a higher rate of complete resection, but no survival benefit. However, results of the largest trial to date[25] have demonstrated a survival advantage. The Medical Research Council Oesophageal Cancer Working Party[25] randomised 802 previously untreated patients with resectable oesophageal carcinoma (33% squamous and 67% adenocarcinoma) to pre-operative chemotherapy with cisplatin and 5-fluorouracil followed by surgery, or surgery alone. At 2 years' follow-up, there was an overall survival advantage in favour of neo-adjuvant chemotherapy (hazard ratio, 0.79; 95% CI, 0.67–0.93) with survival rates of 43% and 34%, respectively.

GASTRIC CARCINOMA

Until recently, the efficacy of adjuvant chemotherapy in gastric cancer, after curative resection, was controversial. A meta-analysis of all trials comparing adjuvant chemotherapy with control after radical resection of gastric cancer[26] concluded that adjuvant chemotherapy results in a significant survival advantage in patients with gastric cancer.

Radiochemotherapy, has also been shown to be effective. In a randomised study of 556 patients[27] with curative resection of the stomach or gastro-oesophageal junction (AJCC stage IB–IVM0), patients were assigned to surgery alone or surgery plus postoperative chemoradiotherapy (local–regional radiotherapy plus 5-fluorouracil and leucovorin chemotherapy, as a combined regimen administered over 16 weeks). Resection of all detectable disease was required for participation in the trial. Interestingly, although an extensive lymph-node dissection was recommended, only 10% of the patients underwent a D2 dissection. The 3-year survival rates were 50% in the chemoradiotherapy group and 41% in the surgery-only group. With a median follow-up of 5 years, the hazard ratios for death (1.35; 95% CI, 1.09–1.66) and relapse (1.52; 95% CI, 1.23–1.86) in the chemoradiotherapy group as compared with the surgery-only group were significantly increased. Adjuvant treatment with 5-fluorouracil plus leucovorin and radiation should be considered for all patients with high-risk gastric cancer.

LAPAROSCOPIC REPAIR FOR PERFORATED PEPTIC ULCER

Laparotomy for peritonitis secondary to a perforated peptic ulcer is a prime example of a technically simple operation, requiring significant access. In a randomised controlled study of 121 patients,[28] the laparoscopic approach was quicker and was associated with significantly less postoperative pain and reduced parenteral analgesic use. The laparoscopic to open conversion rate was 15% and 2 patients in the laparoscopic group developed intra-abdominal collections.

Key point 7

- GTN administered prior to ERCP improves cannulation success rates and reduces the occurrence of pancreatitis.

Key point 8

- For cholecystectomy, laparoscopy rather than mini-laparotomy should be the preferred approach until further comparative research is undertaken to evaluate the comparative reproducibility of mini-laparotomy.

Key point 9

- In patients with gastric cancer, adjuvant chemotherapy results in a significant survival advantage.

COLORECTAL SURGERY

PROPHYLACTIC ANTIBIOTICS

Administration of only prophylactic intravenous antibiotics in patients undergoing colonic surgery, appears to be counter-intuitive. Lewis *et al.*[29] randomised 215 patients undergoing elective colonic surgery to either oral neomycin and metronidazole or placebo on the last pre-operative day. All patients received amikacin and metronidazole intravenously at induction. Significant reductions were observed in wound infection rates (RR, 0.29; $P <$ 0.01) and positive bacterial wound swabs ($P < 0.001$). A meta-analysis of all 13 published comparative randomised controlled studies, by the same authors,[29] was in favour of the combined antibiotic approach (RR, 0.51; $P < 0.001$).

PENETRATING COLONIC INJURY

A recent Cochrane systematic review[30] of studies comparing primary repair to faecal diversion following penetrating colonic injury favoured primary repair. Total complications (OR, 0.28; 95% CI, 0.18–0.42), total infections (OR, 0.41; 95% CI, 0.27–0.63), abdominal sepsis (OR, 0.52; 95% CI, 0.31–0.86), wound complications including dehiscence (OR, 0.55; 95% CI, 0.34–0.89) were significantly reduced with primary repair. Mortality was not significantly different between the two groups. Another randomised controlled study of 240 patients presenting with delayed penetrating abdominal injury was also in favour of primary repair.[31]

PREVENTION AND SCREENING

A Cochrane systematic review and meta-analysis, evaluated the effect of dietary fibre on the incidence of colorectal adenomas or colorectal cancer. In 5 trials with 4349 patients that met the methodological criteria, there was no evidence that increased dietary fibre intake reduced the incidence or recurrence of adenomatous polyps within 2–4 years. The incidence of colorectal cancer was not a predefined outcome in any of the studies; only two studies reported it and numbers were too small for firm conclusions.

Using screening for faecal occult blood, to date three trials have demonstrated significant reductions in mortality from colorectal cancer. One of these, the Danish group, published their results at 13 years of follow-up. A total of 61,933 patients were randomised to biennial screening with Haemoccult-II or no screening. Mortality from colorectal cancer was significantly reduced in the screened group (RR, 0.82; 95% CI, 0.69–0.97).

Screening for polyps and chemoprevention have also been used for the primary prevention of colorectal cancer. To date, trials of screening with colonoscopy or flexible sigmoidoscopy have not demonstrated a reduction in mortality from colorectal cancer. The UK Flexible Sigmoidoscopy Screening Trial has completed recruitment and is now underway.[32] A total of 170,432 patients were randomised and will be followed up for 15 years.

The APACC study[33] is underway and will determine if 160 or 300 mg/day of aspirin is effective in reducing colorectal adenoma recurrence. So far, 274 patients were enrolled and 618 polyps excised at baseline colonoscopy.

FOLLOW-UP OF PATIENTS WITH COLORECTAL CANCER

Patients with colorectal cancer are usually followed up, but intensity of follow-up varies and has not been shown to achieve a survival advantage. A Cochrane review[34] of all randomised controlled trials comparing different follow-up strategies, found five trials that met methodological quality. Meta-analysis demonstrated a survival benefit at 5 years for patients undergoing intensive follow-up (OR, 0.67; 95% CI, 0.53–0.84); no difference in the number of recurrences was seen. Study difference and significant study heterogeneity precluded further comparisons or a clear recommendation. Another systematic review[35] also found five suitable trials and came to similar conclusions.

ADJUVANT CHEMOTHERAPY IN THE ELDERLY

Adjuvant chemotherapy is standard treatment for patients with resected colorectal cancer who are at high risk of recurrence; but, for patients over the age of 70 years, the risks are believed to exceed any potential benefit. However, pooled analysis of 7 phase III randomised controlled trials[36] with 3351 patients, found a significant improvement in overall survival (HR, 0.76; $P < 0.001$) and time-to-recurrence (HR, 0.68; $P < 0.001$). Overall 5-year survival was 71% with chemotherapy and 64% without.

PRE-OPERATIVE RADIOTHERAPY FOR RECTAL CANCER

Two large randomised controlled trials provide strong evidence to support the treatment of all patients with primary radiotherapy followed by surgery. Five days of pre-operative radiotherapy (25 Gy) to rectum and pararectal tissues has been shown to reduce local recurrence[37,38] and improve survival in patients who underwent curative resections.[37] The Dutch Colorectal Cancer Group[38] reported results of their 1861 patients with resectable rectal cancer, randomised to a 5-day course of pre-operative radiotherapy followed by total mesorectal excision or total mesorectal excision alone, with a follow-up of at least 2 years. Overall survival (82.0% *versus* 81.8%; $P = 0.84$) was equivalent, but the rate of local recurrence was significantly reduced in the group that had received pre-operative radiotherapy (2.4% *versus* 8.2%; $P < 0.001$). Univariate subgroup analysis demonstrated that this benefit was not significant in those patients who had tumours with an inferior margin more than 10 cm from the anal verge. More recently, a subgroup analysis of 1530 patients who underwent total mesorectal excision (TME) confirmed that TME and pre-operative radiotherapy was superior to TME alone.[39] Although there was a significant increase in total number of complications and intra-operative blood loss with pre-operative radiotherapy, mortality was no different (4.0% *versus* 3.3%).

In the Stockholm II study,[37] 557 patients with biopsy proven rectal carcinoma judged as being operable were randomised to pre-operative radiotherapy followed by surgery within a week, or surgery alone. All patients were followed up for a minimum of 5.6 years and a median of 8.8 years. It is not clear what proportion of patients underwent total mesorectal excision, but a curative resection was achieved in 481 patients (86%). Of those who underwent curative resection, the incidence of pelvic recurrence (12% *versus*

25%; $P < 0.001$) was reduced and overall survival (46% *versus* 39%; $P < 0.03$) improved in the irradiated patients. However, for all included patients, overall survival was equivalent (39% *versus* 36%) and intercurrent death was increased in the irradiated group (19% *versus* 12%; $P = 0.1$). The introduction of total mesorectal excision has led to a reduction of local recurrence rates in the 1990s, and it is important to note here that in neither study did the investigators test the benefit or otherwise, of the technique. The demonstrated benefit of radiotherapy compared to the clinical benefit of improved surgical technique remains unknown. Another clinical implication regards the use of a lower dose of radiotherapy (25 Gy) as well as the use of pre-operative rather than postoperative radiotherapy. It has been suggested that the dose-response ratio and patient compliance are higher with pre-operative radiotherapy. The Colorectal Cancer Collaborative Group reviewed 22 randomised trials and concluded that pre-operative radiotherapy significantly reduces risk of local recurrence and death from colorectal cancer. The optimal timing of surgery after radiotherapy (within 1 week or after 4–8 weeks) is not known and the Stockholm III trial was launched in 1999 to address this question. At present, a compromise would be sensible: to administer pre-operative radiotherapy to all patients with locally advanced or large operable disease, and offer primary surgery to patients with early disease or to those with high rectal tumours.

LAPAROSCOPIC-ASSISTED COLECTOMY

The role of laparoscopic-assisted surgery in the treatment of colorectal cancer is as yet unclear, but positive evidence is emerging. A recent randomised controlled study of 219 patients followed up for 4 years was in favour of the laparoscopic approach.[40] Time to first peristalsis, time to first oral intake, and hospital stay were all significantly reduced in the laparoscopic group. Overall mortality was no different, but morbidity was lower in the laparoscopic group ($P = 0.001$). Interestingly, the probability of cancer-related survival was increased in the laparoscopic group ($P = 0.02$), and risk of recurrence was reduced (HR, 0.39; 95% CI, 0.19–0.82). This primarily reflected results obtained in patients with stage III disease, who appeared to benefit the most. Only 1 patient developed a port-site metastasis.

Several large, randomised, controlled trials are currently underway including the UK MRC CLASICC (Conventional *versus* Laparoscopic-assisted Surgery in Colorectal Cancer) trial,[41] a similar trial in the US and the multicentre international COLOR (COlon carcinoma Laparoscopic or Open Resection) trial in Sweden.[42] Major questions remain unsolved with respect to port-site implantation, immune response and cost-effectiveness.

HAEMORRHOIDECTOMY

Gencosmanoglu *et al.*[43] compared open with closed haemorrhoidectomy in a randomised study of 80 patients with III/IV degree haemorrhoids. The open approach was associated with a significantly shorter operating time, lower analgesic requirements on day 1, and lower morbidity rate. Healing time was significantly shorter with the closed approach. Length of hospital stay and time off work, were similar.

Stapled haemorrhoidectomy is gaining support over conventional haemorrhoidectomy. Shalaby et al.[44] randomised 200 patients with grade II–IV haemorrhoids to either Milligan-Morgan haemorrhoidectomy or stapled haemorrhoidectomy (33 mm circular stapling device). In the stapled group, operating time was shorter (9 versus 19 min; $P < 0.001$), postoperative pain and analgesic requirements were reduced, hospital stay was reduced (1.1 versus 2.2; $P < 0.001$) with earlier return to normal activity. Ho et al.[45] randomised 119 patients with grade III/IV haemorrhoids to either stapled haemorrhoidectomy or to open diathermy haemorrhoidectomy. Open diathermy haemorrhoidectomy was quicker to perform (11.4 versus 17.6 min) but more painful, with more bleeding – 85.5% of wounds were unhealed at 2 weeks and patients resumed work later compared with stapled haemorrhoidectomy (22.9 versus 17.1 days; $P < 0.05$). The authors scored faecal incontinence and performed anorectal manometry as well as endo-anal ultrasound, but the complication rate was similar in the two groups.

The Ligasure diathermy system allows accurate application of bipolar diathermy to vascular structures. Two small randomised trials[46,47] compared Ligasure to conventional diathermy haemorrhoidectomies with similar results. Reduced operative time,[46,47] reduced blood loss,[46] no difference in postoperative pain,[46,47] reduced analgesic use,[47] and more same-day discharges.[46]

Key point 10

- The Dutch Colorectal Cancer Group and Stockholm II trials provide strong evidence that 5 days of pre-operative radiotherapy, in patients with operable rectal carcinoma, significantly reduces local recurrence rate.

HEPATOBILIARY AND PANCREATIC SURGERY

ENTERAL FEEDING FOR ACUTE PANCREATITIS

Pancreatic rest, by discontinuation of oral intake or parenteral nutrition, is standard practice for the treatment of acute pancreatitis. As an alternative approach, hypocaloric jejunal feeding was compared to parenteral nutrition in consecutive patients who failed to respond to 48 h conservative management.[48] Of 156 patients, 52 were randomised to either enteral or parenteral nutrition. Although enteral nutrition was less effective at meeting nutritional requirements, duration of feeding and cost were significantly reduced. Septic complications were also reduced in the enteral group. Hypocaloric jejunal feeding is a safe and less expensive alternative to parenteral nutrition in patients with acute pancreatitis who do not respond to 48 h pancreatic rest.

DRAINS FOLLOWING PANCREATIC RESECTION

Intraperitoneal drains are routinely used after pancreatic resection. In a randomised study of 179 patients undergoing pancreatic resection (pancreaticoduodenectomy, $n = 139$; distal pancreatectomy, $n = 40$), 108 patients (59%) developed a postoperative complication and overall 30-day mortality was 2%.[49] There was no significant difference in the rate or type of complications observed in the two groups. Thus, following pancreatic resection, closed suction drainage should not be considered mandatory or standard practice.

RADIOFREQUENCY ABLATION FOR HEPATOCELLULAR CARCINOMA

The only curative treatment for hepatocellular carcinoma remains hepatectomy. However, in a significant proportion of patients, resection is not indicated since disease is inoperable, is associated with underlying severe liver cirrhosis, or because of significant co-morbidity. Even after liver resection, long-term outcome is poor with a high incidence of local recurrence in the liver remnant. Several therapeutic interventional radiological techniques have been used to treat patients who are not suitable for surgical resection. A Cochrane systematic review of the efficacy of radiofrequency thermal ablation for hepatocellular carcinoma, was recently updated.[50] Only interim analysis of one randomised controlled trial was available for review. In 102 patients randomised to either ethanol injection or radiofrequency ablation, no significant difference was seen.

PANCREATIC CARCINOMA

Pylorus-preserving pancreaticoduodenectomy (PPPD) is a more conservative, alternative operation to a Whipple, in patients with peri-ampullary and pancreatic head lesions. However, the radicality of this operation in pancreatic cancer has been questioned. In a recent, large, single-institution trial,[51] 299 patients were randomised to standard (86% PPPD) or radical pancreaticoduodenectomy (standard resection plus distal gastrectomy and retroperitoneal lymphadenectomy). The standard group had a significantly shorter operating time (5.9 *versus* 6.4 h; $P = 0.02$) and a significantly reduced complication rate (29% *versus* 43%; $P = 0.01$). There was no difference in intra-operative blood loss or transfusion requirement. Patients in the radical group had a significantly higher rate of delayed gastric emptying, pancreatic fistulae and increased mean postoperative stay. At a mean patient follow-up of 24 months, there was no difference in overall survival. With respect to the need for pre-operative biliary drainage in patients with jaundice, a systematic review and meta-analysis of all published comparative studies, including 5 randomised controlled studies, concluded that pre-operative drainage procedures significantly increase morbidity without reducing mortality.[52]

Key point 11

- Hypocaloric jejunal feeding is a safe and less expensive alternative to parenteral nutrition in patients with acute pancreatitis who do not respond to 48 h pancreatic rest.

Key point 12

- Following pancreatic resection, closed suction drainage should not be considered mandatory or standard practice.

Key point 13

- Compared to pylorus-preserving pancreaticoduodenectomy, radical pancreaticoduodenectomy is associated with increased morbidity, but no survival benefit.

Key point 14

- In patients with obstructive jaundice undergoing tumour resection, pre-operative biliary drainage significantly increases morbidity without reducing mortality.

THYROID DISEASE

VIDEO-ASSISTED THYROID LOBECTOMY

Video-assisted thyroid lobectomy, developed in Italy in 1998,[53] is a technique for minimally invasive, totally gasless thyroid lobectomy. Using a 5-mm 30 degrees laparoscope, the procedure is undertaken using both endoscopic and conventional instruments. A small horizontal skin incision is used to extract the resected thyroid. Bellantone et al.[54] randomised 62 patients with thyroid nodules (<= 3 cm) to conventional or video-assisted thyroid lobectomy. No significant difference in complication rates (including recurrent nerve damage) was observed, demonstrating the feasibility of this approach. Cosmetic outcome, postoperative pain in the first 2 days and hospital stay were all significantly reduced in the video-assisted group. In a different randomised trial with similar entrance criteria and 49 patients randomised, significant differences in postoperative pain and cosmesis were observed in favour of the video-assisted technique.[55] However, operative time was significantly longer in the video-assisted group. Clearly, prior to considering video-assisted thyroid lobectomy as a viable alternative to the open approach, a larger randomised controlled trial is required.

Key point 15

- Video-assisted thyroid lobectomy can improve cosmetic result and reduce postoperative pain; however, prior to considering it as a viable alternative to the open approach, a larger randomised controlled trial is required.

MELANOMA

Surgical resection with an excision margin of 2 cm, is safe for the majority of patients with cutaneous melanoma and this approach enables closure of most defects by simple skin flap techniques. Outcome in malignant melanoma is primarily dependent upon stage at presentation. Lymph node status in melanoma patients is a powerful prognostic indicator and it is reliably predicted by sentinel node biopsy. A meta-analysis of studies comparing elective with delayed lymphadenectomy (performed at the time of local recurrence) showed no significant overall-survival benefit. It is thus sufficient to perform sentinel node biopsy in the majority of patients and lymphadenectomy should be limited to patients with sentinel lymph node involvement.

The clinical relevance of micrometastatic involvement of sentinel nodes, as detected by reverse transcriptase polymerase chain reaction (RT-PCR) is still a subject for research. The value of additional therapy (including elective lymph node dissection and interferon therapy) is currently being investigated by the national multicentre Sunbelt Melanoma Trial in the US.[56]

The American Joint Committee on Cancer staging (AJCC) recently published the sixth edition of the *AJCC Cancer Staging Manual*,[57] with significant changes to the staging of cancer at various anatomical sites, including breast and melanoma. The new classification of cutaneous malignant melanoma includes melanoma thickness and ulceration (but not level of invasion) in the T category, and distinguishes between macroscopic and microscopic lymph node metastases.[58]

Key point 16

- The American Joint Committee on Cancer staging (AJCC) recently published the sixth edition of the *AJCC Cancer Staging Manual*, with significant changes to the staging of cancer at various anatomical sites, including breast and melanoma.

Key points for clinical practice

- After surgery for abdominal or pelvic cancer, prophylaxis with Enoxaparin for 1 month significantly reduces the incidence of venographically proven deep venous thrombosis.

- In hospitals where laparoscopic expertise is available, laparoscopy has several advantages over open appendicectomy. However, in the presence of perforation, the risk of residual intra-abdominal sepsis is higher with laparoscopy and thus the open approach should be preferred.

- Repair of groin hernia with synthetic mesh reduces the risk of recurrence by about 50%, irrespective of the placement method. Mesh repair reduces the chance of developing persistent groin pain.

Key points for clinical practice (continued)

- The latest overview of all the Swedish screening trials demonstrated a survival benefit of mass screening for breast cancer. However, the number of mastectomies is increased by 20% and wide local excisions by 30% in the screened group.

- Following breast conserving surgery for early breast cancer, standard adjuvant postoperative radiotherapy with additional dose to the tumour bed reduces the risk of local recurrence, especially in women under 50 years of age.

- Early results of the UK ATAC trial (anastrazole, tamoxifen or the combination) demonstrated that anastrazole monotherapy was superior to tamoxifen and also to the combination. However, a 5-year course of adjuvant tamoxifen remains the standard therapy for women with hormone receptor-positive breast cancer.

- GTN administered prior to ERCP improves cannulation success rates and reduces the occurrence of pancreatitis.

- For cholecystectomy, laparoscopy rather than mini-laparotomy should be the preferred approach until further comparative research is undertaken to evaluate the comparative reproducibility of mini-laparotomy.

- In patients with gastric cancer, adjuvant chemotherapy results in a significant survival advantage.

- The Dutch Colorectal Cancer Group & Stockholm II trials provide strong evidence that 5 days of pre-operative radiotherapy, in patients with operable rectal carcinoma, significantly reduces local recurrence rate.

- Hypocaloric jejunal feeding is a safe and less expensive alternative to parenteral nutrition, in patients with acute pancreatitis who do not respond to 48 h pancreatic rest.

- Following pancreatic resection, closed suction drainage should not be considered mandatory or standard practice.

- Compared to pylorus-preserving pancreaticoduodenectomy, radical pancreaticoduodenectomy is associated with increased morbidity, but no survival benefit.

- In patients with obstructive jaundice undergoing tumour resection, pre-operative biliary drainage significantly increases morbidity without reducing mortality.

- Video-assisted thyroid lobectomy can improve cosmetic result and reduce postoperative pain; however, prior to considering it as a viable alternative to the open approach, a larger randomised controlled trial is required.

- The American Joint Committee on Cancer staging (AJCC) recently published the sixth edition of the *AJCC Cancer Staging Manual*, with significant changes to the staging of cancer at various anatomical sites, including breast and melanoma..

References

1. Bergqvist D, Benoni G, Bjorgell O et al. Low-molecular-weight heparin (enoxaparin) as prophylaxis against venous thromboembolism after total hip replacement. *N Engl J Med* 1996; **335**: 696–700.

2. Bergqvist D, Agnelli G, Cohen AT et al. Duration of prophylaxis against venous thromboembolism with enoxaparin after surgery for cancer. *N Engl J Med* 2002; **346**: 975–980.

3. Sauerland S, Lefering R, Neugebauer EA. Laparoscopic *versus* open surgery for suspected appendicitis. *Cochrane Database Syst Rev* 2002; CD001546.

4. Kaiser S, Frenckner B, Jorulf HK. Suspected appendicitis in children: US and CT – a prospective randomized study. *Radiology* 2002; **223**: 633–638.

5. The EU hernia Trialists Collaboration. Repair of groin hernia with synthetic mesh: meta-analysis of randomized controlled trials. *Ann Surg* 2002; **235**: 322–332.

6. Voyles CR, Hamilton BJ, Johnson WD, Kano N. Meta-analysis of laparoscopic inguinal hernia trials favors open hernia repair with preperitoneal mesh prosthesis. *Am J Surg* 2002; **184**: 6–10.

7. Douek M, Smith G, Oshowo A, Stoker DL, Wellwood J. Prospective randomized controlled trial of laparoscopic *versus* open hernia mesh repair: 5 year follow-up. *Br J Surg* 2002; **89**: 37.

8. Arroyo A, Garcia P, Perez F, Andreu J, Candela F, Calpena R. Randomized clinical trial comparing suture and mesh repair of umbilical hernia in adults. *Br J Surg* 2001; **88**: 1321–1323.

9. Lewis SJ, Egger M, Sylvester PA, Thomas S. Early enteral feeding versus 'nil by mouth' after gastrointestinal surgery: systematic review and meta-analysis of controlled trials. *BMJ* 2001; **323**: 773–776.

10. Olsen O, Gotzsche PC. Cochrane review on screening for breast cancer with mammography. *Lancet* 2001; **358**: 1340–1342.

11. Olsen O, Gotzsche PC. Screening for breast cancer with mammography. *Cochrane Database Syst Rev* 2001; CD001877.

12. Nystrom L, Andersson I, Bjurstam N, Frisell J, Nordenskjold B, Rutqvist LE. Long-term effects of mammography screening: updated overview of the Swedish randomised trials. *Lancet* 2002; **359**: 909–919.

13. Clarke D, Khonji NI, Mansel RE. Sentinel node biopsy in breast cancer: ALMANAC trial. *World J Surg* 2001; **25**: 819–822.

14. Grube BJ, Giuliano AE. Observation of the breast cancer patient with a tumor-positive sentinel node: implications of the ACOSOG Z0011 trial. *Semin Surg Oncol* 2001; **20**: 230–237.

15. Keshtgar MR, Ell PJ. Clinical role of sentinel-lymph-node biopsy in breast cancer. *Lancet Oncol* 2002; **3**: 105–110.

16. Bartelink H, Horiot JC, Poortmans P et al. Recurrence rates after treatment of breast cancer with standard radiotherapy with or without additional radiation. *N Engl J Med* 2001; **345**: 1378–1387.

17. The ATAC Trialists' Group. Anastrozole alone or in combination with tamoxifen *versus* tamoxifen alone for adjuvant treatment of postmenopausal women with early breast cancer: first results of the ATAC randomised trial. *Lancet* 2002; **359**: 2131–2139.

18. Winer EP, Hudis C, Burstein HJ et al. American Society of Clinical Oncology technology assessment on the use of aromatase inhibitors as adjuvant therapy for women with hormone receptor-positive breast cancer: status report 2002. *J Clin Oncol* 2002; **20**: 3317–3327.

19. Early Breast Cancer Trialists' Collaborative Group. Multi-agent chemotherapy for early breast cancer. *Cochrane Database Syst Rev* 2002; CD000487.

20. van der Hage JA, van de Velde CJ, Julien JP, Tubiana-Hulin M, Vandervelden C, Duchateau L. Preoperative chemotherapy in primary operable breast cancer: results from the European Organization for Research and Treatment of Cancer trial 10902. *J Clin Oncol* 2001; **19**: 4224–4237.

21. Sudhindran S, Bromwich E, Edwards PR. Prospective randomized double-blind placebo-controlled trial of glyceryl trinitrate in endoscopic retrograde cholangiopancreato-graphy-induced pancreatitis. *Br J Surg* 2001; **88**: 1178–1182.

22. Ghori A, Hallisey M, Nwokolo C, Loft D, Fraser I. The secret (GTN) of successful ERCP cannulation: a prospective randomised controlled study. *J R Coll Surg Edinb* 2002; **47**: 634–637.

23. Ros A, Gustafsson L, Krook H *et al*. Laparoscopic cholecystectomy *versus* mini-laparotomy cholecystectomy: a prospective, randomized, single-blind study. *Ann Surg* 2001; **234**: 741–749.

24. Urschel JD, Urschel DM, Miller JD, Bennett WF, Young JE. A meta-analysis of randomized controlled trials of route of reconstruction after esophagectomy for cancer. *Am J Surg* 2001; **182**: 470–475.

25. Medical Research Council Oesophageal Cancer Working Group. Surgical resection with or without preoperative chemotherapy in oesophageal cancer: a randomised controlled trial. *Lancet* 2002; **359**: 1727–1733.

26. Panzini I, Gianni L, Fattori PP *et al*. Adjuvant chemotherapy in gastric cancer: a meta-analysis of randomized trials and a comparison with previous meta-analyses. *Tumori* 2002; **88**: 21–27.

27. Macdonald JS, Smalley SR, Benedetti J *et al*. Chemoradiotherapy after surgery compared with surgery alone for adenocarcinoma of the stomach or gastroesophageal junction. *N Engl J Med* 2001; **345**: 725–730.

28. Siu WT, Leong HT, Law BK *et al*. Laparoscopic repair for perforated peptic ulcer: a randomized controlled trial. *Ann Surg* 2002; **235**: 313–319.

29. Lewis RT. Oral *versus* systemic antibiotic prophylaxis in elective colon surgery: a randomized study and meta-analysis send a message from the 1990s. *Can J Surg* 2002; **45**: 173–180.

30. Nelson R, Singer M. Primary repair for penetrating colon injuries. *Cochrane Database Syst Rev* 2002; CD002247.

31. Kamwendo NY, Modiba MC, Matlala NS, Becker PJ. Randomized clinical trial to determine if delay from time of penetrating colonic injury precludes primary repair. *Br J Surg* 2002; **89**: 993–998.

32. UK Flexible Sigmoidoscopy Screening Trial Investigators. Single flexible sigmoidoscopy screening to prevent colorectal cancer: baseline findings of a UK multicentre randomised trial. *Lancet* 2002; **359**: 1291–1300.

33. Benamouzig R, Yoon H, Little J *et al*. APACC, a French prospective study on aspirin efficacy in reducing colorectal adenoma recurrence: design and baseline findings. *Eur J Cancer Prev* 2001; **10**: 327–335.

34. Jeffery GM, Hickey BE, Hider P. Follow-up strategies for patients treated for non-metastatic colorectal cancer. *Cochrane Database Syst Rev* 2002; CD002200.

35. Renehan AG, Egger M, Saunders MP, O'Dwyer ST. Impact on survival of intensive follow up after curative resection for colorectal cancer: systematic review and meta-analysis of randomised trials. *BMJ* 2002; **324**: 813–816.

36. Sargent DJ, Goldberg RM, Jacobson SD *et al*. A pooled analysis of adjuvant chemo-therapy for resected colon cancer in elderly patients. *N Engl J Med* 2001; **345**: 1091–1097.

37. Martling A, Holm T, Johansson H, Rutqvist LE, Cedermark B. The Stockholm II trial on preoperative radiotherapy in rectal carcinoma: long-term follow-up of a population-based study. *Cancer* 2001; **92**: 896–902.

38. Kapiteijn E, Marijnen CA, Nagtegaal ID *et al*. Preoperative radiotherapy combined with total mesorectal excision for resectable rectal cancer. *N Engl J Med* 2001; **345**: 638–646.

39. Marijnen CA, Kapiteijn E, van de Velde CJ *et al*. Acute side effects and complications after short-term preoperative radiotherapy combined with total mesorectal excision in primary rectal cancer: report of a multicenter randomized trial. *J Clin Oncol* 2002; **20**: 817–825.

40. Lacy AM, Garcia-Valdecasas JC, Delgado S *et al*. Laparoscopy-assisted colectomy *versus* open colectomy for treatment of non-metastatic colon cancer: a randomised trial. *Lancet* 2002; **359**: 2224–2229.

41. Stead ML, Brown JM, Bosanquet N *et al*. Assessing the relative costs of standard open surgery and laparoscopic surgery in colorectal cancer in a randomised controlled trial in the United Kingdom. *Crit Rev Oncol Hematol* 2000; **33**: 99–103.

42. Hazebroek EJ. COLOR: a randomized clinical trial comparing laparoscopic and open resection for colon cancer. *Surg Endosc* 2002; **16**: 949–953.

43. Gencosmanoglu R, Sad O, Koc D, Inceoglu R. Hemorrhoidectomy: open or closed technique? A prospective, randomized clinical trial. *Dis Colon Rectum* 2002; **45**: 70–75.

44. Shalaby R, Desoky A. Randomized clinical trial of stapled *versus* Milligan-Morgan haemorrhoidectomy. *Br J Surg* 2001; **88**: 1049–1053.

45. Ho YH, Seow-Choen F, Tsang C, Eu KW. Randomized trial assessing anal sphincter injuries after stapled haemorrhoidectomy. *Br J Surg* 2001; **88**: 1449–1455.

46. Jayne DG, Botterill I, Ambrose NS, Brennan TG, Guillou PJ, O'Riordain DS. Randomized clinical trial of Ligasure *versus* conventional diathermy for day-case haemorrhoidectomy. *Br J Surg* 2002; **89**: 428–432.

47. Palazzo FF, Francis DL, Clifton MA. Randomized clinical trial of Ligasure *versus* open haemorrhoidectomy. *Br J Surg* 2002; **89**: 154–157.

48. Abou-Assi S, Craig K, O'Keefe SJ. Hypocaloric jejunal feeding is better than total parenteral nutrition in acute pancreatitis: results of a randomized comparative study. *Am J Gastroenterol* 2002; **97**: 2255–2262.

49. Conlon KC, Labow D, Leung D *et al*. Prospective randomized clinical trial of the value of intraperitoneal drainage after pancreatic resection. *Ann Surg* 2001; **234**: 487–493.

50. Galandi D, Antes G. Radiofrequency thermal ablation versus other interventions for hepatocellular carcinoma. *Cochrane Database Syst Rev* 2002; CD003046.

51. Yeo CJ, Cameron JL, Lillemoe KD *et al*. Pancreaticoduodenectomy with or without distal gastrectomy and extended retroperitoneal lymphadenectomy for periampullary adenocarcinoma, part 2: randomized controlled trial evaluating survival, morbidity, and mortality. *Ann Surg* 2002; **236**: 355–366.

52. Sewnath ME, Karsten TM, Prins MH, Rauws EJ, Obertop H, Gouma DJ. A meta-analysis on the efficacy of preoperative biliary drainage for tumors causing obstructive jaundice. *Ann Surg* 2002; **236**: 17–27.

53. Bellantone R, Lombardi CP, Raffaelli M, Rubino F, Boscherini M, Perilli W. Minimally invasive, totally gasless video-assisted thyroid lobectomy. *Am J Surg* 1999; **177**: 342–343.

54. Bellantone R, Lombardi CP, Bossola M *et al*. Video-assisted vs conventional thyroid lobectomy: a randomized trial. *Arch Surg* 2002; **137**: 301–304.

55. Miccoli P, Berti P, Raffaelli M, Materazzi G, Baldacci S, Rossi G. Comparison between minimally invasive video-assisted thyroidectomy and conventional thyroidectomy: a prospective randomized study. *Surgery* 2001; **130**: 1039–1043.

56. Davis EG, Chao C, McMasters KM. Polymerase chain reaction in the staging of solid tumors. *Cancer J* 2002; **8**: 135–143.

57. American Joint Committee on Cancer. *AJCC: Cancer Staging Manual*. New York: Springer, 2002.

58. Thompson JA. The revised American Joint Committee on Cancer staging system for melanoma. *Semin Oncol* 2002; **29**: 361–369.

Index

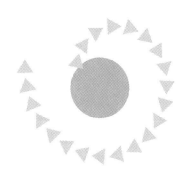

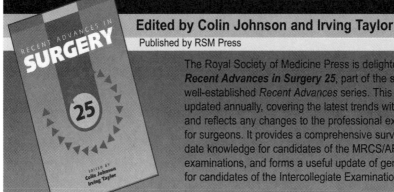